Lab Values
Interpretation

The ultimate laboratory tests manual
of Reference Ranges and what they mean

Dr. Gabriel J. Connor

CONTENTS

INTRODUCTION

Laboratory studies are essential components of a full assessment of the patient. After taking an individual's history and physical examination, laboratory data provide evidence of health status. Nurses are more and more expected to integrate an understanding of laboratory procedures and expected outcomes into the assessment, implementation, planning, and evaluation of nursing care. The data helps to develop and promote nursing diagnosis, treatments, and results.

This book is penned to help health care providers understand and interpret clinical and diagnostic procedures and their outcomes. Just as significant, it is devoted to all healthcare professionals who witness the miracles of laboratory science and testing, conducted and presented compassionately and efficiently.

This book is a guide for nurses, nursing students, and other health experts.

It is a useful clinical tool as well as a helpful text to supplement clinical courses. It can be utilized by nursing students at all levels in academic courses, by combining laboratory data as one property of nursing care; by practicing nurses to update information; and in clinical settings as a quick. This book provides detail and comprehensive to the user, allowing easy access to information on laboratory tests and procedures. Tests are described in a specific category or according to the body system. Each monograph shall be presented in a standardized format for easy identification of specific details briefly. For each laboratory and diagnostic test, the following information is provided:

- The test Name for every monograph is given as a widely used name.
- Synonyms / Acronyms for each test are also specified, if applicable.
- The technique of specimen collection includes the amount of specimen usually collected and, where appropriate, the method of tube or container that is commonly recommended.
- Normal values for each monograph are also included,
- Explanation of the intention of the study and insight into how and why the test results may have an impact on health.
- Indications are a list of the tests used for assessment, evaluation, monitoring, screening, identification, or assistance in diagnosing a clinical condition.
- Results present a list of conditions under which values may be increased or decreased.
- Impending causes are substances or circumstances that may influence the results of the test, rendering the results invalid or unreliable.

Even though I have aimed my best to provide updated knowledge, medicine is still a very dynamic and evolving field. Different tests are adding on the list with the improvement in the previous one. This book is a small effort to help understand that what laboratory tests provide are essential, and to provide a foundation for the building of knowledge.

CARDIOVASCULAR SYSTEM

The cardiovascular system is often known as a blood-vascular system, or merely a circulatory system. It comprises the heart, a mechanical pumping unit, and a closed system of blood vessels, arteries, veins, and capillaries. As the term suggests, the blood found in the circulatory system is pumped by the heart through the closed-loop or circuit of the vessels as it travels through the different "circulations" of the body.

It transfers nutrients (such as amino acids, fats, cholesterol, and electrolytes), Oxygen, hormones, Drugs, and immune blood cells to and from the different body's cells to feed and help combat disease, regulate temperature and pH, and sustain homeostasis by removing carbon dioxide and other waste products.

Following are the list of important laboratory tests done to evaluate the circulatory system

Test to detect heart attack
- Creatine kinase (CK)
- Creatine kinase-MB (CKMB)
- Myoglobin
- Cardiac troponin I or cardiac troponin T

Test to measure Heart failure
- Atrial natriuretic peptide

Tests for detection of future cardiac risks:
- Apo Lipoprotein A
- Apo-Lipoprotein B
- Cholesterol
- HDL Cholesterol
- LDL Cholesterol
- Triglycerides
- Lipid Panel
- High-sensitivity C-reactive Protein (hs-CRP)

Also, certain Drug levels like that of digoxin can be important too.

APOLIPOPROTEIN A (Apo A)

SAMPLING: 1 mL of serum is collected in a red- or tiger-top tube.
TECHNIQUE: Immunonephelometric
NORMAL VALUES:

Sex/Age	Conventional Units	SI Units (Conversion Factor 0.01)
Male		
Newborn	41–93 mg/dL	0.41–0.93 g/L
6 mo–4 y	67–163 mg/dL	0.67–1.63 g/L
Adult	81–166 mg/dL	0.81–1.66 g/L
Female		
Newborn	38–106 mg/dL	0.38–1.06 g/L
6 mo–4 y	60–148 mg/dL	0.60–1.48 g/L
Adult	80–214 mg/dL	0.80–2.14 g/L

EXPLAINATION:

Apolipoprotein A (Apo A), the main component of high-density lipoprotein (HDL), is synthesized in the liver and intestines. Apolipoproteins help regulate lipid metabolism by activating and inhibiting the enzymes required for this process. Apo A-I stimulates the enzyme lecithin-cholesterol acyltransferase (LCAT), while Apo A-II inhibits LCAT.

Apolipoproteins also help to keep the lipids in the solution while they flow in the blood and guide the lipids to the correct target organs and tissues in the body.

It is believed that measurements of Apo A may be more important than measurements of HDL cholesterol as a predictor of coronary artery disease (CAD). There is an inverse relationship between the level of Apo A and the risk of developing CAD. Due to difficulties with the standardization of procedures, the comparison ranges listed above should be used as a rough guide in estimating abnormal conditions. The values for African Americans are 5 to 10 mg / dL higher than those for whites.

INDICATIONS:

Evaluation for risk of coronary artery disease

RESULT

Increased in:
Familial hyper-α-lipoproteinemia
Weight reduction
Decreased in:
A-β-lipoproteinemia
Cholestasis
Diet high in carbohydrates or polyunsaturated fats
Chronic renal failure
Diabetes (uncontrolled)

Familial deficiencies of related enzymes and lipoproteins
Hepatocellular disorders
Hypertriglyceridemia
Nephrotic syndrome
Premature coronary heart disease
Smoking

IMPEDING FACTORS:
- Medications and substances that may increase Apo A levels include anticonvulsants, beclobrate, bezafibrate, ciprofibrate, estrogens, furosemide, lovastatin, pravastatin, prednisolone, simvastatin, and ethanol (abuse).
- Drugs that may reduce Apo A levels comprise androgens, beta-blockers, diuretics, and probucol.

APOLIPOPROTEIN B (Apo B)

SAMPLING: 1 mL of serum is collected in a red- or tiger-top tube.
TECHNIQUE: Immunonephelometric
NORMAL VALUES:

Age	Conventional Units	SI Units (Conversion Factor X0.01)
Newborn–5 y	11–31mg/dL	0.11–0.31 g/L
5–17 y		
Male	47–139 mg/dL	0.47–1.39 g/L
Female	41–96 mg/dL	0.41–0.96 g/L
Adult		
Male	46–174 mg/dL	0.46–1.74 g/L
Female	46–142 mg/dL	0.46–1.42 g/L

EXPLAINATION:
Apolipoprotein B (Apo B), the main component of low-density lipoproteins (chylomicrons, LDLs, and very-low-density lipoproteins), is synthesized in the liver and intestines. Apolipoproteins help regulate lipid metabolism by activating and inhibiting the enzymes required for this process. Apolipoproteins also help to keep the lipids in the solution while they flow in the blood and guide the lipids to the appropriate target organs and tissues in the body.
INDICATIONS: Assessment for risk of coronary artery disease (CAD).

RESULT

Increased in:
Diabetes
Dysglobulinemia
Anorexia nervosa
Cushing's syndrome
Emotional stress
Porphyria
Pregnancy
Premature CAD
Hepatic disease
Hepatic obstruction
Hyperlipoproteinemia
Hypothyroidism
Infantile hypercalcemia
Nephrotic syndrome
Renal failure
Werner's syndrome
Decreased in:
Alpha lipoprotein deficiency (Tangier disease)
Acute stress (burns, illness)
Chronic anemias
Chronic pulmonary disease
Inflammatory joint disease
Intestinal malabsorption
Malnutrition
Familial deficiencies of related enzymes and lipoproteins
Hyperthyroidism
Myeloma
Reye's syndrome
Weight reduction

IMPEDING FACTORS:

- Medications that may raise Apo B levels include amiodarone, androgens, beta-blockers, catecholamines, cyclosporine, diuretics, ethanol (abuse), etretinate, glucogenic corticosteroids, oral contraceptives, and phenobarbital.
- Medications that may reduce Apo B levels are fibrates, beclobrate, cholestyramine, captopril, ketanserin, lovastatin, niacin, nifedipine, pravastatin, prazosin, probucol, and simvastatin.

ATRIAL NATRIURETIC FACTOR

(Atrial natriuretic, Atrial natriuretic hormone, peptide, ANF, ANH)

SAMPLING:1 ml of plasma is collected in a chilled, lavender-top tube. Specimens should be moved in a tightly capped container and an ice slurry.

TECHNIQUE: Radioimmunoassay

NORMAL VALUE:

Conventional Units	SI Units (Conversion Factor1)
20–77 pg./mL	20–77 ng/L

EXPLAINATION:

Atrial natriuretic factor (ANF) is an enzyme secreted by cells in the right atrium of the heart when the right atrial pressure increases. The production of this cardiac peptide is triggered by a rise in the atrial wall caused by a rise in blood pressure or blood volume. Elevated sodium levels also activate ANF receptors.

The extremely potent hormone increases the excretion of salt and water by suppressing the release of aldosterone and renin. ANF reduces angiotensin II and vasopressin, resulting in vasodilation and reduced blood volume and blood pressure.

INDICATIONS:

- Assist in verifying congestive heart failure (CHF), as indicated by an increased level.

- Identify asymptomatic cardiac volume overload, as suggested by the increased level.

RESULT

Increased in:
Asymptomatic cardiac volume overload
CHF
Elevated cardiac filling pressure
Paroxysmal atrial tachycardia
Decreased in:
Not any specific disease

IMPEDING FACTORS:

- Medications that may increase the levels of ANF include atenolol, candoxatril, captopril, carteolol, dopamine, morphine, oral contraceptives, vasopressin, and verapamil.

- Medications that may decrease the levels of ANF include clonidine, prazosin, and urapidil.

- Recent radioactive scans or radiation exposure within one week of the test can conflict with the test results when radioimmunoassay is the desired test method.

Hs-CRP test

C-reactive protein (CRP) is a protein that grows in the blood with inflammation and injury after a heart attack, surgery, or trauma. The hs-CRP test specifically tests low CRP levels to classify low yet steady-state inflammation levels and helps determine a person's risk of developing CVD.

Two main tests measure CRP, and each test defines a particular set of CRP levels in the blood for other purposes:

- The standard CRP test tests dramatically elevated protein levels to recognize diseases that induce pronounced inflammation. It tests CRP in the range of 10 to 1000 mg / L. This test can be used to diagnose inflammation.

- The hs-CRP test specifically measures lower protein levels than the normal CRP test. It tests CRP in the range of 0.5 to 10 mg / L. This procedure is used to assess people at risk of CVD.

CHOLESTEROL, HDL, LDL

(α1-Lipoprotein cholesterol, high-density cholesterol, HDLC, β-lipoprotein cholesterol, low-density cholesterol, LDLC)

SAMPLING: 2 ml of serum is collected in a red- or tiger-top tube.

TECHNIQUE: Spectrophotometry

NORMAL VALUE:

HDLC	Conventional Units	SI Units (Conversion Factor 0.0259)
Birth	6–56 mg/dL	0.16–1.45 mmol/L
Children and adults	40–65 mg/dL	0.9–1.7 mmol/L
LDLC	Conventional Units	SI Units (Conversion Factor 0.0259)
Birth	20–56 mg/dL	0.52–1.45 mmol/L
5–19 y		
Male	65–130 mg/dL	1.68–3.37 mmol/L
Female	65–140 mg/dL	1.68–3.63 mmol/L
20–29 y		
Male	65–165 mg/dL	1.68–4.27 mmol/L
Female	55–160 mg/dL	1.42–4.14 mmol/L
30–44 y		
Male	80–185 mg/dL	2.07–4.79 mmol/L
Female	70–175 mg/dL	1.81–4.53 mmol/L
>45 y		
Male	90–185 mg/dL	2.33–4.79 mmol/L
Female	80–215 mg/dL	2.07–5.57 mmol/L

EXPLAINATION:

The main transport proteins for cholesterol in the body are high-density lipoprotein cholesterol (HDLC) and low-density lipoprotein cholesterol (LDLC). It is suspected that HDLC may have protective properties in that its function involves the transfer of cholesterol from the blood circulation to the liver.

LDLC is the most important transport protein for cholesterol from the liver to the arteries. LDLC can be measured using total cholesterol, total triglyceride, and HDLC levels.

HDLC levels below 40 mg / dL in males and females constitute a coronary risk factor. There is an inverse link between HDLC and the risk of coronary artery disease (CAD) (i.e., lower HDLC rates face a higher risk of CAD). The LDLC risk levels for CAD are directly proportional to the risk and vary by age group. The LDLC can be anticipated using the following formula for Fried Ewald:

LDLC = (Total Cholesterol) -HDLC) - (VLDLC)

Very low-density lipoprotein cholesterol (VLDL-C) is estimated by dividing the triglycerides (conventional units) by 5. Triglycerides in SI units would be separated by 2.18 to calculate VLLDC. It is important to mention that the formula is only accurate if the triglycerides are < 400 mg / dL or 4.52 mmol / L.

INDICATIONS:
- Determine the risk of cardiovascular disease.
- Evaluate the response to dietary and drug treatment for hypercholesterolemia.
- Investigate hypercholesterolemia given the family history of cardiovascular disease.

RESULT:

Risk	Units Conventional	SI Units (Conversion Factor X 0.0259)
Optimal	< 2.59 mmol/L	
Near optimal	100–129 mg/dL	2.59–3.34 mmol/L
Borderline high	130–159 mg/dL	2.67–4.11 mmol/L
High	160–189 mg/dL	4.14–4.90 mmol/L
Extremely high	>4.92 mmol/L	

HDLC increased in:	HDLC decreased in:
Exercise	A- β -lipoproteinemia
Familial hyper-β -lipoproteinemia	Fisheye disease
Alcoholism	Genetic predisposition or enzyme/cofactor deficiency
Biliary cirrhosis	Hypertriglyceridemia
Chronic hepatitis	

LDLC Recommended Levels

HDLC increased in:
• Exercise
• Familial hyper-α-lipoproteinemia
• Alcoholism
• Biliary cirrhosis
• Chronic hepatitis
HDLC decreased in:
• A-β-lipoproteinemia
• Fish-eye disease
• Genetic predisposition or enzyme/ cofactor deficiency
• Hypertriglyceridemia
• Obesity
• Sedentary lifestyle
• Smoking
• Tangier disease
• Chronic renal failure
• Cholestasis
• Uncontrolled diabetes
• Hepatocellular disorders
• Nephrotic syndrome
• Premature CAD
LDLC increased in:
• Corneal arcus
• Hyperlipoproteinemia types IIa and IIb
• Premature CAD
• Tendon and tuberous xanthomas
• Anorexia nervosa
• Chronic renal failure
• Cushing's syndrome
• Diabetes
• Diet high in cholesterol and saturated fat
• Dysglobulinemia
• Hepatic disease

	HDLC increased in:
•	Hepatic obstruction
•	Hypothyroidism
•	Nephrotic syndrome
•	Porphyria
•	Pregnancy
	LDLC decreased in:
•	Genetic predisposition or enzyme/cofactor deficiency
•	Hypolipoproteinemia and a-β-lipoproteinemia
•	Tangier disease
•	Acute stress (severe burns, illness)
•	Chronic anemias
•	Chronic pulmonary disease
•	Hyperthyroidism
•	Inflammatory joint disease
•	Myeloma
•	Reye's syndrome
•	Severe hepatocellular destruction or disease

IMPEDING FACTORS:
- Medications that may raise HDLC levels include albuterol, anticonvulsants, cholestyramine, cimetidine, clofibrate, and other fibric acid derivatives, niacin, estrogens, ethanol (moderate use), lovastatin oral contraceptives, pravastatin, pindolol, prazosin, and simvastatin.
- Medications that may reduce HDLC levels include acebutolol, atenolol, nonselective-adrenergic blocking agents, danazol, diuretics, etretinate, interferon, isotretinoin, linseed oil, metoprolol, neomycin, probucol, progesterone, thiazides, and steroids.
- Medications that may raise LDLC levels include androgens, catecholamines, chenodiol, cyclosporine, danazol, diuretics, glucogenic corticosteroids, etretinate, and progestins.
- Medications that may reduce LDLC levels include aminosalicylic acid, cholestyramine, colestipol, estrogens, fibric acid derivatives, niacin, pravastatin, interferon, lovastatin, neomycin prazosin, probucol, simvastatin, terazosin, and thyroxine.
- Some of the drugs used to reduce total cholesterol and LDLC or increase HDLC may cause liver damage.

- Grossly extremely high triglyceride levels invalidate the Fried Ewald formula for LDLC mathematical estimation, and if the triglyceride is >400 mg / dL, the formula should not be used.
- Fasting before collection of specimens is highly recommended. Preferably, the patient should be on a stable diet for three weeks and fast 12 hours before the specimen is obtained.

CHOLESTEROL, TOTAL

SAMPLING: 1 mL of serum is collected in a red- or tiger-top tube. 1 ml of plasma collected in a green-top (heparin) tube is also acceptable. It is vital to use the same tube type when serial specimen collections are anticipated for consistency in testing.

TECHNIQUE: Spectrophotometry

NORMAL VALUE:

Risk	Conventional Units	SI Units (Conversion Factor X 0.0259)
Desirable	< 200 mg/dL	< 5.18 mmol/L
Borderline	200–239 mg/dL	5.18–6.19 mmol/L
High	>240 mg/dL	>6.22 mmol/L

EXPLAINATION:

Cholesterol is a lipid required to form cell membranes and a part of the materials that make the skin waterproof. It also helps to form bile salts, adrenal corticosteroids, estrogens, and androgens. Cholesterol is attained from the diet (exogenous cholesterol) and is also synthesized (endogenous cholesterol). Although most body cells form some cholesterol, it is produced mainly by the liver, and the plasma values maybe 10 % lower than the serum values. Intestinal mucosa Cholesterol is an essential component of cell membrane maintenance and hormonal production. Even low levels of cholesterol, as is sometimes seen in critically ill patients, can be as life-threatening as exceedingly high levels.

According to the National Cholesterol Education Program, keeping cholesterol levels below 200 mg /dL significantly reduces the risk of coronary heart disease. No age or gender stratification is presented as part of its guidance.

Numerous studies have been conducted, and there are inconsistencies between the studies to target "normal" separated by age and gender. Many important risk factors must be considered in addition to total cholesterol and high-density lipoprotein cholesterol (HDLC).

Most myocardial infarctions arise even in patients whose cholesterol levels are deemed to be within acceptable limits or who are in a low-risk category. The blend of risk factors and lipid values helps identify individuals at risk so that appropriate interventions can be taken. If the cholesterol level is higher than 200 mg / dL, repeat testing after 12 to 24 hours is recommended.

INDICATIONS:
- Assist in the assessment of cardiovascular disease risk.
- Help in the treatment of nephrotic syndrome, hepatic diseases, pancreatitis, and thyroid disorders.
- Evaluate dietary response and hypercholesterolemia drug therapy.
- Investigate hypercholesterolemia considering the family history of cardiovascular disease.

RESULT:

Increased in:
Acute intermittent porphyria
Alcoholism
Anorexia nervosa
Cholestasis
Chronic renal failure
Diabetes (with poor control)
Diets high in cholesterol and fats
Familial hyperlipoproteinemia
Glomerulonephritis
Glycogen storage disease (von Gierke disease)
Gout
Hypothyroidism (primary)
Ischemic heart disease
Nephrotic syndrome
Obesity
Pancreatic and prostatic malignancy
Pregnancy
Werner's syndrome
Decreased in:
Burns
Chronic myelocytic leukemia
Chronic obstructive pulmonary disease
Hyperthyroidism
Liver disease (severe)
Malabsorption and malnutrition syndromes
Myeloma

| Pernicious anemia |
| Polycythemia vera |
| Severe illness |
| Sideroblastic anemias |
| Tangier disease |
| Thalassemia |
| Wald Enstrom's macroglobulinemia |

IMPEDING FACTORS:

- Drugs that may raise cholesterol levels include amiodarone, androgens, catecholamines, cyclosporine, danazol, diclofenac, disulfiram, glucogenic corticosteroids, ibuprofen, isotretinoin, levodopa, methyclothiazide, miconazole (due to castor oil, not to the drug), nafarelin, nandrolone, certain oral contraceptives, phenobarbital, phenothiazine, oxymetholone, prochlorperazine, and sotalol
- Drugs that may lower cholesterol levels include acebutolol, amiloride, aminosalicylic acid, ascorbic acid, asparaginase, atenolol, atorvastatin, beclobrate, bezafibrate, carbetamide, cerivastatin, cholestyramine, ciprofibrate, clofibrate, clonidine, colestipol, dextrothyroxine, doxazosin, enalapril, estrogens, fenofibrate, fenfluramine, Fluvastatin, gemfibrozil, haloperidol, hydralazine.
- Alcohol ingestion 12 to 24 hours before the test can falsely increase the results.
- Ingestion of medicines that can change cholesterol levels within 12 hours of the examination may give a false impression about cholesterol levels unless the test is performed to evaluate such effects.

LIPOPROTEIN ELECTROPHORESIS

α1-lipoprotein cholesterol, high-density lipoprotein (HDL); β-lipoprotein cholesterol, Lipid fractionation; lipoprotein phenotyping; low-density lipoprotein (LDL); pre- β -lipoprotein cholesterol, very-low-density lipoprotein (VLDL)

SAMPLING: 3 mL of serum is collected in a red- or tiger-top tube.

TECHNIQUE: Electrophoresis and 4oC test for specimen appearance

NORMAL VALUE:

There is no quantitative definition of the test. The appearance of the specimen and the electrophoretic sequence was visually interpreted.

Hyperlipoproteinemia: Fredrickson Type	Specimen Appearance	Electrophoretic Pattern
Type I	Clear with a creamy top layer	Heavy chylomicron band
Type IIa	Clear	Heavy β band
Type IIb	Clear or faintly turbid	Heavy β and preβ-band
Type III	Slightly to moderately turbid	Heavy β band
Type IV	Slightly to moderately turbid	Heavy pre-β band
Type V	Slightly to moderately turbid with creamy top layer	Intense chylomicron band and heavy pre-β band

EXPLAINATION:
Lipoprotein electrophoresis analyzes lipoprotein fractions to assess the pathological distribution and concentration of lipoproteins in the blood, an important risk factor for coronary artery disease (CAD). They are named in order of increasing density of lipoprotein fractions are (1) chylomicrons, (2) very-low-density lipoprotein (VLDL), (3) low-density lipoprotein (LDL), and (4) high-density lipoprotein (HDL). Chylomicrons and VLDL contain the maximum levels of triglycerides and lower levels of cholesterol and protein. LDL and HDL have the lowest triglyceride levels and relatively higher cholesterol and protein content.

INDICATIONS:
- Evaluate known or suspected conditions associated with elevated lipoprotein levels.
- Evaluate patients with serum cholesterol levels higher than 250 mg / dL, indicating a high risk for CAD.
- Analyze response to high cholesterol medication and decide the need for drug therapy.
RESULT:
Type I: Hyperlipoproteinemia or elevated chylomicrons may be primarily due to an inherited lipoprotein lipase deficiency; or secondary due to uncontrolled diabetes, systemic lupus erythematosus, and dysgammaglobulinemia. Overall, cholesterol is normal to mildly elevated, and triglycerides (mainly exogenous chylomicrons) are extremely elevated. If the disorder is inherited, signs may begin in infancy.

Type IIa: Hyperlipoproteinemia may be primarily due to genetic or secondary symptoms caused by nephrotic syndrome, hypothyroidism, and dysgammaglobulinemia. Total cholesterol level is higher, triglycerides are normal, and LDL cholesterol (LDLC) is decreased. If the disease is inherited, signs may begin in infancy.

Form IIb: Hyperlipoproteinemia can occur for the same reasons as in Type IIa. Total cholesterol, triglycerides, and LDLCs are all elevated.

Type III: Hyperlipoproteinemia may be primary, due to inherited characteristics; or secondary, due to hypothyroidism, uncontrolled diabetes, alcoholism, and dysgammaglobulinemia. Total cholesterol and triglycerides are elevated, while LDLC is normal.

Type IV: Hyperlipoproteinemia may be primarily due to inherited characteristics; or secondary due to poorly controlled diabetes, hypertension, nephrotic syndrome, chronic renal failure, and dysgammaglobulinemia. Total cholesterol is low to elevated mildly, triglycerides are mild to severely elevated, and LDLC is normal.

Form V: Hyperlipoproteinemia may be primarily due to inherited characteristics; or secondary due to uncontrolled diabetes, depression, nephrotic syndrome, and dysgammaglobulinemia. Overall, cholesterol is low to mildly elevated, triglycerides are high, and LDLC is normal.

CRITICAL VALUES: N/A

IMPEDING FACTORS:

- Failure to follow the usual diet for two weeks before the test will result in findings that do not accurately reflect the cholesterol levels of the patient.
- Ingestion of alcohol 24 hours before the test, intake of food 12 hours ahead of the test, and extreme exercise 12 hours before the test alters the tests.
- Various medicines have the potential to alter the findings.

MYOGLOBIN (MB)

SAMPLING: 1 mL of serum is collected in a red- or tiger-top tube.

TECHNIQUE: Nephelometry

NORMAL VALUE:

Conventional Units	SI Units (Conversion Factor X1)
5–70 µg/dL	5–70 µg/dL

EXPLAINATION:

Myoglobin is an oxygen-binding muscle protein commonly found in the skeletal and cardiac muscles. It is discharged into the bloodstream following muscle damage due to ischemia, trauma, or inflammation. While myoglobin testing is more sensitive than creatinine kinase and isoenzyme testing, it does not indicate the specific location.

INDICATIONS:
- Help in predicting flare-up of polymyositis.
- Possible risk of skeletal muscle damage or myocardial infarction.

RESULT:

Increased in:
• Exercise
• Malignant hyperthermia
• Myocardial infarction
• Shock
• Thrombolytic therapy
• Progressive muscular dystrophy
• Cardiac surgery
• Cocaine use
• Renal failure
• Rhabdomyolysis
Decreased in:
• Myasthenia gravis
• Rheumatoid arthritis
• The occurrence of antibodies to myoglobin as seen in patients with polymyositis

IMPEDING FACTORS:
Not any

PERICARDIAL FLUID ANALYSIS

SAMPLING: 5 mL of pericardial fluid is collected in a lavender-top (ethylenediamine tetra-acetic acid [EDTA]) tube for cell count, a red- or a green-top (heparin) tube for glucose, and sterile containers for microbiology specimens. Make sure that there is an equivalent amount of fluid to fixative in a clear vessel for cytology.

TECHNIQUE: Glucose spectrophotometry, electronic or manual cell count, macroscopic analysis of cultured organisms, and microscopic examination of specimens for microbiology, cytology, and cultured microorganisms

NORMAL VALUE:

Pericardial Fluid	NORMAL Value
Appearance	Clear
Color	Pale yellow

Glucose	Parallel serum values
Red blood cell count	None has seen
White blood cell count	< 1000/mm^3
Culture	No growth
Gram stain	No organisms are seen
Cytology	No abnormal cells are seen

EXPLAINATION:

The heart is situated inside a protective membrane known as the pericardium. The fluid between the two pericardial membranes is called fluid. Usually, only a small amount of fluid is present because the rate of fluid production and absorption is roughly the same. Some unhealthy conditions can lead to fluid build-up in the pericardium. Different tests are usually performed in addition to a general set of tests used to differentiate a transudate from an exudate. *Transudates are effusions which form because of a systemic disease that disrupts fluid balance regulation, such as presumed perforation.*

Exudates are caused by conditions affecting the membrane tissue itself, such as inflammation or malignancy. The fluid is extracted from the pericardium by needle aspiration and evaluated, as shown in the tables below.

Characteristic	Transudate	Exudate
Appearance	Clear	Cloudy or turbid
Specific gravity	< 1.015	>1.015
Total protein	< 2.5 g/dL	>3.0 g/dL
Fluid-to-serum protein ratio	< 0.5	>0.5
LDH	Parallels serum value	< 200 U/L
Fluid-to-serum LDH ratio	< 0.6	>0.6
Fluid cholesterol	< 55 mg/dL	>55 mg/dL
White blood cell count	< 100/mm^3	>1000/mm^3

INDICATIONS:

- Determine the effusion of unknown etiology.
- Investigate suspected bleeding immune disease malignancy or infection.

RESULT:

Increased in (condition/test showing increased result):
• Bacterial pericarditis (red blood cell count [RBC], white blood cell count [WBC] with a predominance of neutrophils)
• Hemorrhagic pericarditis (RBC count, WBC count)
• Malignancy (RBC count, anomalous cytology)
• Post myocardial infarction syndrome, also termed Dressler Syndrome (RBC count, WBC count with most neutrophils)

•	Rheumatoid disease like systemic lupus erythematosus (RBC count, WBC count)
•	Tuberculosis or fungal pericarditis (RBC count, WBC count with a high proportion of lymphocytes)
•	Viral pericarditis (RBC count and WBC count with a high proportion of neutrophils)
Decreased in (condition/test showing decreased result):	
•	Bacterial pericarditis (glucose)
•	Malignancy (glucose)
•	The rheumatoid or systemic lupus erythematosus (glucose)

IMPEDING FACTORS:
- Bloody fluid may be the consequence of a traumatic tap.
- Unknown hyperglycemia or hypoglycemia may be confusing when comparing fluid and plasma glucose levels. It is therefore advisable to collect comparative serum samples a few hours before pericardiocentesis is performed.

TRIGLYCERIDES (Trigs, TG)
SAMPLING: 1 mL of serum is collected in a red- or tiger-top tube. 1 mL of plasma collected in a green-top (heparin) tube is also acceptable.
TECHNIQUE: Spectrophotometry
NORMAL VALUE:

Age	Conventional Units	SI Units (Conversion Factor 0.0113)	Risk
0–9 y			
Male	30–100 mg/dL	0.34–1.13 mmol/L	
Female	35–110 mg/dL	0.40–1.24 mmol/L	
10–20 y			
Male	32–148 mg/dL	0.36–1.67 mmol/L	
Female	37–124 mg/dL	0.42–1.40 mmol/L	
Adult	< 150 mg/dL	< 1.70 mmol/L	Normal
	150–199 mg/dL	1.70–2.25 mmol/L	Borderline high
	200–499 mg/dL	2.26–5.64 mmol/L	High
	>500 mg/dL	>5.65 mmol/L	Exceedingly high

EXPLAINATION:

Triglycerides are a blend of three fatty acids and one molecule of glycerol. They are required to provide energy for a variety of metabolic processes. Excess triglycerides are contained in adipose tissue, and fatty acids provide the raw materials needed for conversion to glucose (gluconeogenesis) or direct use as a source of energy. While fatty acids occur in the diet, many are also derived from unused glucose and amino acids that the liver transforms into stored energy.

Triglyceride levels differ by age, sex, weight, and race: they increase with age. The rates in men are higher than in women (among women, those who take oral contraceptives are 20 to 40 mg / dL > those who do not). The percentages of overweight and obese people are > those of normal weight. The rates in African Americans are approximately 10 to 20 mg / dL lower than in Caucasians.

INDICATIONS:

- Evaluate known or suspected conditions associated with elevated triglyceride levels.
- Identify hyperlipoproteinemia (hyperlipidemia) in individuals with a family history of illness.
- Monitor exposure to drugs known to change triglyceride levels.
- Survey adults over 40 years of age or obese to assess the likelihood of atherosclerotic cardiovascular disease.

RESULT:

Increased in:
• Nephrotic syndrome
• Obesity
• Pancreatitis (acute and chronic)
• Acute myocardial infarction
• Alcoholism
• Glycogen storage disease
• Gout
• Hyperlipoproteinemia
• Anorexia nervosa
• Chronic ischemic heart disease
• Cirrhosis
• Hypertension
• Hypothyroidism
• Impaired glucose tolerance
• Pregnancy
• Renal failure
• Respiratory distress syndrome
• Stress
• Viral hepatitis
• Werner's syndrome

Decreased in:
• Brain infarction
• Chronic obstructive lung disease (COPD)
• End-stage liver disease
• Hyperparathyroidism
• Hyperthyroidism
• Malabsorption disorders
• Malnutrition
• Hypolipoproteinemia and a-β -lipoproteinemia
• Intestinal lymphangiectasia

IMPEDING FACTORS:

- Medications that may raise triglyceride levels include acetylsalicylic acid, aldatense, atenolol, Bendroflumethiazide, cyclosporine, danazol, glucocorticoids, oral contraceptives, oxprenolol, pindolol, prazosin, propranolol, tamoxifen, and timolol.

- Drugs and substances that may lower the triglyceride levels include ascorbic acid, bezafibrate, captopril, ciprofibrate, clofibrate, colestipol, dextrothyroxine, doxazosin, enalapril, carvedilol, cicloprolol, chenodeoxycholic acid, cholestyramine, cilazapril, eptastatin, fenofibrate, flaxseed oil, gemfibrozil, glucagon, halofenate, medroxyprogesterone, metformin, nafenopin, niacin, niceritrol, pinacidil, pindolol, pravastatin, prazosin, probucol, insulin, levonorgestrel, lovastatin, simvastatin, and verapamil.

TROPONINS I AND T

(Cardiac troponin I (cTnI), Cardiac troponin, Cardiac troponin T (cTnT))

SAMPLING: 1 mL of serum is collected in a red- or tiger-top tube. 1ml of plasma collected in a green-top (heparin) tube is also acceptable. Serial sampling is highly suggestive. Attention must be given to use the same kind of collection container if serial measurements are taken.

TECHNIQUE: Enzyme immunoassay

NORMAL VALUE:

Troponin I	< 0.35 ng/mL
Troponin T	< 0.20 g/L

EXPLAINATION:

Troponin is a complex molecule of three contractile proteins that adjust the relationship between actin and myosin. Troponin C is a calcium-binding subunit; it does not have a heart muscle-specific subunit. However, Troponin I and Troponin T have cardiac muscle-specific subunits. These are observable a few hours to seven days after the onset of symptoms. Troponin I am a more specific marker for cardiac damage than Troponin T.

Heart troponin I begin to rise 2 to 6 hours after myocardial infarction (MI). It has a biphasic interval that initially occurs at 15 to 24 hours after the MI and then has a lower average at 60 to 80 hours. Cardiac troponin T levels increase up to 2 to 6 hours after MI and stay elevated. All proteins are returned to the NORMAL range seven days after MI

INDICATIONS:

- Help in establishing a diagnosis of MI.
- Assess myocardial cell damage.

RESULT:

Increased in:
• Acute MI
• Slight myocardial damage
• Unstable angina pectoris
• Myocardial damage after coronary artery bypass surgery or percutaneous transluminal coronary angioplasty
Decreased in:
Not any specific disease

IMPEDING FACTORS: Not any

NOTES

_____

_____

_____

_____

_____

_____

_____

_____

_____

HEMATOLOGY AND ONCOLOGY

Hematology includes the study of blood, in specific how blood can impact general health or illness. Hematology studies comprise blood tests, blood proteins, and blood-producing organs.

These tests can assess several blood conditions, including infection, anemia, inflammation, hemophilia, blood clotting disorders, leukemia, and the body's responsiveness to chemotherapy. Testing may be normal and regular, or it may be required to identify medical problems in emergencies. In certain cases, the findings of a blood test may provide a reliable measure of the body's conditions and how internal or external factors may impact the health of the patient.

Tests to aid in diagnosing anemia, certain cancers of the blood, inflammatory diseases, and to monitor blood loss and infection
- Complete blood count (CBC)
- White blood cell count (WBC)
- Red blood cell count (RBC)
- Hemoglobin concentration (HB).
- Platelet count
- Hematocrit red blood cell volume (HCT)
- Differential white blood count
- Red blood cell indices (measurements)

Tests to diagnose and/or to monitor certain types of bleeding and clotting disorders
- Platelet count

Tests to evaluate bleeding and clotting disorders and to monitor anticoagulation (anticlotting) therapies
- Prothrombin time (PT)
- Partial Thromboplastin Time (PTT)
- International Normalized Ratio (INR)

Tests to Check for the tumor marker.
- Tumor markers are compounds created by tumor cells that can be found in the blood.
- But tumor markers are often produced by certain normal cells, and levels can be slightly higher under non-cancer conditions.

δ-AMINOLEVULINIC ACID (δ-ALA):

SAMPLING: 25 ml of urine is collected from a timed specimen in a dark plastic container and hydrochloric acid as a preservative.

TECHNIQUE: Spectrophotometry

NORMAL VALUE:

Conventional Units	SI Units (Conversion Factor X7.626)
1.5–7.5 mg/24 h	11.4–57.2 mol/24 h

EXPLAINATION:

δ-Aminolaevulinic acid (δ-ALA) is engaged in the formation of porphyrins. Disturbances in the metabolism of porphyrin can cause increased excretion of δ-ALA in the urine. While lead poisoning may cause increased urinary excretion, the δ-ALA test is not useful to indicate lead toxicity because it is not observable in the urine until the blood lead level is reached and reaches 40 µg / dL.

INDICATIONS:

- Help in the diagnosis of porphyria.

RESULT:

Increased in:
• Aminolaevulinic acid dehydrase deficiency
• Acute porphyria's
• Hereditary tyrosinemia
• Lead poisoning
Decreased in:
• Liver disease (alcoholic)

IMPEDING FACTORS:

- Drugs that may rise δ-ALA levels include ammonia, glucosamine, and penicillin.
- Cisplatin may reduce δ-ALA levels.
- Various drugs are suspected as possible initiators of attacks of acute porphyria. However, those classified as unsafe for high-risk individuals include antipyrine, aminopyrine, aminoglutethimide, barbiturates, carbamazepine, carbromal, chlorpropamide, danazol, dapsone, diclofenac, diphenylhydantoin, ergot preparations, ethchlorvynol, ethinamate, glutethimide, griseofulvin, mephenytoin, meprobamate, methyprylons, N-isopropyl meprobamate, novobiocin, phenylbutazone, primidone, pyrazalone preparations, succinimides, sulfonamides, sulfonethylmethane, sulfamethazine, synthetic estrogens and progestins, tolazamide, tolbutamide, trimethadione, and valproic acid.

HEPARIN COFACTOR ASSAY, AT-III.

SAMPLING: 1 mL of plasma is collected in the blue-top (sodium citrate) tube.
TECHNIQUE: Radio immunodiffusion
NORMAL VALUE:

	Conventional Units	SI Units
Functional assay	85–115% of standard	(Conversion Factor 0.01) 0.85–1.15
Immunologic assay	21–30 mg/dL	(Conversion Factor 10) 210–300 mg/L

EXPLAINATION:
Antithrombin III (AT-III) can hinder thrombin and factors IX, X, XI, and XII. It is a cofactor of heparin, associated with heparin and thrombin. AT-III serves to increase the rate of thrombin neutralized or inhibited and reduces the total amount of thrombin inhibited. Low-level patients show considerable aversion to heparin therapy.

Indications: Explore the tendency for thrombosis.

RESULT

Increased in:
• Acute hepatitis
• Inflammation
• Menstruation
• Obstructive jaundice
• Renal transplant
• Vitamin K deficiency
Decreased in:
• Congenital deficiency
• Disseminated intravascular coagulation
• Carcinoma
• Chronic liver failure
• Cirrhosis
• Liver transplant or partial hepatectomy
• Nephrotic syndrome
• Pulmonary embolism

IMPEDING FACTORS:
- Medicines that may increase the levels of AT-III include anabolic steroids, gemfibrozil, and warfarin.
- Pharmaceuticals that may decrease AT-III levels include asparaginase, heparin, estrogens, gemstone, and oral contraceptives.
- Placing the tourniquet for more than 1 minute can result in venous stasis and alter the strength of the plasma proteins to be tested. Activation of the platelet may also occur under these conditions, resulting in inaccurate measurements.

CLOT RETRACTION

SAMPLING: Whole blood is collected in a full 5-mL red-top tube.

TECHNIQUE: Macroscopic observation of the sample

NORMAL VALUE: A normal clot, gently separated from the side of the test tube and incubated at 37°C, shrinks to about half of its initial size within 1 hour. The result is a fibrin clot that is firm and cylindrical. It consists of red blood cells and is distinguished from the serum by clear demarcation. Complete clot retraction may take up to 6 to 24 hours.

EXPLAINATION: The clot retraction test determines the adequacy of the platelet function by measuring the speed and degree of the retraction of the clot when blood clots in the test tube are removed from the sidewalls of the tube. Platelets play a dynamic role in the process of retraction of clots. When platelets are diminished, or the function is compromised, the serum in the tube becomes scarce, and the clot is thick, plump, and poorly demarcated. In addition to normal platelets, the retraction of clots depends on the contractile protein thrombasthenia, adenosine triphosphate (ATP), magnesium, and pyruvate kinase. Clot retraction is also affected by hematocrit and fibrinogen structure and concentration.

INDICATIONS:
- Investigate the expected abnormalities of fibrinogen or fibrinolytic activity.
- Evaluate the adequacy of platelet function.
- Evaluate the thrombocytopenia of unknown origin.
- Investigate the possibility of Glanzmann's disease.

RESULT:

Increased in: N/A	
Decreased in: Glanzmann's thrombasthenia	

IMPEDING FACTORS:
- Drugs that may result in decreased outcomes include apronalide, carbenicillin, and plicamycin.

- Platelet count < 100,000/ µL, acetylsalicylic acid therapy, altered fibrinogen/fibrin structure, polycythemia, hemoconcentration, hypofibrinogenemia, and multiple myeloma are conditions in which atypical clot retraction may occur, limiting the ability to form a valid platelet function assessment.
- Fast and proper processing, storage, and analysis of specimens are important for achieving accurate results. Specimens obtained in the laboratory more than 1 hour after selection should be rejected.

COAGULATION FACTORS

SAMPLING: Whole blood in a filled 5-mL blue-top (sodium citrate) tube.
NORMAL VALUE: Activity from 50 to 150 percent

	Preferred Name	Synonym
Factor I	Fibrinogen	—
Factor II	Prothrombin	Pre-thrombin
Factor III	Tissue factor	Tissue thromboplastin
Factor IV	Calcium	Ca^2
Factor V	Proaccelerin	Labile factor, accelerator globulin (AcG)
Factor VII	Proconvertin	Stabile factor, serum prothrombin conversion accelerator, auto-prothrombin I
Factor VIII:C	Antihemophilic factor	Antihemophilic globulin
	(AHF)	(AHG), antihemophilic factor A, platelet cofactor 1
Factor IX	Plasma thromboplastin	Christmas factor,
	component (PTC)	Antihemophilic factor B, platelet cofactor 2
Factor X	Stuart-Prower factor	Autoprothrombin III, thrombokinase

Factor XI	Plasma thromboplastin antecedent (PTA)	Antihemophilic factor C

Factor XII	Hageman factor	Glass factor, contact factor
Factor XIII	Fibrin-stabilizing factor (FSF)	Laki-Lorand factor (LLF), fibrinase, plasma transglutinase
	Prekallikrein	Fletcher factor
	High-molecular-weight kininogen (HMWK)	Fitzgerald factor, contact activation cofactor, Williams factor, Falujenc factor

EXPLAINATION:

Coagulation proteins respond to injury to the blood vessel in a chain of events. Intrinsic and extrinsic mechanisms of secondary hemostasis are a series of reactions involving substrate protein fibrinogen, coagulation factors (also identified as enzyme precursors or zymogens), non-enzyme cofactors (Ca2), and phospholipids. Roman numerals were applied to the variables in the order of their discovery, not their position in the coagulation series. Factor VI was thought to be a separate coagulation factor. Subsequently, it was shown to be the same as the modified form of Factor V, and therefore the number is no longer used.

In the liver, the coagulation factors are produced. They can be sub-divided into three groups based on their common characteristics:

1. The contact group became activated in vitro by surfaces such as glass and activated in vivo by collagen. The factors included in the contact group are factor XI, factor XII, prekallikrein, and high molecular weight kininogen.
2. The prothrombin or vitamin K-dependent category comprises factors II, VII, IX, and X.
3. The fibrinogen group consists of factors I, V, VIII, and XIII. They are the most labile factors and are consumed during the coagulation process. The factors listed in the table are those most measured.

INDICATIONS:

- Identify the presence of genetic bleeding disorders.
- Identify the presence of a qualitative or quantitative cause deficiency.

RESULT:

Increased in: N/A
Decreased in:
• Congenital deficiency

•   Disseminated intravascular coagulation
•   Liver disease

IMPEDING FACTORS:

- Medications that may increase the level of factor II include fluoxymesterone, methandrostenolone, nandrolone, and oxymetholone.
- Medications that may decrease the level of factor II include warfarin.
- Medications that may increase factors V, VII, and X include anabolic steroids, fluoxymesterone, methandrostenolone, nandrolone, oral contraceptives, and oxymetholone.
- Drugs that may reduce the amount of factor V include streptokinase.
- Medications that may decrease the level of factor VII include asparaginase, acetylsalicylic acid, cefamandole, ceftriaxone, dextran, dicumarol, gemfibrozil, oral contraceptives, and warfarin.
- Medicines that may increase the level of factor VIII include chlormadinone.
- Medications that may decrease the level of factor VIII include asparaginase.
- Drugs that may increase the level of factor IX include chlormadinone and oral contraceptives.
- Drugs that may reduce the amount of factor IX include asparaginase and warfarin.
- Medications that may decrease the level of factor X include chlormadinone, dicumarol, oral contraceptives, and warfarin.
- Medications that may decrease the level of factor XI include asparaginase and captopril.
- Medications that may decrease the level of factor XII include captopril.
- The test results of patients on anticoagulant therapy are not accurate.
- Placing the tourniquet for more than 1 minute can cause venous stasis and changes in the concentration of plasma proteins to be measured.
- Activation of the platelet may also occur under these conditions, resulting in incorrect results.
- Vascular injury during phlebotomy may trigger platelets and coagulation factors, resulting in incorrect results.
- Hemolyzed samples must be refused because hemolysis is an indication of platelet activation and coagulation factor activation.
- Incompletely filled tubes mixed with heparin or clotted specimens shall be refused.
- Icteric or lipemic specimens' conflict with optical test methods and yield incorrect results.
- Incompletely filled collection tubes, heparin-contaminated specimens, clotted specimens, or unprocessed specimens not delivered to the laboratory within 1 hour of collection should be refused.

COMPLETE BLOOD COUNT (CBC)

SAMPLING: Whole blood from one full lavender tube (ethylenediaminetetraacetic acid [EDTA]) or microtainer. Whole blood from a green-top tube (lithium or sodium heparin tube) may be sent. Still, the following automated values may not be stated: white blood cell count (WBC), WBC differential, platelet count, and mean platelet volume.

TECHNIQUE: Automated, multichannel, computerized analyzers that sort and size cells based on changes in either electrical impedance or light signals as the cells pass in front of the laser. Many of these analyzers can determine a 5-part WBC differential.

NORMAL VALUE:

This set of tests includes hemoglobin, hematocrit, red blood cell count (RBC), RBC morphology, RBC indexes, RBC distribution width index (RDW), platelet size, platelet count, WBC count, and WBC differential. The five-part automated WBC differentiation recognizes and lists neutrophils, lymphocytes, monocytes, eosinophils, and basophils.

Age	Conventional Units	SI Units (Conversion Factor 10)
Cord blood	13.5–20.5 g/dL	135–205 mmol/L
2 wk	13.4–19.8 g/dL	134–198 mmol/L
1 mo	10.7–17.1 g/dL	107–171 mmol/L
6 mo	11.1–14.4 g/dL	111–144 mmol/L
1 y	11.3–14.1 g/dL	113–141 mmol/L
9–14 y	12.0–14.4 g/dL	120–144 mmol/L
Adult		
Male	13.2–17.3 g/dL	132–173 mmol/L
Female	11.7–15.5 g/dL	117–155 mmol/L
Older adult (65–74 y)		
Male	12.6–17.4 g/dL	126–174 mmol/L
Female	11.7–16.1 g/dL	117–161 mmol/L

Age	Conventional Units (%)	SI Units (Conversion Factor 0.01) *
Cord blood	47–57	0.47–0.57
1 d	51–65	0.51–0.65
2 wk	47–57	0.47–0.57
1 mo	38–52	0.38–0.52
6 mo	35–41	0.35–0.41
1 y	37–41	0.37–0.41
10 y	36–42	0.36–0.42
Adult		
Male	43–49	0.43–0.49
Female	38–44	0.38–0.44

White Blood Cell Count and Differential

Age	SI Units (C.F 10⁹cells/L)	Neutrophils	Lymphocytes	Monocytes	Eosinophils	Basophils		
	WBC $10^3/mm^3$ or cells/µL	Total (Absolute) and %	Bands (Absolute) and %	Segments (Absolute) and %	(Absolute) and %	(Absolute) and %	(Absolute) and %	(Absolute) and %
Birth	0.0–30.0	(6.0–26.0) 61%	(1.65) 9.1%	(9.4) 52%	(2.0–11) 31%	(0.4–3.1) 5.8%	(0.02–0.85) 2.2%	(0–0.64) 0.6%
1 d	9.4–34.0	(5.0–21.0) 61%	(1.75) 9.2%	(9.8) 52%	(2.0–11.5) 31%	(0.2–3.1) 5.8%	(0.02–0.95) 2.0%	(0–0.30) 0.5%
2 wk	5.0–20.0	(1.0–9.5) 40%	(0.63) 5.5%	(3.9) 34%	(2.0–17.0) 48%	(0.2–2.4) 8.8%	(0.07–1.0) 3.1%	(0–0.23) 0.4%
1 mo	5.0–19.5	(1.0–9.0) 35%	(0.49) 4.5%	(3.3) 30%	(2.5–16.5) 56%	(0.15–2.0) 6.5%	(0.07–0.90) 2.8%	(0–0.20) 0.5%
6 mo	6.0–17.5	(1.0–8.5) 32%	(0.45) 3.8%	(3.3) 28%	(4.0–13.5) 61%	(0.1–1.3) 4.8%	(0.07–0.75) 2.5%	(0–0.20) 0.4%
1 y	6.0–17.5	(1.5–8.5) 31%	(0.35) 3.1%	(3.2) 28%	(4.0–10.5) 61%	(0.05–1.1) 4.8%	(0.05–0.70) 2.6%	(0–0.20) 0.4%
10 y	4.5–13.5	(1.8–8.0) 54%	(1.8–7.0) 3.0%	(1.8–7.0) 51%	(1.5–6.5) 38%	(0–0.8) 4.3%	(0–0.60) 2.4%	(0–0.20) 0.5%
Adult	4.5–11.0	(1.8–7.7) 59%	(0–0.7) 3.0%	(1.8–7.0) 56%	(1.0–4.8) 34%	(0–0.8) 4.0%	(0–0.45) 2.7%	(0–0.20) 0.5%

Red Blood Cell Count

Age	Conventional Units	SI Units
Cord blood	4.14–4.69 10^6 cells/mm^3	4.14–4.69 10^{12} cells /L
1 d	5.33–5.47 10^6 cells/mm^3	5.33–5.47 10^{12} cells /L
2 wk	4.32–4.98 10^6 cells/mm^3	4.32–4.98 10^{12} cells /L
1 mo	3.75–4.95 10^6 cells/mm^3	3.75–4.95 10^{12} cells /L
6 mo	3.71–4.25 10^6 cells/mm^3	3.71–4.25 10^{12} cells /L
1 y	4.40–4.48 10^6 cells/mm^3	4.40–4.48 10^{12} cells /L
10 y	4.75–4.85 10^6 cells/mm^3	4.75–4.85 10^{12} cells /L
Adult		
Male	4.71–5.14 10^6 cells/mm^3	4.71–5.14 10^{12} cells /L
Female	4.20–4.87 10^6 cells/mm^3	4.20–4.87 10^{12} cells /L

Age	MCV (fl)	MCH (pg/cell)	(MCHCg/dL)	RDW
Cord blood	107–119	35–39	32–34	14.9–18.7
1 d	104–116	35–39	32–34	14.9–18.7
2 wk	95–117	29–35	28–32	14.9–18.7
1 mo	93–115	29–35	28–34	14.9–18.7
6 mo	82–100	24–30	28–32	14.9–18.7
1 y	81–95	25–29	29–31	11.6–14.8
10 y	75–87	25–31	33–35	11.6–14.8
Adult				
Male	85–95	28–32	33–35	11.6–14.8
Female	85–95	28–32	33–35	11.6–14.8

Morphology	Normal Limits	1+	2+	3+	4+
Size					
Anisocytosis	0–5+	5–10	10–20	20–50	>50
Macrocytes	0–5+	5–10	10–20	20–50	>50
Microcytes	0–5+	5–10	10–20	20–50	>50

Morphology	Normal Limits	1	2	3	4
Shape					
Poikilocytes	0–2+	3–10	10–20	20–50	>50
Burr cells	0–2+	3–10	10–20	20–50	>50
Acanthocytes	< 1+	2–5	5–10	10–20	>20
Schistocytes	< 1+	2–5	5–10	10–20	>20
Dacryocytes (teardrop cells)	0–2+	2–5	5–10	10–20	>20
Codocytes (target cells)	0–2+	2–10	10–20	20–50	>50
Spherocytes	0–2+	2–10	10–20	20–50	>50
Ovalocytes	0–2+	2–10	10–20	20–50	>50
Stomatocytes	0–2+	2–10	10–20	20–50	>50
Drepanocytes (sickle cells)	Absent	Reported as present or absent			
Helmet cells	Absent	Reported as present or absent			
Agglutination	Absent	Reported as present or absent			
Rouleaux	Absent	Reported as present or absent			
Hemoglobin Content					
Hypochromia	0–2+	3–10	10–50	50–75	>75
Polychromasia					
Adult	< 1+	2–5	5–10	10–20	>20
Newborn	1–6+	7–15	15–20	20–50	>50

Inclusions	Normal Limits	1	2	3	4
Heinz bodies	Absent	Reported as present or absent			
Hemoglobin C crystals	Absent	Reported as present or absent			
Pappenheimer bodies	Absent	Reported as present or absent			
Intracellular parasites	Absent	Reported as present or absent			

Inclusions	Normal Limits	1	2	3	4
Cabot rings	Absent	Reported as present or absent			
Basophilic stippling	0–1	1–5	5–10	10–20	>20
Howell-Jolly bodies	Absent	1–2	3–5	5–10	>10

Age	Conventional Units	SI Units (Conversion Factor 106)	MPV (fl)
1–5 y	217–497 $10^3/$ µL/ mm^3	217–497 $10^9/L$	7.2–10.0
Adult	150–450 $10^3/$ µL/ mm^3	181–521 $10^9/L$	7.0–10.2

EXPLAINATION:

Complete blood count (CBC) is a collection of tests used for specific screening purposes. It is probably the most widely distributed laboratory test. Results include the enumeration of cellular blood elements, the calculation of RBC indices, and the evaluation of cell morphology by automation and assessment of staining. The results can provide valuable diagnostic information on the overall health of the patient and the patient's reaction to the disease and treatment.

INDICATIONS:

- Detecting hematological disease, neoplasm, leukemia, or immunological abnormality.
- Determining the existence of inherited hematological abnormality.
- Evaluating known or suspected anemia and correlated treatment.
- Observe the effects of physical or emotional stress.
- Monitor blood loss and reaction to blood replacement.
- Monitor fluid imbalances or medication for fluid imbalances.
- Monitor hematological status during pregnancy.
- Monitor the progression of non-hematological disorders such as chronic obstructive pulmonary disease, malabsorption syndrome, cancer, and renal disease.
- Monitor chemotherapy response and assess undesired reactions to medications that may cause blood dyscrasias.
- Include screening as part of a general physical examination, particularly after entry to a health care facility or before surgery.

RESULT:

Hemoglobin:
• < 6 g/dL
• >18 g/dL
Hematocrit:
• < 18 percent
• >54 percent
WBC count (on admission):
• < 2500/mm3
• >30,000/mm3
Platelet:
• < 20,000/mm3
• More than 1,000,000 / mm3

The appearance of abnormal cells, other morphological characteristics, or cellular inclusions can indicate a potentially life-threatening or severe health condition and, therefore, should be investigated. Examples are the presence of sickle cells, mild spherocyte counts, marked schistocytosis, oval macrocytes, basophilic stippling, eosinophilic counts >10%, monocytosis >15%, nucleated RBCs (if the patient is not a baby), malaria, bacteria, agranular neutrophils, hypersegmented neutrophils, blasts or other immature cells, Auer rods Döhle bodies marked toxic granulation and plasma cells.

IMPEDING FACTORS:

- Failure to fill the tube adequately (< three-fourths full) can result in insufficient sample volume for automated analyzers and may be a cause for the rejection of the specimen.

- Hemolyzed or clotted samples should be rejected for examination.

- Elevated serum glucose or sodium levels may cause elevated mean body volume values due to swelling of erythrocytes.

- A recent history of transfusion should be considered when assessing the CBC.

COOMBS' ANTIGLOBULIN, DIRECT (Direct antiglobulin testing (DAT))

SAMPLING: 1 mL of serum is collected in a red-top tube. 1 mL of whole blood is collected in a lavender-top (ethylenediaminetetra-acetic acid [EDTA]) tube.

TECHNIQUE: Agglutination

NORMAL VALUE: Negative (no agglutination).

EXPLAINATION:

Direct antiglobulin therapy (DAT) detects in vivo red blood cell sensitization antibodies (RBCs). Immunoglobulin G (IgG) formed in certain disease states or responses to certain medications can coat the surface of RBCs, resulting in cell damage and hemolysis. When DAT is done, RBCs are obtained from a patient's bloodstream, cleaned with salt to remove residual globulins, and combined with an anti-human globulin reagent. If the anti-human globulin reagent induces agglutination of the RBCs of the patient, specific antiglobulin reagents may be used to assess whether the RBCs of the patient are coated with IgG, substitute, or both.

INDICATIONS:

- Predict autoimmune hemolytic anemia or fetal hemolytic disorder.
- Assess suspected drug-induced hemolytic anemia.
- Assess transfusion reactions.

RESULT:

Positive in:
• Anemia (autoimmune hemolytic, drug-induced)
• Infectious mononucleosis
• Hemolytic disease of the newborn
• SLE (Systemic lupus erythematosus) and other connective tissue immune disorders
• Lymphomas
• Mycoplasma pneumonia
• Passively acquired antibodies from plasma products
• Post–cardiac vascular surgery
• Transfusion reactions (blood incompatibility)
• Paroxysmal cold hemoglobinuria (idiopathic or disease-related)
Negative in:
Specimens in which sensitization of erythrocytes has not occurred

IMPEDING FACTORS:
- Medicines and substances that may cause a positive DAT include acetaminophen, dipyrone, ethosuximide, fenfluramine, hydralazine, hydrochlorothiazide, ibuprofen, insulin, isoniazid, levodopa, cephalosporins, chlorinated hydrocarbon insecticides, chlorpromazine, aminosalicylic acid, aminopyrine, ampicillin, antihistamines, aztreonam, chlorpropamide, cisplatin, clonidine, mefenamic acid, melphalan, methadone, methicillin, methyldopa, moxalactam, penicillin, phenytoin, probenecid, procainamide, quinidine, quinine, rifampin, streptomycin, stibophen, sulfonamides, and tetracycline.
- Wharton's jelly can cause a false positive DAT.
- Cold agglutinins and massive quantities of paraproteins in the specimen can yield false-positive results.
- Newborn cells may have negative effects on hemolytic ABO disease.

COOMBS' ANTIGLOBULIN, INDIRECT (Indirect antiglobulin test (IAT), antibody screen)
SAMPLING: 1 mL of serum is collected in a red-top tube.
TECHNIQUE: Agglutination
NORMAL VALUE: no agglutination, -ve, Negative.
EXPLAINATION:
The IAT or Indirect Antiglobulin Test detects and recognizes unwanted circulating molecules or antibodies in the patient's serum. The first use of this study was to detect and identify anti-D using an indirect method. The test is now widely used to scan a patient's serum for antibodies that may lead to transfusion of red blood cells (RBCs). The serum of the patient may be incubated with reagent RBCs during processing. The RBC reagents used are from group O donors, and most clinically significant antigens are present (D, C, K, E c, e, M, N, S, s, Fya, Fyb, Jka, and Jkb). Antibodies are found in the RBC membrane serum coat of the patient. The reagent cells are sprayed with salt to eliminate any unbound antibody. In the final step of the test, anti-human globulin is applied. If the patient's serum contained antibodies, anti-human globulin might allow RBCs to hold together or agglutinate.
INDICATIONS:
- Discover any maternal blood antibodies that may be potentially harmful to the fetus.
- Determine antibody titers in Rh-negative people who are sensitized to the Rh-positive fetus.
- Monitor for antibodies before blood transfusion.
- Test for defective Rh variant Du antigen.

RESULT:

	Positive in:
•	Hemolytic disease of the newborn
•	Incompatible crossmatch
•	Maternal-fetal Rh incompatibility
•	Hemolytic anemia (drug-induced or autoimmune)
	Negative in:
•	Specimens in which sensitization of erythrocytes has not arisen (complete absence of antibodies)
•	Specimens in which reagent erythrocyte antigens are unable to detect low prevalence antibodies
•	Samples in which patient antibodies show dosage effects (i.e., more homozygous than heterozygous antibody reactions) and reagent erythrocyte antigens contain single dose

IMPEDING FACTORS:
- Drugs that can cause positive IAT include quinidine, penicillin, phenacetin, and rifampin.
- Recent dispensation of dextran, whole blood or fractions, or intravenous contrast media can result in a false-positive reaction.

BLEEDING TIME

Mielke bleeding time, Surgicutt, Ivy bleeding time, Simplate bleeding time, Template bleeding time.
SAMPLING: Whole blood.
TECHNIQUE: Timed observation of incision
NORMAL VALUE:
Template: 2.5 to 10 minutes
Ivy: 2 to 7 minutes
There are slight differences between the disposable devices being used to make the incision. While Mielke or Prototype bleeding time is claimed to provide more standardization to a subjective technique, both methods are equally sensitive and reproducible.
EXPLAINATION:
Bleeding time is used to test platelet and capillary activity.
INDICATIONS:
- Evaluate platelet and capillary function
- Assess ecchymosis, unexplained bleeding or bruising, and tendency to bleed

- Screen for coagulopathy
RESULT:
This test does not predict unwarranted bleeding during a surgical procedure.

Prolonged in:
•   Hereditary telangiectasia
•   Liver disease
•   Macroglobulinemia
•   Some myeloproliferative disorders
•   Renal disease
•   Thrombocytopenia
•   von Willebrand's disease
•   Bernard-Soulier syndrome
•   Fibrinogen disorders
•   Glanzmann's thrombasthenia
Decreased in:
Not any specific disease

IMPEDING FACTORS:
- Drugs that may prolong bleeding time consist of acetylsalicylic acid, aminocaproic acid, ampicillin, asparaginase, flurbiprofen, fluroxene, halothane, heparin, ketorolac, mezlocillin, carbenicillin, cefoperazone, cilostazol, dextran, diltiazem, ethanol, moxalactam, nafcillin, naproxen, nifedipine, nonsteroidal anti-inflammatory drugs, penicillin, piroxicam, plicamycin, propranolol, streptokinase, sulindac, ticarcillin, tolmetin, urokinase, valproic acid, and warfarin.
- Drugs that may reduce bleeding time include desmopressin and erythropoietin.
- The test should not be done on patients who need restraint, who have excessively cold or edematous arms, who have a platelet count of < 50,000 / mm3, who have an infectious skin disease, or who cannot have a blood pressure cuff placed on the arm.

HEMATOCRIT
Packed cell volume (PCV), Hct
SAMPLING: Whole blood from one full tube with lavender top (ethylenediaminetetraacetic acid [EDTA]), microtainer, or capillary. Whole blood from a green tube (lithium or sodium heparin) can also be obtained.
TECHNIQUE: Automated, computerized, multichannel analyzers

NORMAL VALUE:

Age	Conventional Units (%)	SI Unit (Volume Fraction, Conversion Factor X 0.01)
Baby Cord blood	47–57	0.47–0.57
1 d	51–65	0.51–0.65
2 wk	47–57	0.47–0.57
1 mo	38–52	0.38–0.52
6 mo	35–41	0.35–0.41
1 y	37–41	0.37–0.41
10 y	36–42	0.36–0.42
Adult		
Male	43–49	0.43–0.49
Female	38–44	0.38–0.44

EXPLAINATION:

Blood consists of a fraction of liquid (plasma) and a solid part of red blood cells (RBCs), white blood cells, and platelets. Hematocrit, or packed cell volume, is the number of RBCs in whole blood. For example, 45 percent hematocrit (Hct) means that a 100-mL blood sample contains 45 mL of RBCs. Although Hct is largely dependent on the number of RBCs, the average size of the RBCs plays a role.

Conditions that cause RBCs to swell, such as when the serum sodium concentration is raised, can increase the level of Hct. Hct volume is included in the complete blood count (CBC) and is usually measured together with hemoglobin (Hgb). Both rates are like each other and are the best determinant of the degree of anemia or polycythemia. Polycythemia is a concept used in connection with symptoms resulting from abnormal changes in Hgb, Hct, and RBC counts. *Anemia is a concept associated with conditions resulting from abnormal reductions in Hgb, Hct, and RBC levels. The findings of the Hgb, Hct, and RBC measurements should be tested at the same time as the same underlying conditions influence this triad of measures. The RBC number multiplied by three will represent the Hgb concentration. The Hct should be three times the Hgb if the RBC population is average in size and shape.* The Hct plus six is supposed to equal the first two RBC counts within three (e.g., Hct is 40%; thus, 40 + 6 = 46, and RBC is expected to be 4.3–4.9). There are some cultural variations in the standards of Hgb and Hct (H&H). After the first decade of life, the median Hgb in African Americans is 0.5 to 1.0 g lower than in Caucasians. Mexican Americans and Asian-Americans have higher H&H values than Caucasians did.

INDICATIONS:

- Detecting hematological disease, neoplasm, or immunological abnormality.
- Determining the existence of inherited hematological abnormality.

- Evaluating documented or presumed anemia and related treatment in conjunction with Hgb.
- Monitor blood loss and blood replacement response in conjunction with Hgb.
- Monitor physical or emotional stress effects.
- Monitor fluid imbalances or their management.
- Monitor hematological status during pregnancy in conjunction with Hgb.
- Monitor the occurrence of non-hematological disorders such as chronic obstructive pulmonary disease, malabsorption syndrome, cancer, and renal disease.
- Monitor response to medications or chemotherapy and determine undesired reactions to drugs that may cause blood dyscrasias.
- Include screening as part of a general physical examination of the CBC, particularly after entry to a hospital or before surgery.

RESULT:

Increased in:
• Erythrocytosis
• Hemoconcentration
• Polycythemia
• Shock
Decreased in:
• Anemia
• Blood loss (acute and chronic)
• Bone marrow hyperplasia
• Burns (severe)
• Chronic disease
• Hemolytic reactions

CRITICAL VALUES:
< 18 percent, more than 54 percent = Identify and document some seriously increased or decreased values and indications to the health care practitioner:
- Extreme hemodilution can lead to heart failure and death. Symptoms of hemodilution include rales, anxiety, irritability, edema, hypertension, jugular venous distention, and shortness of breath. Possible interventions include diuretics, fluid and sodium restriction, and careful monitoring of input and output monitoring. Symptoms of loss of blood include hypotension, bleeding, and hypoxia. Once the source of blood loss has been recognized, possible interventions may include blood transfusion and giving vasopressin, omeprazole, or isotonic fluids.

- Severe hemoconcentration can lead to unplanned instant blood clotting. Symptoms of hemoconcentration include reduced pulse pressure and volume, skin turgor loss, dry mucous membranes, orthostatic hypotension, low central venous pressure, tachycardia, thirst, and exhaustion. Possible interventions include intravenous fluids and diuretic cessation if they are suspected of leading to severely elevated Hct. Symptoms of polycythemic overload crises include symptoms of thrombosis, discomfort, and redness in the extremities, facial flushing, and anxiety. Potential interventions include surgical phlebotomy and intravenous fluids.

IMPEDING FACTORS:
- Drugs and substances that may cause a reduction in Hct include those that cause hemolysis as a result of drug sensitivity or enzyme deficiency, such as aminopyrine, amphetamine, anticonvulsants, antimalarials, antipyretics, cephalothin, aminosalicylic acid, dipyrone, dapsone, dimercaprol, diphenhydramine, glucosulfone, glycerin, gold, mephytoin, methyldopa, nalidixic acid, neomycin, niridazole, nitrobenzene, nitrofurantoin, novobiocin, penicillin, phenacemide, propranolol, pyrazolones, quinines, streptomycin, sulfamethizole, sulfamethoxypyridazine, chloroquine, chlorothiazide, chlorpromazine, colchicine, corticosteroids, sulfisoxazole, suramin, tolbutamide, trimethadione, pipobroman (intended effect for polycythemia), primaquine, probenecid, and tripelennamine.
- Other medications may also influence Hct values by increasing or decreasing the RBC count.
- The outcomes of RBC counts may differ depending on the position of the patient: Hct may decrease when the patient is a recumbent position due to hemodilution and may increase when the patient rises due to hemoconcentration.
- Keeping the tourniquet in position for more than 60 seconds can wrongly increase the level by 2 to 5 percent.
- Traumatic venipuncture and hemolysis can result in a false decrease in values.
- Failure to fill the tube adequately (i.e., tube < three-quarters full) may result in insufficient sample volume for automatic analyzers and may be a factor for the decline of the specimen.
- Clotted specimens must be refused for analysis.
- Care should be taken when measuring Hct during the first few hours after transfusion or acute blood loss, as the value may appear to be normal and may not be a reliable indicator of anemia.
- RBC size defects (macrocytes, microcytes) or form anomalies (spherocytes, sickle cells) may change values such as hereditary spherocytosis, sickle cell anemia, and iron deficiency.
- In case of diseases and conditions such as elevated blood glucose or serum sodium levels may cause elevated levels due to swelling of the erythrocytes.

HEMOGLOBIN (Hgb)

SAMPLING: Whole blood from one full tube with the lavender-top (ethylenediaminetetraacetic acid [EDTA]), microtainer, or capillary. Whole blood from a green tube (lithium or sodium heparin) can also be obtained.

TECHNIQUE: Spectrophotometry

NORMAL VALUE:

Age	Conventional Units	SI Units (Conversion Factor 10)
Cord blood	13.5–20.5 g/Dl	135–205 mmol/L
2 wk	13.4–19.8 g/dL	134–198 mmol/L
1 mo	10.7–17.1 g/dL	107–171 mmol/L
6 mo	11.1–14.4 g/dL	111–144 mmol/L
1 y	11.3–14.1 g/dL	113–141 mmol/L
9–14 y	12.0–14.4 g/dL	120–144 mmol/L
Adult		
Male	13.2–17.3 g/dL	132–173 mmol/L
Female	11.7–15.5 g/dL	117–155 mmol/L
Older adult (65–74 y)		
Male	12.6–17.4 g/dL	126–174 mmol/L
Female	11.7–16.1 g/dL	117–161 mmol/L

EXPLAINATION:

Hemoglobin (Hgb) is the central erythrocyte intracellular protein. This holds oxygen (O_2) and eliminates carbon dioxide (CO_2) from red blood cells (RBCs). It also serves as a buffer to preserve the acid-base balance of the extracellular fluid. Each Hgb molecule is made up of heme and globulin. Copper is a cofactor essential for the enzymatic absorption of iron molecules in the heme. Heme contains iron (Fe) and porphyrin molecules that have a high O_2 affinity. The affinity of Hgb molecules to O_2 is affected by 2,3-diphosphoglycerate (2,3-DPG), a material produced by anaerobic glycolysis to generate RBC energy. Once Hgb binds to 2,3-DPG, the affinity of O_2 reduces. An oxyhemoglobin dissociation curve can graphically represent Hgb's ability to bind and release O_2. The expression change to the left is used to define a rise in Hgb's affinity to O_2.

Factors that may trigger this shift to the left include decreased body temperature, decreased 2,3-DPG, decreased CO_2 concentration, or increased pH. Conversely, a shift to the right reflects a reduction in the sensitivity of Hgb to O_2. Conditions that may induce a right shift include an increase in body temperature, an increase in 2,3-DPG levels, an increase in CO_2 concentration, or a drop in pH. Hgb levels are a direct indication of the O_2-combining potential of the blood. It is the mixture of heme and O_2 that gives blood its distinctive red color. RBC counts like the O_2-combining power of Hgb, but because some RBCs produce more Hgb than other cells, the association is not directly proportional.

When CO2 diffuses into RBCs, an enzyme called carbonic anhydrase transforms CO2 to bicarbonate and hydrogen ions. Hgb that is not bound to O2 binds for free hydrogen ions, raising pH. As this binding happens, bicarbonate leaves RBC in exchange for chloride ions. Hgb is incorporated in the complete blood count (CBC) and is generally performed with a hematocrit (Hct). These amounts are parallel and are often used to test anemia.

Polycythemia is a term used in connection with symptoms resulting from abnormal changes in Hgb, Hct, and RBC levels. Anemia is a concept associated with conditions resulting from abnormal reductions in Hgb, Hct, and RBC counts. The findings of the Hgb, Hct, and RBC counts should be tested at the same time as the same underlying conditions influence this triad of measures.

The RBC number multiplied by three will equal the Hgb concentration. The Hct should be three times the Hgb if the RBC population is average in size and shape. Hct plus six will approximate the first two RBC counts within three (e.g., Hct is 40%; so, 40 + 6 = 46, and RBC should be 4.6 or 4.3–4.9). There are some cultural variations in the levels of Hgb and Hct (H&H). After the first decade of life, the median Hgb in African Americans is 0.5 to 1.0 g lower than in Caucasians. Mexican Americans and Asian-Americans have higher values of Hgb and H&H than Caucasians.

INDICATIONS:
- Detecting hematological disease, neoplasm, or immunological abnormality.
- Determining the existence of inherited hematological abnormality.
- Evaluating documented or presumed anemia and related treatment in conjunction with Hct.
- Monitor blood loss and blood replacement response in combination with Hct.
- Monitor the impact of physical or emotional stress on the patient.
- Monitor hematological status during pregnancy following Hct.
- Monitor the development of non-hematological disorders, such as chronic obstructive pulmonary disease (COPD), malabsorption syndrome, cancer, and kidney disease.
- Monitor response of chemotherapy or medications and assess undesired responses to medicines that may cause blood dyscrasias.
- Include screening as part of a general physical examination of the CBC, particularly upon admission to a health care facility or before surgery.

RESULT:

Increased in:
• **Congestive heart failure**
• **Burns**
• **COPD**
• **Dehydration**
• **Erythrocytosis**
• **Polycythemia vera**
• **Hemoconcentration**

•	**High altitudes**
Decreased in:	
•	**Hemorrhage (acute and chronic)**
•	**Hodgkin's disease**
•	Anemias
•	**Carcinoma**
•	**Fluid retention**
•	**Hemolytic disorders**
•	**Hemoglobinopathies**
•	**Incompatible blood transfusion**
•	**Intravenous overload**
•	**Leukemia**
•	**Pregnancy**
•	**Splenomegaly**
•	**Lymphomas**
•	**Nutritional deficit**

CRITICAL VALUES:

< 6.0 g/dL

>18.0 g/dL

Note and record critically higher or lower values and symptoms to the health care provider:

- Severe hemodilution can lead to heart failure and death. Symptoms of hemodilution include rales, agitation, irritability, edema, hypertension, jugular venous distention, and shortness of breath. Possible interventions include diuretics, fluid and sodium control, and careful monitoring of input and output. Symptoms of loss of blood include hypotension, bleeding, and hypoxia. Once the source of blood loss has been detected, possible interventions may include blood transfusion and initiation of vasopressin, omeprazole, or isotonic fluids.
- Serious hemoconcentration can lead to spontaneous blood clotting. Signs of hemoconcentration include reduced pulse pressure and volume, skin turgor loss, dry mucous membranes, orthostatic hypotension, low central venous pressure, tachycardia, thirst, and exhaustion. Possible interventions include intravenous fluids and diuretic discontinuation if they are suspected of leading to severely elevated Hct. Symptoms of polycythemic stress crises include symptoms of thrombosis, discomfort, and redness in the extremities, facial flushing, and irritability. Potential interventions include surgical phlebotomy and intravenous fluids.

IMPEDING FACTORS:
- Medicines and substances that may cause a reduction in Hgb levels include those that induce hemolysis because of drug sensitivity or enzyme deficiency, such as acetaminophen, aminopyrine, aminosalicylic acid, amphetamine, dipyrone, glucosulfone, gold, hydroflumethiazide, indomethacin, antipyrine, arsenicals, benzene, busulfan, cephalothin, chemotherapy, chlorate, chloroquine, chlorothiazide, chlorpromazine, anticonvulsants, carbenicillin, colchicine, diphenhydramine, mephenytoin, nalidixic acid, neomycin, nitrofurantoin, penicillin, phenacemide, phenazopyridine, phenothiazines; and those that result in anemia, such as miconazole and penicillamine, phenylhydrazine, streptomycin, sulfamethizole, sulfamethoxypyridazine, sulfisoxazole, primaquine, probenecid, pyrazolones, pyrimethamine, quinines, trimethadione, suramin, thioridazine, tolbutamide, and tripelennamine.
- Certain medications may also influence Hgb values by increasing or decreasing the RBC count.
- The outcomes of RBC counts may differ depending on the position of the patient: Hct may decrease when the patient is recumbent due to hemodilution and may increase when the patient rises due to hemoconcentration.
- The use of neutraceutical liver extract is highly contraindicated in iron storage conditions, such as hemochromatosis, because it is high in heme (Hgb iron-containing pigment).
- Severe copper deficiency can result in lower Hgb levels.
- Cold agglutinins can falsely increase the mean corpuscular concentration of Hgb (MCHC) and decrease the RBC count, affecting Hgb values. This can be fixed by warming the blood or by replacing the plasma with warm saline and by repeating the test.
- Keeping the tourniquet in position for more than 60 seconds can wrongly increase the level by 2 to 5 percent.
- Failure to fill the tube adequately (i.e., tube < three-quarters full) may result in insufficient sample volume for automatic analyzers and may be a cause for the rejection of the specimen.
- Clotted specimens must be declined for analysis.
- The assessment of Hct should be done carefully during the first few hours of transfusion or acute blood loss, as this may tend to be normal.
- Lipemia would wrongly increase the amount of Hgb, even impacting the mean corpuscular volume (MCV) and mean corpuscular Hgb (MCH). This can be resolved by mixing plasma with saline, repeated measurements, and manually correcting Hgb, MCH, and MCHC using complex mathematical formulas.

HEMOGLOBIN ELECTROPHORESIS

SAMPLING:1 mL of whole blood is collected in a lavender-top (ethylene-diamine-tetra-acetic acid [EDTA]) tube.

TECHNIQUE: Electrophoresis

NORMAL VALUE:

Hgb A	
Adult	>95%
Hgb A$_2$	
Adult	1.5–3.7%

Hgb F	
Newborns and infants	
1 d–3 wk	70–77%
6–9 wk	42–64%
3–4 mo	7–39%
6 mo	3–7%
8–11 mo	0.6–2.6%
Adult	< 2%

EXPLAINATION:

Hemoglobin (Hgb) electrophoresis is a split-up process used to distinguish normal and abnormal sources of Hgb. Hgb A is the primary form of Hgb in a normal adult. Hgb F is the most important form of Hgb in the fetus, the remainder of which consists of Hgb A1 and A2. Small amounts of Hgb F are usual in adults. Hgb D, E, H, S, and C is the result of abnormal amino acid substitutions during Hgb development and are hereditary hemoglobinopathies.

INDICATIONS:

. Aid in the diagnosis of Hgb C Disease.

- Aid in the diagnosis of thalassemia, especially in patients with a positive family history of the disease.

- Differentiation between types of thalassemia.

- Assess hemolytic anemia of unknown cause.

- Assess a positive sickle cell screening test to distinguish sickle cell trait from sickle cell disease.

RESULT:

Increased:

• Hgb A2:

- Megaloblastic anemia
- Thalassemias

• Hgb F:

- Acquired aplastic anemia
- Hereditary persistence of fetal Hgb

- Hyperthyroidism
- Leakage of fetal blood into
- Maternal circulation
- Leukemia (acute or chronic)
- Myeloproliferative disorders
- Sickle cell disease
- Thalassemias

β-Chain substitutions:
- Hgb C leading to Hgb C disease
- Hgb D leading to Splenomegaly without other significant clinical implications
- Hgb E leading to Thalassemia-like condition
- Hgb S leading to Sickle cell trait or disease

α-Chain substitutions:
Hgb H:
- α- Thalassemias

Bart's Hgb:
- α-Thalassemias
- Hgb Bart's hydrops fetalis syndrome

Decreased:
Hgb A2:(Erythroleukemia)
- Hgb H disease
- Iron-deficiency anemia (untreated)
- Sideroblastic anemia

IMPEDING FACTORS:
- At high altitude and dehydration values can increase.
- Iron deficiency can decrease Hgb A2, C, and S.
- False-negative results for Hgb S happen in coincidental polycythemia in patients < 3 months of age.
-Red blood cell transfusion may mask abnormal levels of Hgb within four months of the study.

HEMOSIDERIN

Hemosiderin stain, Pappenheimer body stain, iron stain.

SAMPLING: 5 mL of urine from a random first-morning sample is collected in a clean, plastic collection container.

TECHNIQUE: Microscopic examination of Prussian blue-stained specimen

NORMAL VALUE: None has seen.

EXPLAINATION:

Hemosiderin stain is used to signify the presence of iron storage granules called *hemosiderin* by microscopic examination of urine sediment. Granules of hemosiderin taint blue when potassium ferrocyanide is added up to the sample. Hemosiderin is usually found in the liver, spleen, and bone marrow, but not in the urine. Under normal conditions, hemosiderin is captured by the renal tubules; however, in extensive hemolysis, renal tubule damage, or an iron metabolism condition, hemosiderin filters out through the urine. The Prussian blue stain may be used as well to detect siderocytes (iron-containing red blood cells [RBCs]) in peripheral blood. The occurrence of siderocytes in circulating RBCs is atypical.

INDICATIONS:

- Aid in the diagnosis of hemochromatosis (tissue damage caused by iron toxicity).
- Detection of excessive RBC hemolysis within the systemic circulation.
- Evaluation of renal tubular dysfunction.

RESULT:

Increased in:
• **Burns**
• **Cold hemagglutinin disease**
• **Hemochromatosis**
• **Hemolytic transfusion reactions**
• **Mechanical trauma to RBCs**
• **Megaloblastic anemia**
• **Microangiopathic hemolytic anemia**
• **Paroxysmal nocturnal hemoglobinuria**
• **Pernicious anemia**
• **Sickle cell anemia**
• **Thalassemia major**

HAM'S TEST FOR PAROXYSMAL NOCTURNAL HEMOGLOBINURIA

Acid hemolysis test for PNH.

SAMPLING: 5 mL of whole blood is collected in lavender-top (ethylene-diamine-tetra- acetic acid [EDTA]) top tube, and 3 ml of serum is collected in a red-top tube.

TECHNIQUE: Acidified hemolysis

NORMAL VALUE: No hemolysis seen.

EXPLAINATION:

Paroxysmal nocturnal hemoglobinuria (PNH) is an ailment in which the patient develops nocturnal hemoglobinuria, chronic hemolytic anemia, reduced or absent generation of new red blood cells (RBCs), and susceptibility to thrombosis. This is triggered by an inherited deficiency in hematopoietic stem cells. In patients with PNH, erythrocytes have increased susceptibility to treatment and will lyse when combined with a complement of acidified serum. Patient RBCs are also combined with fresh, natural blood that is ABO compliant with the patient's cells.

A little of the control serum is acidified, and some are heated to inactivate the complement. The result is considered positive if 10 to 50 percent of cell lyses appear in samples mixed with the patient and controlled serum acidification. There should be no hemolysis in the heated control serum. The sugar water test may also be performed to investigate the existence of PNH. Platelet and granulocyte membranes are also impaired, but the positive test of RBC hemolysis is clear evidence of PNH.

INDICATIONS:

- Assess hemolytic anemia, especially with haemosiderinuria.
- Assess suspected congenital dyserythropoietic anemia, type II (also known as HEMPAS (hereditary erythroblastic multinuclearity with a positive acidified serum test)).
- Assess suspected PNH.

RESULT:

Increased in:
• **Congenital dyserythropoietic anemia, type II**
• **Paroxysmal nocturnal hemoglobinuria**
Decreased in: Not any

IMPEDING FACTORS:
- Results may be falsely-positive in the presence of other conditions such as aplastic anemia, HEMPAS, inherited or acquired spherocytosis, leukemia, and myeloproliferative syndromes. False positives may also occur with aged RBCs. The test for sugar water in HEMPAS is negative.
- False-negative results can occur if the patient's serum sample comprises a low level of complement

IRON (Fe)

SAMPLING: 1 mL of serum is collected in a red- or tiger-top tube.
TECHNIQUE: Spectrophotometry
NORMAL VALUE:

Age	Conventional Units	SI Units (Conversion Factor X0.179)
Newborn	100–250 µg/dL	17.9–44.8 µmol/L
Infant–9 y	20–105 µg/dL	3.6–18.8 µmol/L
10–14 y	20–145 µ g/dL	3.6–26.0 µmol/L
Adult		
Male	65–175 µg/dL	11.6–31.3 µmol/L
Female	50–170 µg/dL	9–30.4 µmol/L

EXPLAINATION:
Iron plays a key role in erythropoiesis. Iron is essential for the distribution and maturation of red blood cells and is needed for the synthesis of hemoglobin. The body normally has 4 g of iron, out of which nearly 65 percent of iron is hemoglobin and 3 percent is myoglobin. A small amount is also present in cellular enzymes that catalyze oxidation and reduce iron. Most of the iron is stored in the liver, bone marrow, and spleen as ferritin or haemosiderin. The iron found in the serum is in transit between the food tract, the bone marrow, and the sufficient sources of iron preservation. Iron moves through the bloodstream bound to transferrin, a protein produced by the liver. Usually, iron enters the body by oral ingestion; about 10% is consumed, but 20% can be ingested in patients with iron deficiency anemia. Freed iron is highly toxic, but there is usually an excess of transferrin available to prevent the build-up of unbound iron in circulation. Iron overload is as clinically considerable as iron deficiency, particularly in children's accidental poisoning caused by excessive intake of iron-containing multivitamins.

INDICATIONS:
- Assist in the diagnosis of blood loss caused by decreased serum iron.
- Help in the diagnosis of hemochromatosis or other diseases of iron metabolism and storage.
- Determine the presence of disorders involving decreased protein synthesis or iron absorption defect.
- Help to determine the differential diagnosis of anemia.
- Evaluate unintended iron deficiency.

- Evaluate iron toxicity in dialysis patients or patients with transfusion-dependent anemia.
- Evaluate thalassemia and sideroblastic anemia.
- Monitor hematological reactions during pregnancy when serum iron is normally lowered.
- Monitor exposure to anemia.

RESULT:

Increased in:
• Pernicious anemias
• Sideroblastic anemias
• Thalassemia
• Acute iron poisoning (children)
• Acute leukemia
• Acute liver disease
• Aplastic anemia
• Excessive iron therapy
• Hemochromatosis
• Hemolytic anemias
• Lead toxicity
• Nephritis
• Transfusions (repeated)
• Vitamin B6 deficiency
Decreased in:
• Acute and chronic infection
• Carcinoma
• Hypothyroidism
• Iron-deficiency anemia
• Nephrosis
• Postoperative state
• Protein malnutrition (kwashiorkor)
• Chronic blood loss (gastrointestinal, uterine)
• Remission of pernicious anemia

CRITICAL VALUES:
Ingestion by the child of 30 mg/kg of elemental iron may be sufficient to induce toxicity. More than 400 g / dL is suggestive of possible toxicity. Intervention may include chelation therapy with deferoxamine mesylate (Desferal).

IMPEDING FACTORS:
- Medications that may raise iron levels include blood transfusions, chemotherapy, iron (intramuscular), iron dextran, iron-protein succinylate, methimazole, methotrexate, oral contraceptives, and rifampin.

- Products that may decrease iron levels include allopurinol, acetylsalicylic acid, cholestyramine, corticotropin, cortisone, deferoxamine, and metformin.
- Failure to withhold iron-containing medicine 24 hours before the check can falsely increase the value.

IRON-BINDING CAPACITY (TOTAL), TRANSFERRIN, & IRON
SATURATION (TIBC, Fe Sat)
SAMPLING: 1 mL of serum is collected in a red- or tiger-top tube.
TECHNIQUE: nephelometry for transferrin and Spectrophotometry for TIBC
NORMAL VALUE:

Test	Conventional Units	SI Unit
TIBC	250–350 µ g/dL	(Conversion Factor X0.179) 45–63 µmol/L
		(Conversion Factor 0.01)
Transferrin	200–380 mg/dL	2–3.8 g/L
Iron saturation	20–50%	

EXPLAINATION:
Iron plays a key role in erythropoiesis. It is essential for the proliferation and maturation of red blood cells and the synthesis of hemoglobin. Of the body's normal 4 g for iron (less in women), about 65 percent is present in hemoglobin, and about 3 percent is present in myoglobin. A small amount is also present in cellular enzymes that catalyze oxidation and reduce iron. Most of the iron is stored in the liver, bone marrow, and spleen as ferritin or haemosiderin. The iron present in the serum is in transit between the food tract, the bone marrow, and the available sources of iron preservation. Iron travels through the bloodstream used to transport proteins. Transferrin is the major iron transport protein, holding between 60 and 70 percent of the body's iron. For this function, complete iron-binding capacity (TIBC) and transferrin are sometimes referred to interchangeably, even though other proteins bear iron and participate in the TIBC. Free iron is highly toxic, but there is usually an excess of transferrin sufficient to prevent the build-up of unbound iron in circulation. The level of iron saturation shall be calculated by dividing the serum iron content by the TIBC value and multiplying by 100.
INDICATIONS:
- Help diagnose iron-deficiency anemia.
- Differentiate between iron deficiency anemia and chronic disease secondary anemia.
- Control hematological response to pregnancy medication and iron deficiency anemia.

- Assist in the treatment of hemochromatosis or disorders of the metabolism and preservation of iron.

RESULT:

Increased in:
• **Acute liver disease**
• **Late pregnancy**
• **Hypochromic (iron-deficiency) anemias**

Decreased in:
• **Renal disease**
• **Sideroblastic anemias**
• **Thalassemia**
• **Chronic infections**
• **Cirrhosis**
• **Hemochromatosis**
• **Hemolytic anemias**
• **Protein depletion**
• **Neoplastic diseases**

IMPEDING FACTORS:
- Products that may raise the TIBC level include mestranol and oral contraceptives.
- Products that may decrease TIBC levels include asparaginase, chloramphenicol, corticotropin, cortisone, and testosterone.

KLEIHAUER-BETKE TEST

hemoglobin F, Fetal hemoglobin, acid elution slide test

SAMPLING: 1 mL of whole blood is collected in a lavender-top (ethylenediaminetetra-acetic acid [EDTA]) tube. Freshly prepared blood smears are also suitable. Cord blood may be demanded to use as a positive control.

TECHNIQUE: Microscopic examination of treated as well as stained peripheral blood smear

NORMAL VALUE: < 1 percent.

EXPLAINATION:

The Kleihauer-Betke test is used to establish the degree of fetal-maternal hemorrhage and to help calculate the dosage of RhoGAM to be administered to Rh-negative mothers in some cases. The procedure may also be used to differentiate other types of thalassemia from the inherited presence of fetal hemoglobin. Still, flow-cytometry and hemoglobin electrophoresis techniques are more widely used for this reason.

INDICATIONS:
- Help in the diagnosis of certain types of anemia.

- Calculating dosage of RhoGAM.
- Screening postpartum maternal blood for the incidence of fetal-maternal hemorrhage.

RESULT:

Positive in:
• **Fetal-maternal hemorrhage**
• **Hereditary persistence of fetal hemoglobin**
Negative in: N/A

IMPEDING FACTORS:
Specimens must be obtained before blood transfusion.

LEUKOCYTE ALKALINE PHOSPHATASE

LAP, LAP score, LAP smear

SAMPLING: 1 mL of whole blood is collected in a lavender-top (ethylenediaminetetraacetic acid [EDTA]) tube.

TECHNIQUE: Microscopic assessment of specially stained blood smears

NORMAL VALUE:
32 to 182 (this score is based on 0 to 4+rating of 100 neutrophils)

EXPLAINATION:
Enzyme Alkaline phosphatase is important for intracellular metabolic processes. It is present in the neutrophilic granulocyte cytoplasm from the metamyelocyte to the segmented level. Leukocyte alkaline phosphatase (LAP) concentrations may be impaired by infection, pain, chronic inflammatory diseases, Hodgkin's disease, and hematological disorders. The levels are low in leukemic leukocytes and high in normal white blood cells (WBCs), making this measure effective as a helpful test for the differential diagnosis of leukemia. It should be considered that the test results must be consistent with the patient's condition because LAP levels increase to normal in response to therapy.

INDICATIONS:
Differentiate chronic myelocytic leukemia from other diseases that raise the WBC count.
Monitor Hodgkin's disease response to therapy.

RESULT

Increased in:
• **Down syndrome**
• **Hodgkin's disease**
• **Hairy cell leukemia**
• **Leukemia (acute and chronic lymphoblastic)**
• **Aplastic leukemia**
• **Chronic inflammation**

• Myelofibrosis with myeloid metaplasia
• Stress
• Thrombocytopenia
• Multiple myeloma
• Polycythemia vera
• Pregnancy
Decreased in:
• Paroxysmal nocturnal hemoglobinuria
• Chronic myelogenous leukemia
• Hereditary hypophosphatemia
• Idiopathic thrombocytopenic purpura
• Nephrotic syndrome
• Sickle cell anemia
• Sideroblastic anemia

IMPEDING FACTORS: Drugs that may raise the LAP score include steroids.

METHEMOGLOBIN (Hemoglobin, hemoglobin M, MetHb, Hgb M)

SAMPLING: 1 mL of whole blood is collected in a green-top (heparin) tube. Specimens should be transported tightly capped and in an ice slurry.

TECHNIQUE: Spectrophotometry

NORMAL VALUE:

Conventional Units	SI Units (Conversion Factor X155)
0.06–0.24 g/dL*	9.3–37.2 µmol/L*

* Percentage of total hemoglobin = 0.41–1.15 %.

EXPLAINATION:

Methemoglobin is a structural hemoglobin variant founded when the heme portion of deoxygenated hemoglobin is oxidized to a ferric state, which renders it incapable of combining with and transporting oxygen to tissues. Visible cyanosis can result in an approaching 10 to 15 % of total hemoglobin levels.

INDICATIONS:

- Assist in the diagnosis of inherited methemoglobinemia due to toxic effects of chemicals and medications.

- Assist in the identification of congenital methemoglobinemia, demonstrated by loss of red blood cell nicotinamide adenine dinucleotide (NADH)-methemoglobin reductase or methemoglobin.

- To assess cyanosis in the presence of normal blood gases.

RESULT:

Increased in:

- Acquired methemoglobinemia (drugs, cigarettes containing tobacco or ionizing radiation)

- Carbon monoxide poisoning

- Hereditary methemoglobinemia (NADH-methemoglobin reductase or hemoglobinopathy deficiency)

Decreased in: N/A

CRITICAL VALUES:

Cyanosis can occur at rates >10%.

Dizziness, headache, fatigue, and tachycardia can occur at rates >30%.

Symptoms of central nervous system depression that appear at levels >45%.

Death can occur at rates >70%.

Possible interventions include airway management, oxygen delivery, hourly neurological evaluation, constant pulse oximetry, hyperbaric oxygen therapy, and exchange transfusion. The utilization of activated charcoal or gastric lavage may be successful if it is done immediately after the ingestion of the toxic agent. Emesis should never be triggered in people with no gag reflex due to the risk of aspiration. Methylene blue may be utilized to reverse the methemoglobin formation process, but it should be used with caution when methemoglobin levels are >30%. The use of methylene blue in the case of glucose-6-phosphate dehydrogenase deficiency is contraindicated.

IMPEDING FACTORS:

- Medications that may raise methemoglobin levels include acetanilide, amyl nitrate, aniline derivatives, benzocaine, chlorate, chloroquine, lidocaine, phenacetin, dapsone, glucosulfone, isoniazid, phenytoin, primaquine, nitroglycerin, resorcinol, sulfonamides, and thiazolsulfone.

- Nitrate-containing water from well is the most common cause of methemoglobinemia in children.

- Breastfeeding infants are competent of converting inorganic nitrate from traditional topical anesthetic applications containing nitrate to nitrite ion, resulting in nitrite toxicity and decreased methemoglobin.

- Prompt and proper processing, storage, and analysis of specimens are important for the achievement of accurate results. Methemoglobin is unstable and should be transferred with ice within a few hours of collection, or the specimen should be discarded.

OSMOTIC FRAGILITY

Red blood cell osmotic fragility, OF

SAMPLING: 1 mL of whole blood is collected in a green-top (heparin) tube and two peripheral blood smears.

TECHNIQUE: Spectrophotometry

NORMAL VALUE: Hemolysis begins at 0.5 w/v sodium chloride (NaCl) solution and is complete at 0.3 w/v NaCl solution. Results are compared to a normal curve.

EXPLAINATION:

In this test, RBCs are held in graded sodium chloride dilutions. Cell swelling occurs at lower concentrations of NaCl as it absorbs water in the hypotonic solution. Thicker cells, such as spherocytes, have increased OF; thinner cells have decreased OF.

INDICATIONS: Assess hemolytic anemia.

RESULT:

Increased in:
• **Hemolytic disease of the newborn**
• **Hereditary spherocytosis**
• **Malaria**
• **Pyruvate kinase deficiency**
• **Acquired immune hemolytic anemias**
• ***Decreased in:***
• **Asplenia**
• **Hemoglobinopathies**
• **Iron deficiency anemia**
• **Liver disease**
• **Reticulocytosis**
• **Thalassemias**

IMPEDING FACTORS:

- Medications that may improve osmotic fragility include dapsonine.

- Parasitic infestations, such as malaria, may individually cause cell hemolysis.

- Samples should be sent directly after collection for analysis.

PARTIAL THROMBOPLASTIN TIME, ACTIVATED (APTT)

SAMPLING: 1 mL of plasma is collected in a filled blue-top (sodium citrate) tube.
TECHNIQUE: Clot detection
NORMAL VALUE: 25 to 39 seconds, usually compared X10 seconds to normal control.

EXPLAINATION:

APTT or the activated partial thromboplastin time test assesses the activity of the intrinsic factors (factors XII, XI, IX, and VIII) & common factors (factors V, X, II, and I) coagulation sequence pathways, primarily the intrinsic thromboplastin system. This represents the time needed for a firm fibrin clot to form after thromboplastin tissue, or phospholipid reagents like thromboplastin and calcium have been introduced to the specimen. APTT is dysfunctional in 90% of patients with coagulation disorders and is useful for observing the inactivation of factor II impact of heparin therapy.

The measure is prolonged when there is a deficit of 30 to 40 percent in one of the factors needed or when factor inhibitors (e.g., antithrombin III, protein C, or protein S) are present. APTT has additional activators, such as kaolin, ellagic acid, or celite, which activate factor XII more quickly, making this test quicker and more reproducible than the partial thromboplastin time (PTT). A similarity between the findings of the APTT and the prothrombin time (PT) tests may make it possible to make certain inferences that a factor deficiency exists.

Normal APTT with prolonged PT could only occur in factor VII deficiency. A prolonged APTT with normal PT may suggest a deficit in factors XII, XI, IX, VIII, and VIII: C (von Willebrand factor). Factor deficiencies can also be detected by correction or replacement trials using the regular serum. Such tests are easy to perform and are carried out by applying plasma from a normal patient to a specimen of a patient suspected of having a factor deficiency. When the APTT is repeated and corrected, or within the NORMAL range, it can be concluded that a factor deficiency causes prolonged APTT. Serial monitoring of APTT is not needed for the administration of prophylactic low-dose heparin.

INDICATIONS:

- Diagnose congenital defects of clotting factors as seen in conditions such as hemophilia (factor VIII) and hemophilia B (factor IX).
- Assess reaction to heparin or coumarin-derived anticoagulant therapy.
- Identify people who may be vulnerable to bleeding during surgical, obstetric, dental, or invasive diagnostic procedures.
- Identify possible causes of abnormal bleeding, such as epistaxis, hematoma, gingival bleeding, hematuria, and menorrhagia.
- Evaluate the hemostatic effects of diseases such as liver disease, protein deficiency, and malabsorption of fat.

RESULT:

Prolonged in:
Afibrinogenemia
Disseminated intravascular coagulation
Factor deficiencies
Hemodialysis patients
Polycythemia
Severe liver disease
Vitamin K deficiency
Von Willebrand's disease
Circulating products of fibrin and fibrinogen degradation

CRITICAL VALUES: More than 70 seconds.

Important signs to remember including excessive bleeding, venipuncture site hematoma, hemorrhage, blood in stool, gum bleeding, and shock. Monitor vital signs and neurological changes until levels are within the normal range. Protamine sulfate administration may be needed. The health care provider should also be alerted if the APTT is < 53 seconds in a patient receiving heparin therapy. Lower values indicate that there is inadequate anticoagulation therapy

IMPEDING FACTORS:

- Medications and substances such as anistreplase, antihistamines, chlorpromazine, salicylates, and ascorbic acid can cause prolonged APTT.
- Anticoagulant treatment with heparin can prolong the duration of APTT.
- Copper is a factor V component, and serious copper deficiencies may result in prolonged APTT values.
- Painful venipunctures can trigger the coagulation sequence by contamination of the sample with tissue thromboplastin, and it may produce false shortened tests.
- Failure to fill the tube enough to achieve a correct blood-to-anticoagulant ratio invalidates the tests and is a cause for the rejection of the test.
- Excessive activity that induces hemolysis of the sample may wrongly decrease APTT levels because hemolyzed cells stimulate plasma clotting factors.
- Inadequate mixing of the tube can yield incorrect results.
- Samples left unprocessed for more than 4 hours should be refused for review.
- High platelet count or insufficient centrifugation can result in lower values.
- Hematocrit >55% can produce incorrectly prolonged results due to anticoagulant excess. Excessive anticoagulant chelates the calcium reagent in the test system, making it impossible to react properly with the patient sample.

PLASMINOGEN (Profibrinolysin, PMG)

SAMPLING:1 mL of plasma is collected in the blue-top (sodium citrate) tube.
TECHNIQUE: Chromogenic substrate
NORMAL VALUE: 80 to 120 percent of normal for plasma.
EXPLAINATION:
Plasminogen is a plasma glycoprotein, which is a circulating inactive precursor to plasmin. Damaged tissues discharge a substance called a plasminogen activator that initiates plasminogen conversion to plasmin. Plasmin is active in fibrinolysis and is capable of degrading fibrin, factor I (fibrinogen), factor V and factor VIII.
INDICATIONS:
- Estimate the level of circulating plasminogen in patients with thrombosis or prolonged intravascular coagulation (DIC).
RESULT

Increased in:
• **Pregnancy (late)**
• **Decreased in:**
• **DIC**
• **Postsurgical period**
• **Hereditary deficiency**
• **Liver disease**
• **Neonatal hyaline membrane disease**
• **Fibrinolytic therapy with tissue plasminogen activators like streptokinase or urokinase**

IMPEDING FACTORS:
Drugs that may decrease plasminogen values include streptokinase and urokinase.

PLATELET ANTIBODIES (ANTIPLATELET ANTIBODY, PLATELET-BOUND IGG/IGM DIRECT AND INDIRECT)

SAMPLING:1 mL of serum is collected in a red-top tube for indirect IgG antibody. 7 mL of whole blood is collected in a lavender-top (ethylenediaminetetraacetic acid [EDTA]) tube for direct antibody.
TECHNIQUE: Solid phase hemagglutination and flow cytometry
NORMAL VALUE: Negative.
EXPLAINATION:
Platelet antibodies may be produced by an autoimmune response, or maybe developed in response to transfusion products.

Platelet autoantibodies are immunoglobulins proteins of autoimmune origin (i.e., immunoglobulin G) and are common in multiple autoimmune disorders, including thrombocytopenia.

Platelet alloantibodies evolve in patients who become sensitized to transfused blood platelet antigens. Therefore, both the donor and the native platelets are demolished along with a reduced survival time of the platelets in the transfusion recipient. The platelet antibody detection assessment is also used for platelet sorting, which allows suitable platelets to be administered to patients with disorders such as aplastic anemia and cancer. Platelet typing reduces the risk of alloimmunization resulting from repeated transfusions from anonymous donors. Platelet typing may also provide added support for post-transfusion purpura diagnosis.

INDICATIONS:

- Aid in the detection of platelet alloimmune disorders.
- Help to determine platelet type for refractory patients.

RESULT:

Increased in:
• **Acute myeloid leukemia**
• **Idiopathic thrombocytopenic purpura**
• **Immune complex diseases**
• **Multiple blood transfusions**
• **Multiple myeloma**
• **Neonatal immune thrombocytopenia**
• **Acquired immunodeficiency syndrome (AIDS)**
• **Paroxysmal hemoglobinuria**
• **Rheumatoid arthritis**
• **Systemic lupus erythematosus**
• **Thrombocytopenias provoked by drugs**
Decreased in: N/A

IMPEDING FACTORS: Hemolyzed or clotted samples will affect results.

PLATELET COUNT (Thrombocytes)

SAMPLING: Whole blood from one full tube with lavender-top (ethylenediaminetetraacetic acid [EDTA]).

TECHNIQUE: Automated, computerized multichannel analyzers that sort out and size cells based on either change in light pulses or electrical impedance as the cells pass in front of a laser beam

NORMAL VALUE:

Age	Platelet Count*	SI Units (Conversion Factor 106)	MPV (fl)
1–5 y	217–497 10^3/ L/mm^3	217–497 10^9/L	7.2–10.0
Adult	150–450 10^3/ L/mm^3	181–521 10^9/L	7.0–10.2

EXPLAINATION:

Platelets are non-nucleated, cytoplasmic, round, or oval disks formed by the budding of massive, multinucleated cells (megakaryocytes). Platelets have an essential function in the development of coagulation, hemostasis, and blood thrombus. Thrombocytosis is a rise in platelet counts. In reactive thrombocytosis, the change is acute and short-lived and typically does not pose a health risk. One exception may be aggressive thrombocytosis following coronary bypass surgery. This disease has been identified as an important risk factor for postoperative infarction and thrombosis. The definition of thrombocythemia is used to describe platelet development in chronic myeloproliferative disorders. Thrombocytopenia is used to identify platelet counts of < 140 X10^6/ µL. Decreased platelet counts happen whenever the body's need for platelets reaches the platelet production rate; this will occur if the production rate reduces or the lack of platelets increases. The extent of bleeding is related to platelet count and platelet function. Platelet counts may be within normal limits, but the patient may show signs of internal bleeding; this condition usually indicates an imbalance in platelet function. Abnormal scatterplot results by automated cell counters may signify the need for a peripheral blood test for platelet estimation. Abnormally large or giant platelets can result in underestimated automatic counts of 30 to 50 percent. A massive difference between the automatic count and the estimate requires a manual count. The importance of platelet size is becoming more widely known, as modern cell counters are capable of reporting platelet indexes that are equivalent to red blood cell (RBC) indices. Platelet size, expressed by mean platelet volume (MPV) and cellular age, is inversely related; that is, younger platelets tend to be larger. The increase in MPV indicates an increase in the turnover of the platelet. Therefore, the platelet count and the MPV have an inverse relationship in a normal patient. Abnormal platelet size can also indicate the presence of a disease. In idiopathic thrombocytopenic purpura, both MPV and platelet distribution width (PDW) are raised. MPV also rises in May-Hegglin disease, Bernard-Soulier syndrome, myeloproliferative conditions, hyperthyroidism, and preeclampsia. MPV has declined in Wiskott-Aldrich Syndrome, septic thrombocytopenia, and hypersplenism.

INDICATIONS:

- Verify low platelet count (thrombocytopenia) that may be associated with bleeding.
- Validate high platelet count (thrombocytosis) that may cause enhanced clotting.
- Detect the probable cause of abnormal bleeding, like epistaxis, hematuria, hematoma, gingival bleeding, and menorrhagia.
- Contain screening as part of a complete blood count for general physical examination, mainly after admission to a hospital or before surgery.

RESULT:

Increased in:
Rebound recovery from thrombocytopenia
Acute infections
After exercise (transient)
Chronic heart disease
Cirrhosis
Essential thrombocythemia
Leukemias (chronic)
Pancreatitis (chronic)
Polycythemia vera
Anemias (post hemorrhagic, hemolytic, iron-deficiency)
Rheumatic fever (acute)
Rheumatoid arthritis
Splenectomy (2 months post procedure)
Ulcerative colitis
Malignancies (carcinoma, Hodgkin's, lymphomas)
Trauma
Tuberculosis
Surgery (2 weeks post procedure)
Decreased in (due to megakaryocytic hyperproliferation):
Alcohol toxicity
Aplastic anemia
Congenital conditions (Fanconi's, Wiskott-Aldrich, May-Hegglin, Gaucher's, Bernard-Soulier, Chédiak-Higashi syndromes)
Drug toxicity
Prolonged hypoxia
Decreased in the count (due to ineffective thrombopoiesis):
Megaloblastic anemia (B12/folate deficiency)

Iron-deficiency anemia
Paroxysmal nocturnal hemoglobinuria
Thrombopoietin deficiency
Viral infection
Ethanol abuse without malnutrition
Decreased in the count (because of bone marrow replacement):
Myelofibrosis
Granulomatous infections
Metastatic carcinoma
Lymphoma
Increased destruction (as a result of increased loss/ consumption):
Interaction with foreign surfaces (artificial organs, dialysis membranes, grafts, prosthetic devices)
Severe hemorrhage
Extensive transfusion
Disseminated intravascular coagulation
Thrombotic thrombocytopenic purpura
Uremia
Increased destruction in (due to immune reaction):
Refractory reaction to platelet transfusion
Hemolytic disease of the newborn (HDN) (aim is platelets in place of RBCs)
Antibody/human leukocyte antigen reactions
Idiopathic thrombocytopenic purpura (ITP)
Increased destruction in (due to immune reaction secondary to infection):
Bacterial infections
Burns
Rocky Mountain spotted fever
Histoplasmosis
Malaria
Congenital infections (cytomegalovirus, syphilis, herpes, toxoplasmosis)
Increased destruction (because of other causes):
Splenomegaly due to liver disease
Radiation

CRITICAL VALUES:
< 50,000 K/ µL or mm3
>1,000,000 K/µL or mm3

Possible interventions for reduced platelet count may include transfusion of platelets.

IMPEDING FACTORS:

- Drugs that may reduce platelet counts include acetohexamide, acetophenazine, azathioprine, barbiturates, benzene, dactinomycin, dextromethorphan, diethylstilbestrol, ethinamate, ethoxzolamide, busulfan, butaperazine, chlordane, chlorophenothane, chlortetracycline, amphotericin B, antazoline, anticonvulsants, antimony compounds, apronalide, arsenicals, hydroflumethiazide, hydroxychloroquine, iproniazid, mechlorethamine, nystatin, phenolphthalein, phenothiazine, pipamazine, plicamycin, thiouracil, tolazamide, tolazoline, floxuridine, hexachlorobenzene, hydantoin derivatives, mefenamic acid, mepazine, miconazole, mitomycin, sulfonamides, tetracycline, thiabendazole, nitrofurantoin, novobiocin, procarbazine, pyrazolones, streptomycin, tolbutamide, trifluoperazine, and urethane.
- Medications that may increase the number of platelets include glucocorticoids.
- X-ray therapy may also reduce platelet counts.
- The findings of blood counts can differ depending on the position of the patient. Platelet counts may decrease as the patient recumbents because of hemodilution and may increase as the patient rises because of hemoconcentration.
- Platelet counts usually increase under an array of stressors, such as high altitudes or vigorous exercise.
- Platelet counts are typically reduced before menstruation and during pregnancy.
- The effects can be influenced by leaving the tourniquet in place for more than 60 seconds.
- Owing to the activation of the coagulation cascade, painful venipunctures can lead to misleading results.
- Failure to fill the tube adequately (i.e., tube <three-quarters full) may result in insufficient sample volume for automatic analyzers and may be a cause for the rejection of the specimen.
- Hemolysis or clotted samples are reasons for rejection.
- The complete blood count should be carefully evaluated following transfusion or acute blood loss, as the amount can tend to be normal.
- White blood cell counts >100,000 per mm3, intense RBC fragmentation, and extraneous particles in the fluid used to dilute the sample can change the test results.

PORPHYRINS, URINE (Coproporphyrin, porphobilinogen, urobilinogen, and other porphyrins)

SAMPLING: 10 mL of urine from a random or timed specimen is collected in a clean, amber-colored, plastic collection container with sodium carbonate as a preservative.

TECHNIQUE: Spectrophotometry for δ-aminolevulinic acid, Chromatography for uroporphyrins; urobilinogen, and porphobilinogen

NORMAL VALUE:

Test	Conventional Units	SI Units
Total porphyrins	< 320 μg/24 h	
Coproporphyrin		
Tetracarboxylco protoporphyrin		(Conversion Factor X 1.53)
Male	< 96 μg/24 h	< 147 nmol/24 h
Female	< 60 μg/24 h	< 92 nmol/24 h
Uroporphyrins		
Pentacarboxyl porphyrin		(Conversion Factor X 1.43)
Male	< 4 μg/24 h	< 6 nmol/24 h
Female	< 3 μg/24 h	< 4 nmol/24 h
Hexacarboxyl porphyrin		*(Conversion Factor X 1.34)*
Male	< 5 μg/24 h	< 7 nmol/24 h
Female	< 3 μg/24 h	< 4 nmol/24 h

EXPLAINATION:

Porphyrins are produced during heme synthesis. If heme synthesis is disrupted, these precursors accumulate and are removed from the body in excess amounts in the urine. Conditions that produce increased levels of heme precursors are termed porphyria. The two main categories of genetically determined porphyria are erythropoietic porphyria, in which main abnormalities occur in red blood cell chemistry, and hepatic porphyria, in which heme precursors are found in urine and feces. Erythropoietic and hepatic porphyria are rare. Acquired porphyria is marked by greater concentrations of precursors in stool and urine than the one in red blood cells. Lead poisoning is, by far, the most common cause of porphyria. Porphyrin is a reddish fluorescent substance, depending on the type of porphyrin present; the urine could be reddish, roughly like that of port wine. Porphobilinogen is excreted as a colorless substance. A change of color can occur in a porphobilinogen-containing acid sample if the specimen is open to air over several hours.

INDICATIONS:

- Assist in the evaluation of congenital or acquired porphyria, characterized by abdominal pain, tachycardia, emesis, fever leukocytosis, and neurological abnormalities.

- Identifying possible lead poisoning as demonstrated by elevated porphyrins.

RESULT:

Increased in:
• **Acute hepatic porphyrias**
• **Congenital or acquired porphyrias**
• **Variegated porphyrias**
• **Heavy metal, benzene, or carbon tetrachloride toxicity**
Decreased in: N/A

IMPEDING FACTORS:

- Drugs that may raise porphyrin levels in urine include acriflavine, aminopyrine, ethoxazene, griseofulvin, hexachlorobenzene, oxytetracycline, and sulfonmethane.
- Numerous drugs are identified as possible initiators of acute attacks, but medicines listed as dangerous for high-risk individuals include antipyrine; chlorpropamide, danazol, dapsone, diclofenac, diphenylhydantoin, ergot preparations, ethchlorvynol, ethinamate, aminopyrine, aminoglutethimide, barbiturates, carbamazepine, carbromal, meprobamate, mephenytoin, meprobamate, methyprylon, Nbutylscopolammoniumine glutethimide, griseofulvin, Nisopropyl bromide, novobiocin, phenylbutazone, primidone, sulfonethylmethane, sulfonmethane, synthetic estrogens and progestins, pyrazolone preparations, succinimides, sulfonamide antibiotics, tolazamide, tolbutamide, trimethadione, and valproic acid.
- The exposure of the specimen to light can falsely decrease the values.
- Screening methods are not well standardized and may yield false-negative results.
- Failure to properly capture all urine and preserve the specimen during the 24-hour test period will interact with the tests.

PYRUVATE KINASE (PK assay)

SAMPLING

Whole blood collected in yellow-top (acid-citrate-dextrose [ACD]) tube. Samples collected in a lavender-top (ethylenediaminetetraacetic acid [EDTA]) or a green-top (heparin) tube also may be satisfactory in some laboratories.

TECHNIQUE: Spectrophotometry

NORMAL VALUE: 9–22 U/g hemoglobin.

EXPLAINATION:

- Pyruvate kinase is an enzyme that produces pyruvate and adenosine diphosphate (ADP).

- However, there is also an inherited form of pyruvate kinase deficiency that can be expressed as an autosomal recessive trait.

- Insufficiency of the enzyme could also be obtained via ingestion, medications, or because of liver disease.

- Red blood cells lacking this protein have a membrane malfunction due to low levels of adenosine triphosphate (ATP) and are more vulnerable to hemolysis.

INDICATIONS: Evaluate chronic hemolytic anemia

RESULT:

Increased in:
• **Muscle disease**
• **Myocardial infarction**
• **Carriers of Duchenne's muscular dystrophy**
Decreased in:
• **Acquired pyruvate kinase deficiency: Acute leukemia Other anemias Aplasias**
• **Hereditary pyruvate kinase deficiency: Congenital nonspherocytic hemolytic anemia**

IMPEDING FACTORS:

- Tests after blood transfusion can give a false-normal result.
- The enzyme is not stable. The specimen should be frozen immediately after sampling.

PROTHROMBIN TIME & INTERNATIONAL NORMALIZED RATIO (Pro-time, PT)

SAMPLING: 1 mL of plasma is collected in a blue-top (sodium citrate) tube.
TECHNIQUE: Clot detection
NORMAL VALUE: 10 to 13 seconds.

- International Normalization Ratio (INR) 2.0 to 3.0 for patients receiving medication for pulmonary embolism, venous thrombosis, and valve heart disease.

- INR 2.5 to 3.5 for individuals with mechanical heart valves and medications for reoccurring systemic embolism.

EXPLAINATION:

- Normal APTT and prolonged PT can exist with factor VII deficiency.

- A prolonged APTT with normal PT may imply a deficit of factors XII, XI, IX, and VIII and VIII: C (von Willebrand factor).

- Prothrombin time (PT) is a coagulation study carried out to determine the time required for a stable fibrin clot to develop after adding thromboplastin tissue (factor III) and calcium to the sample.

- It is used to evaluate the extrinsic mechanism of coagulation in patients undergoing oral warfarin or coumarin anticoagulation defects. Prothrombin is a vitamin-K-dependent protein made by the liver.

INDICATIONS:

- Difference between defects of clotting factors II, V, VII, and X that prolong PT; and congenital coagulation disorders such as hemophilia (factor VIII) and hemophilia B (factor IX) that do not modify PT.

- Evaluate exposure to anticoagulant therapy with coumarin derivatives and evaluate the dosage required to achieve therapeutic results.

- Identify possible causes of abnormal bleeding, such as epistaxis, hematoma, gingival bleeding, hematuria, and menorrhagia.

- Identify people who may be vulnerable to bleeding during medical, obstetric, dental, or intrusive diagnostic procedures.

- Monitor the effects of liver disease, protein deficiency and fat malabsorption on hemostasis.

- Prothrombin deficiency monitoring.
- Vitamin K deficiency screen.

RESULT:

Increased in:
• **Hereditary deficiencies of factors like of factors II, V, VII, and X**
• **Afibrinogenemia, dysfibrinogenemia or hypofibrinogenemia**
• **Biliary obstruction**
• **Disseminated intravascular coagulation**
• **Intravascular coagulation**
• **Liver disease**
• **Presence of circulating anticoagulant**
• **Systemic lupus erythematosus**
• **Vitamin K deficiency**
• **Poor fat absorption (tropical sprue, celiac disease, chronic diarrhea)**
Decreased in:
• **Ovarian hyperfunction**
• **Regional enteritis or ileitis**

CRITICAL VALUES:

>20 seconds (uncoagulated)
Three times normal control (anticoagulated)

Important signs to remember including excessive vomiting, puncture site hematoma, hemorrhage, bowel fluid, gum bleeding, and shock. Monitor vital signs and neurological changes until PT is within the normal range. Vitamin K, a potent anticoagulant, may be needed.

IMPEDING FACTORS:

- Medications that may improve PT in patients receiving anticoagulation therapy include acetaminophen, amiodarone, anabolic steroids, anisindione, anistreplase, antibiotics, antipyrin, acetylsalicylic acid (high doses), carbenicillin, erythromycin, glucagon, hydroxyzine, indomethacin, laxatives, mercaptopurine, miconazole, nalidixic acid, clofibrate, corticotropin, demeclocycline, dextrothyroxine, diazoxide, neomycin, niacin, oxyphenbutazone, cathartics, chlorthalidone, cholestyramine, diflunisal, diuretics, doxycycline, phenytoin, quinine, sulfachlorpyridazine, and thyroxine.
- Medications that may reduce PT in patients receiving anticoagulation therapy include amobarbital, anabolic steroids, antacids, antihistamines, barbiturates, carbamazepine, chlorohydrate, chlordane, colchicine, corticosteroids, diuretics, oral contraceptives, penicillin, primidone, rifampin, simethicone, spironolactone, tolbutamide, and vitamin K.
- Traumatic venipunctures can trigger the coagulation sequence by contaminating the tissue thromboplastin sample and creating false shortened PT.
- Failure to fill the tube enough to achieve a suitable blood-to-anticoagulant ratio can cause a false lengthening of the PT; the incompletely filled tube is a reason for the rejection of the specimen.
- Excessive aggression that induces hemolysis of the sample can wrongly shorten the PT because hemolyzed cells release plasma clotting factors.

PROTEIN C (Protein C antigen, protein C functional)

SAMPLING: 1 mL of plasma is collected in the blue-top (sodium citrate) tube.
TECHNIQUE: Chromogenic
NORMAL VALUE: 70 to 140 percent activity (0.7–1.4 U/mL). Values are considerably reduced in children (0.4 to 1.1U/mL) because of liver immaturity.
EXPLAINATION:

Protein C is a vitamin K-dependent protein that originates in the liver and circulates in the plasma. Protein C activation occurs on the endothelial cell surface of the thrombomodulin receptor. Thrombin bound to thrombomodulin receptors ideally activates protein C. Freely circulated thrombin transforms fibrinogen to fibrin. Other steps in the activation process include the binding of calcium and protein S to the cofactor. Activated protein C exhibits potent anticoagulant effects due to the degradation of active factors V and VIII. There are two types of C protein deficiency:

Type I: Reduced antigen and activity, detected by functional and antigenic assays.
Type II: Normal antigen but decreased function, detected only by functional assay. Functional assays are recommended for initial assessment due to increased sensitivity.

INDICATIONS:

- Differentiate inherited deficiency from acquired deficiency.
- Investigate the mechanism of idiopathic venous thrombosis.

RESULT:

Increased in: N/A
Decreased in:
•   Congenital deficiency
•   Liver disease
•   Oral anticoagulant therapy

IMPEDING FACTORS:

- Medications that may increase the level of protein C include desmopressin and oral contraceptives. Medications that may decrease protein C levels include warfarin (Coumadin) and coumarin.
- Placing the tourniquet for more than 1 minute can result in venous stasis and changes in the concentration of plasma proteins to be tested. Activation of the platelet may also occur under these conditions, resulting in incorrect results.
- Vascular injury during phlebotomy can cause platelets and coagulation factors, resulting in incorrect outcomes.
- Hemolyzed specimens must be discarded as hemolysis is an indicator of platelet activation and coagulation factor activation.
- Inadequately filled tubes contaminated with heparin or clotted specimens shall be dismissed.
- Icteric or lipemic specimens interfere with optical test methods and yield incorrect results.

PROTEIN S (Protein S antigen, protein S functional)

SAMPLING: Plasma (1 mL of plasma is collected in the blue-top (sodium citrate) tube.
TECHNIQUE: Clot detection
NORMAL VALUE:

	Conventional Units	SI Units (Conversion Factor .X01)
Total protein S	70–140% activity	0.7–1.4 U/mL
Free protein S	60–120% activity	0.6–1.2 U/mL

EXPLAINATION:
Protein S is a vitamin K-dependent protein that originates in the liver and circulates in the plasma. It is a cofactor necessary for protein C activation. Protein S exists in two forms, free (bioactive) and bound. Approximately 40% of protein S circulates in free form; the rest is bound and functionally inactive. There are two types of protein deficiency:

Type I: Reduced antigen and activity, detected by functional and antigenic assays.
Type II: Normal antigen but decreased function, detected only by functional assa.
y Functional assays are recommended for initial assessment due to increased sensitivity.

INDICATIONS: Investigate the cause of hypercoagulable states.
RESULT:

Increased in: N/A
Decreased in:
• **Congenital deficiency**
• **Coumarin-induced skin necrosis**
• **Diabetic neuropathy**
• **Disseminated intravascular coagulation**
• **Chronic renal failure due to hypertension**
• **Liver disease**
• **Oral anticoagulant therapy**

IMPEDING FACTORS:
- Medications that may minimize protein S levels include oral contraceptives, warfarin (Coumadin), and coumarin.
- Placing the tourniquet for more than 1 minute can result in venous stasis and changes in the concentration of plasma proteins to be tested.
- Activation of the platelet may also occur under these conditions, resulting in incorrect results.
- Vascular injury during phlebotomy can cause platelets and coagulation factors, resulting in incorrect outcomes.
- Hemolyzed specimens must be discarded as hemolysis is an indicator of platelet activation and coagulation factor activation.
- Incompletely loaded tubes contaminated with heparin or clotted specimens shall be dismissed.
- Icteric or lipemic specimens' conflict with optical test methods and yield incorrect results.

PURUVATE KINASE (PK assay)

SAMPLING:
Whole blood collected in yellow-top (acid-citrate-dextrose [ACD]) tube. Samples collected in a lavender-top (ethylenediaminetetraacetic acid [EDTA]) or a green-top (heparin) tube also may be satisfactory in some laboratories.

TECHNIQUE: Spectrophotometry

NORMAL VALUE: 9–22 U/g hemoglobin.

EXPLAINATION:
Pyruvate kinase is an enzyme that produces pyruvate and adenosine diphosphate (ADP). However, there is also an inherited form of pyruvate kinase deficiency that can be expressed as an autosomal recessive trait. Insufficiency of the enzyme could also be obtained via ingestion, medications, or because of liver disease. Red blood cells lacking this protein have a membrane malfunction due to low levels of adenosine triphosphate (ATP) and are more vulnerable to hemolysis.

INDICATIONS: Evaluate chronic hemolytic anemia

RESULT:

Increased in:
• **Muscle disease**
• **Myocardial infarction**
• **Carriers of Duchenne's muscular dystrophy**
Decreased in:
• **Acquired pyruvate kinase deficiency: Acute leukemia Other anemias Aplasias**
• **Hereditary pyruvate kinase deficiency: Congenital nonspherocytic hemolytic anemia**

IMPEDING FACTORS:
- Tests after blood transfusion can give a false-normal result.
- The enzyme is not stable. The specimen should be frozen immediately after sampling.

RETICULOCYTE COUNT (Retic count)

SAMPLING:1 mL of whole blood is collected in a lavender-top (ethylenediaminetetraacetic acid [EDTA]) tube.

TECHNIQUE: Microscopic examination of specially stained peripheral blood smear or automated analyzer

NORMAL VALUE:

Age	Total Erythrocyte Count*
Newborn	3–7%
1–12 mo	0.2–2.8%
Adult	1.5–2.5%

* Values are asserted as a percentage of the red blood cell count.

EXPLAINATION:

Normally, when 15 2.5 matures, the red blood cell (RBC) lacks its nucleus. The residual ribonucleic acid (RNA) can emit a characteristic color as different strains are used, making it easy to recognize and enumerate these cells. The presence of reticulocytes indicates the level of erythropoietic involvement in the bone marrow. Reticulocytes are released into circulation prematurely in unhealthy conditions.

INDICATIONS:

- Assess erythropoietic activity.
- Monitor response to anemia therapy.

RESULT:

The Reticulocyte Production Index (RPI) is a good estimate of RBC production. The estimate corrects the count for anemia and early release of reticulocytes to peripheral blood during cycles of hemolysis or severe bleeding. The RPI also considers the maturation time of large polychromatophilic cells or nucleated RBCs seen on the peripheral film.

Hematocrit (%)	Maturation Time (days)
45	1.0
35	1.5
25	2.0
15	2.5

Increased in:
• Megaloblastic anemia
• Blood loss
• Hemolytic anemias
• Iron-deficiency anemia
Decreased in:
• Sideroblastic anemia
• Alcoholism
• Anemia of chronic disease
• Aplastic anemia
• Bone marrow replacement
• **Endocrine disease**
RBC aplasia
Renal disease

IMPEDING FACTORS:

- Medications that may increase reticulocyte counts include acetanilid, acetylsalicylic acid, amyl nitrate, antimalarial, antipyretic, antipyretic, arsenic, corticotropin, dimercaprol, furaltadone, furazolidone, levodopa, methyldopa, nitrofuran, penicillin, procainamide, and sulphones.

- Medicines that may lower the reticulocyte count include azathioprine, dactinomycin, hydroxyurea, methotrexate, and zidovudine. As the formula indicates, the RPI is inversely proportional to Hct, as follows:

RPI = % reticulocytes X [patient hematocrit (Hct)/normal Hct] X (1/maturation time)

- The number of reticulocytes may be incorrectly raised by the presence of RBC inclusions (Howell-Jolly bodies, Heinz bodies, and Pappenheimer bodies) staining with methylene blue.

- The reticulocyte count may be mistakenly reduced following a recent blood transfusion due to the dilution effect.

RED BLOOD CELL MORPHOLOGY AND INCLUSIONS

SAMPLING: Whole blood from one full tube with lavender-top (ethylenediaminetetraacetic acid [EDTA]) or Wright's-stained, thin-film peripheral blood smear. The laboratory should be discussed as to the necessity of thick-film smears for the evaluation of malarial inclusions.

TECHNIQUE: Microscopic and manual review of stained blood smear

NORMAL VALUE:

Red Blood Cell Morphology	Within Normal Limits	1	2	3	4
Size					
Anisocytosis	0–5	5–10	10–20	20–50	>50
Macrocytes	0–5	5–10	10–20	20–50	>50
Microcytes	0–5	5–10	10–20	20–50	>50
Shape					
Poikilocytes	0–2	3–10	10–20	20–50	>50
Burr cells	0–2	3–10	10–20	20–50	>50
Acanthocytes	< 1	2–5	5–10	10–20	>20
Schistocytes	< 1	2–5	5–10	10–20	>20
Dacryocytes (teardrop cells)	0–2	2–5	5–10	10–20	>20

Codocytes (target cells)	0–2	2–10	10–20	20–50	>50
Spherocytes	0–2	2–10	10–20	20–50	>50
Ovalocytes	0–2	2–10	10–20	20–50	>50
Stomatocytes	0–2	2–10	10–20	20–50	>50

Red Blood Cell Morphology	Within Normal Limits	1	2	3	4
Drepanocytes (sickle cells)	Absent	Reported as present or absent			
Helmet cells	Absent	Reported as present or absent			
Agglutination	Absent	Reported as present or absent			
Rouleaux	Absent	Reported as present or absent			
Hemoglobin (Hgb) content					
Hypochromia	0–2	3–10	10–50	50–75	>75
Polychromasia					
Adult	< 1	2–5	5–10	10–20	>20
Newborn	1–6	7–15	15–20	20–50	>50
Inclusions					
Cabot rings	Absent	Mentioned as present or absent			
Basophilic stippling	0–1	1–5	5–10	10–20	>20
Howell-Jolly bodies	Absent	1–2	3–5	5–10	>10
Heinz bodies	Absent	Mentioned as present or absent			
Hgb C crystals	Absent	Mentioned as present or absent			
Pappenheimer bodies	Absent	Mentioned as present or absent			
Intracellular parasites (e.g., Plasmodium, Trypanosoma Babesia,)	Absent	Mentioned as present or absent			

EXPLAINATION:
The decision to manually review a peripheral blood test for red blood cell irregularities (RBC) shape or size is made based on criteria instituted by the reporting laboratory. Cues in the findings of the complete blood count (CBC) can point to specific abnormalities that can be visually checked by a microscopic examination of the blood sample.

INDICATIONS:
- Assist in the diagnosis of anemia.
- Diagnose hematological disease, neoplasm, or immunological abnormality.
- Determine the presence of inherited hematological abnormality.
- Monitor and observe the effects of physical or emotional stress.
- Monitor the severity of non-hematological disorders such as chronic obstructive pulmonary disease (COPD), malabsorption syndrome, cancer, and kidney disease.
- Monitor drug response or chemotherapy and assess undesired responses to medications that may cause blood dyscrasias.
- Provide screening as part of the CBC, particularly upon admission to a health care facility or before surgery.

RESULT:
Red Blood Cell Size
Cell size increased in:

- Grossly elevated glucose (hyperosmotic)
- Alcoholism
- Aplastic anemia
- Chemotherapy
- Chronic hemolytic anemia
- Hemolytic disease of the newborn
- Vitamin B12/folate deficiency
- Hypothyroidism
- Leukemia
- Lymphoma
- Metastatic carcinoma
- Myelofibrosis
- Myeloma
- Refractory anemia
- Sideroblastic anemia

Cell size decreased in:
- Hemoglobin C disease
- Hemolytic anemias
- Hereditary spherocytosis

- Inflammation
- Iron-deficiency anemia
- Thalassemias

Red Blood Cell Shape

Variations of cell shape are the result of hereditary conditions such as elliptocytosis, sickle cell anemia, spherocytosis, thalassemia, or a hemoglobinopathy (e.g., hemoglobin C disease). Irregularities of cell shape may also arise from acquired conditions, such as physical/mechanical cell damage, exposure to chemicals, or drug reactions.

- Acquired spherocytosis can rise from Heinz body hemolytic anemia, microangiopathic hemolytic anemia, secondary iso-immune hemolytic anemia, and old blood transfusion.

- Acanthocytes are concerned with acquired conditions such as alcoholic cirrhosis with hemolytic anemia, lipid metabolism abnormalities, neonatal hepatitis, malabsorptive conditions, metastatic liver disease, post-splenectomy, and pyruvate kinase deficiency.

- Burr cells are frequently seen in acquired renal failure, burns, heart valve dysfunction, disseminated intravascular coagulation (DIC), intravenous fibrin deposition, hypertension, metastatic malignancy, typical neonatal period, and uremia.

- Codocytes are seen in hemoglobinopathies, iron deficiency anemia, obstructive liver disease, and post-splenectomy.

- Dacryocytes are most often associated with bone marrow metastases, myelofibrosis, myeloid metaplasia, pernicious anemia, and tuberculosis.

- Schistocytes are seen in burns, heart valve disease, DIC, glomerulonephritis, hemolytic anemia, microangiopathic hemolytic anemia, renal grafting rejection, thrombotic thrombocytopenic purpura, uremia, and vasculitis.

Red Blood Cell Hemoglobin Content

RBCs with a normal concentration of hemoglobin (Hgb) level have a clear central pallor and are referred to as normochromic.

- Small Hgb cells with a lack of central pallor are referred to as hypochromic cells. Hypochromia is synonymous with iron deficiency anemia, thalassemias, and sideroblastic anemia.

- Excessive Hgb in red blood cells is referred to as hyperchromic, even though they technically lack central pallor. Hyperchromia is usually associated with elevated mean body concentration of Hgb as well as hemolytic anemia.

- Polychromic cells are young erythrocytes that still have ribonucleic acid (RNA). The Wright's stain picks up the ribonucleic acid RNA. Polychromasia is suggestive of premature release of RBCs from bone marrow secondary to increased stimulation of erythropoietin.

Red Blood Cell Inclusions

RBC inclusions may result from certain types of anemia, abnormal precipitation of Hgb, or parasitic infection.

- Cabot rings can be seen in megaloblastic and other anemia, lead poisoning, and disorders in which RBCs are obliterated before they are released from the bone marrow.

- Basophilic stippling is seen if Hgb synthesis is disturbed, such as thalassemias, megaloblastic anemias, obesity, and lead or arsenic poisoning.

- Howell-Jolly bodies are usually seen in sickle cell anemia, other hemolytic anemia, megaloblastic anemia, congenital loss of spleen, and post-splenectomy.

- Pappenheimer can be seen in cases of sideroblastic anemia, thalassemia, refractory anemia, dyserythropoietic anemia, haemosiderosis, and hemochromatosis.

- Heinz bodies are mostly seen in the blood of patients who have taken medications known to induce the development of these inclusion bodies. People of inherited glucose-6-phosphate dehydrogenase (G-6-PD) deficiency are also seen.

- Hgb C crystals can often be found in peripheral staining in patients with inherited hemoglobin C disease.

- Parasites such as Plasmodium (spread by mosquitoes and inducing malaria) and Babesia (transmitted by ticks), believed to infect human RBCs, can be visualized with Wright's stain and other special peripheral bloodstains.

CRITICAL VALUES:
The involvement of sickle cells or bacterial inclusions should be called to the immediate attention of the patient health care practitioner.

IMPEDING FACTORS:
- Medications and compounds that may increase the production of Heinz body as an immediate precursor to severe hemolysis include acetanilide, acetylsalicylic acid, aminopyrine, antimalaria, antipyretics, furadaltone, furazolidone, methylene blue, naphthalene, and nitrofurans.
- Care in assessing the CBC after transfusion should be considered.
- The results can be influenced by leaving the tourniquet in place for more than 60 seconds.
- Morphology can be assessed to some degree utilizing indices; thus, failure to fill the tube adequately (i.e., tube <three-quarters full) may result in insufficient sample volume for automatic analyzers and may be a cause for the rejection of the specimen.
- Hemolyzed or clotted specimens should be turned down.

RED BLOOD CELL INDICES

mean corpuscular hemoglobin concentration (MCHC), mean corpuscular volume (MCV), red blood cell distribution width (RDW), mean corpuscular hemoglobin (MCH)

SAMPLING: 1 mL of whole blood is collected in a lavender-top (ethylenediaminetetraacetic acid [EDTA]) tube.

TECHNIQUE: Automated, computerized, multi-channel analyzers that sort and measure cells based on changes in either electrical impedance or light pulse as the cells pass through the laser.

NORMAL VALUE:

Age	RDW	MCV (fl)	MCH (pg/cell)	MCHC (g/dL)
Cord blood (at birth)	14.9–18.7	107–119	35–39	32–34
1 day	14.9–18.7	104–116	35–39	32–34
2 weeks	14.9–18.7	95–117	29–35	28–32
1 month	14.9–18.7	93–115	29–35	28–34
6 months	14.9–18.7	82–100	24–30	28–32
1 year	11.6–14.8	81–95	25–29	29–31
10 year	11.6–14.8	75–87	25–31	33–35
Adult male	11.6–14.8	85–95	28–32	33–35
Adult female	11.6–14.8	85–95	28–32	33–35

EXPLAINATION:
Red blood cell (RBC) indices give information on mean corpuscular volume (MCV), mean corpuscular hemoglobin concentration (MCHC), mean corpuscular hemoglobin (MCH), and RBC distribution width (RDW). To evaluate the RBC levels, hematocrit, RBC count, and total hemoglobin measures are used. MCV is established by dividing the hematocrit by the cumulative RBC count and is useful in classifying anemia. MCH is determined by dividing the total concentration of hemoglobin by the RBC count. MCHC shall be measured by dividing the total hemoglobin by hematocrit. Hemoglobin production is defined as normochromic, hypochromic, and hyperchromic. The RDW is a function of the distribution of cell size across the whole RBC population. It is a sign of anisocytosis or excessive cell size variation. Cell size is defined as normocytic, microcytic, and macrocytic.

INDICATIONS:
- Assist in the detection of anemia.
- Predict hematological disease, neoplasm, or immunological abnormality.
- Determine the presence of inherited hematological abnormality.
- Observer the effects of physical or emotional stress.
- Monitor the progress of non-hematological disorders such as chronic obstructive pulmonary disease (COPD), malabsorption syndromes, cancer, and kidney disease.
- Monitor drug response or chemotherapy and determine undesired reactions to medications that may cause blood dyscrasias.
- Include screening as part of a complete blood count (CBC) in general physical examination, particularly on hospital admission and before surgery.

RESULT:

MCV increased in:
• **Vitamin B12/folate anemia**
• **Alcoholism**
• **Antimetabolite therapy**
• **Liver disease**
• **Pernicious anemia**
MCV decreased in:
• **Iron-deficiency anemia**
• **Thalassemias**
MCH increased in:
• **Macrocytic anemias**
MCH decreased in:
• **Hypochromic anemias**
• **Microcytic anemias**
MCHC increased in:
• **Thalassemia**

• Spherocytosis
MCHC decreased in:
• Iron-deficiency anemia
RDW increased in:
• Anemias with heterogeneous cell size
RDW decreased in:
N/A

IMPEDING FACTORS:
- Drugs and substances that may decrease MCHC include styrene (occupational exposure).
- Medications that may reduce MCV include nitrofurantoin.
- Medications that may raise MCV include colchicine, pentamidine, pyrimethamine, and triamterene.
- Medications that may increase MCH and MCHC include oral contraceptives (long-term use).
- Diseases that cause RBC agglutination will change the results of the tests.
- Cold agglutinins will wrongly increase the MCV and decrease the RBC count. This can be resolved by warming the blood or diluting the sample with warmed saline and mathematically correcting the RBC count.
- RBC counts can differ depending on the position of the patient, decrease when the patient is lying due to hemodilution, and increase when the patient rises due to hemoconcentration.
- Safety in the opinion of CBC after transfusion should be considered.
- Venous stasis will falsely increase RBC counts; therefore, the tourniquet should not be left on the arm for more than 60 seconds.
- Failure to fill the tube adequately (i.e., tube <three-quarters full) may result in insufficient sample volume for automated analyzers and may be a reason for the rejection of the specimen.
- Hemolyzed or clotted specimens should be rejected.
- Lipemia and reduced white blood cell count (>50,000 / mm3) can wrongly increase the amount of hemoglobin, which also impacts MCV and MCH.

RED BLOOD CELL COUNT (RBC)

SAMPLING: 1 mL of whole blood is collected in a lavender-top (ethylenediaminetetraacetic acid [EDTA]) tube.

TECHNIQUE: Automated, computerized, multi-channel analyzers that sort and measure cells based on changes in either electrical impedance or light pulse as the cells pass through the laser.

NORMAL VALUE:

Age	Conventional Units	SI Units (Conversion Factor X 1)
Cord Blood (at birth)	4.14–4.69 10^6 cells/mm^3	4.14–4.69 10^{12} cells/L
1 day	5.33–5.47 10^6 cells/mm^3	5.33–5.47 10^{12} cells/L
2 weeks	4.32–4.98 10^6 cells/mm^3	4.32–4.98 10^{12} cells/L
1 month	3.75–4.95 10^6 cells/mm^3	3.75–4.95 10^{12} cells/L
6 months	3.71–4.25 10^6 cells/mm^3	3.71–4.25 10^{12} cells/L
1 year	4.40–4.48 $10^{6\ cells}$/mm3	4.40–4.48 10^{12} cells/L
10 years	4.75–4.85 10^6 cells/mm^3	4.75–4.85 10^{12} cells/L
Adult male	4.71–5.14 10^6 cells/mm^3	4.71–5.14 10^{12} cells/L
Adult female	4.20–4.87 10^6 cells/mm^3	4.20–4.87 10^{12} cells/L

EXPLAINATION:

Component of the complete blood count (CBC) and the red blood cell count (RBC) determines the number of RBCs per cubic millimeter. Since RBCs contain hemoglobin (Hgb), the number of RBCs circulating is significant. Although the life span of normal RBC is 120 days, other factors other than cell age and decreased production may cause decreased values, such as excessive destruction due to intravascular trauma caused by atherosclerosis or increased spleen due to leukemia.Main RBC production sites in healthy adults include the bone marrow of the ribs, skull, sternum, vertebrae, pelvis, and proximal ends of the femur and humerus. Spleen and liver are the leading sites of RBC degradation. Erythropoietin regulates the production of RBC. Normal RBC production and function often rely on sufficient levels of vitamin B12, folic acid, and iron. Vitamin E deficiency may contribute to increased cell destruction. Polycythemia is a term used in association for symptoms resulting from abnormal changes in Hgb, hematocrit (Hct), and RBC counts.

Anemia is a medical term associated with conditions resulting from abnormal decreases in Hgb, Hct, and RBC counts. The findings of the Hgb, Hct, and RBC measurements should be tested at the same time as the same underlying conditions influence this triad of measures. The RBC number multiplied by three will match the Hgb concentration. The Hct should be three times the Hgb if the RBC population is normal in size and shape

INDICATIONS:

- Predict hematological disease-causing RBC degradation (e.g., hemolytic anemia).
- Determine the presence of inherited hematological disorders.
- Monitor the impacts of acute or chronic blood loss.
- Monitor patients with conditions associated with elevated erythrocyte counts (e.g., polycythemia vera, chronic obstructive pulmonary disease [COPD]).
- Observe the effects of physical or emotional stress.
- Monitor the occurrence of non-hematological disorders linked with elevated erythrocyte counts such as COPD, hypothyroidism, adrenal dysfunction, liver disease, bone marrow failure, and malabsorption.
- Monitor response to medications or chemotherapy and assess undesired reactions to drugs that may cause blood dyscrasias.
- Include screening as part of a general physical examination of the CBC, particularly after entry to a hospital or before surgery.

RESULT:

Increased in:
• COPD with hypoxia and secondary polycythemia
• Bone marrow failure
• Anxiety or stress
• High altitude
• Erythremic erythrocytosis
• Polycythemia vera
• Dehydration with hemoconcentration
Decreased in:
• Chemotherapy
• Dietary deficiencies
• Hemorrhage
• Hodgkin's disease
• Chronic inflammatory diseases
• Hemoglobinopathy
• Hemolytic anemia
• Leukemia
• Multiple myeloma
• Organ failure
• Overhydration
• Pregnancy (normal dilutional effect)
• Subacute endocarditis

CRITICAL VALUES:

The appearance of irregular cells, other morphological features, or cellular inclusions may indicate a potentially life-threatening or severe health condition and should be investigated. Examples include the presence of sickle cells, mild spherocyte counts of marked schistocytosis, oval macrocytes, basophilic stippling, RBCs (if the patient is not an infant), or malaria species.

IMPEDING FACTORS:

- Medicines and materials that may decrease RBC count include those causing hemolysis resulting from drug sensitivity or enzyme deficiency, such as acetaminophen, antipyrine, arsenicals, benzene, busulfan, chloroquine, chlorothiazide, aminopyrine, aminosalicylic acid, amphetamine chlorpromazine, colchicine, diphenhydramine, neomycin, nitrofurantoin, penicillin, phenacemide, phenazopyridine, anticonvulsants, carbenicillin, cephalothin, chemotherapy, chlorate, dipyrone, glucosulfone, gold, hydroflumethiazide, indomethacin, mephenytoin, nalidixic acid, and phenothiazine.
- Drugs that may decrease RBC count include those that result in anemia such as miconazole, penicillamine, phenylhydrazine, primaquine, probenecid, pyrazolone, pyrimethamine, quinine, streptomycin, sulfamethizole, sulfamethoxypyridine, sulfisoxazole, suramin, thioridazine, tolbutamide trimethadione, and tripelennamine.
- Drugs that may decrease the RBC count include those that cause bone marrow repressions, such as amphotericin B, floxuridine, and phenylbutazone.
- Medications and vitamins that may improve RBC counts include glucocorticosteroids, pilocarpine, and vitamin B12.
- The use of neutraceutical liver extract is highly contraindicated in patients with iron-storage disorders such as hemochromatosis because it is high in heme (Hgb iron-containing pigment).
- Hemodilution (e.g., unwarranted administration of intravenous fluids, normal pregnancy) in the presence of a normal number of RBCs can lead to false reductions in RBC counts.
- Cold agglutinins can falsely raise the mean corpuscular volume (MCV) and decrease the RBC count. This can be adjusted by warming the blood or diluting the sample with warmed saline and performing the analysis again.
- Excessive exercise, anxiety, pain, and dehydration can cause false increases in RBC counts.
- A massively elevated white blood cell count (more than 500,000 103 / mm3) may cause a falsely elevated RBC count. This can be resolved by diluting the sample with saline to obtain an accurate white blood cell count and mathematically correcting the RBC.
- Consideration in evaluating the CBC following transfusion should be considered.
- RBC counts can differ depending on the position of the patient, decrease when the patient is lying due to hemodilution, and increase when the patient rises due to hemoconcentration.

- Venous stasis can mistakenly raise RBC counts; thus, the tourniquet should not be left on the arm for more than 60 seconds.
- Failure to fill the tube adequately (i.e., tube <three-quarters full) may result in insufficient sample volume for automatic analyzers and may be a cause for the rejection of the specimen.
- Hemolyzed or clotted samples should be rejected for examination.

RED BLOOD CELL CHOLINESTERASE (acetylcholinesterase (ACE), RBC)

SAMPLING:1 mL of whole blood is collected in a lavender-top (ethylenediaminetetraacetic acid [EDTA]) tube.

TECHNIQUE: Spectrophotometry, kinetic

NORMAL VALUE:

Test	Conventional Units	SI Units (Conversion Factor X1)
RBC cholinesterase	5–10 U/mL	5–10 kU/L

EXPLAINATION:

There are two forms of cholinesterase: acetylcholinesterase, which is found in red blood cells (RBCs), the lung, and the brain (nerve) tissue; and cholinesterase, which is located mainly in the plasma, liver, and heart. RBC cholinesterase is used to help identify chronic carbamate or organophosphate insecticide (e.g., parathion, malathion) toxicity. Organophosphate pesticides bind irretrievably to cholinesterase, inhibiting natural enzyme activity. Carbamate insecticides bind reversibly. Serum or plasma pseudocholinesterase is more frequently used to measure acute pesticide toxicity.

Patients of hereditary cholinesterase deficiency are at risk during anesthesia when succinylcholine is used as an anesthetic. Succinylcholine is a reversible acetylcholinesterase inhibitor and is hydrolyzed by cholinesterase resulting in prolonged apnea. This test, together with the pseudocholinesterase test, is also used to identify individuals with atypical types of the enzyme cholinesterase. The prevalence of succinylcholine sensitivity in 1,500 patients is 1. Wide preoperative screening is not routinely performed.

INDICATIONS:

Check alleged exposure to organic phosphate insecticides.
- Track cumulative exposure to biphosphate insecticides.

RESULT:

Increased in:
Sickle cell anemia
Decreased in:
Insecticide exposure (organic phosphate)
Late pregnancy
Paroxysmal nocturnal hemoglobinuria
Relapse of megaloblastic anemia

IMPEDING FACTORS:

- Medications and compounds that may increase RBC cholinesterase levels include echothiophate, parathion, and antiepileptic drugs such as carbamazepine, phenobarbital, phenytoin, and valproic acid.
- Inadequate anticoagulant: fluoride interferes with the calculation and induces a fake decrease in value.

SICKLE CELL SCREEN (Sickle cell test)

SAMPLING: 1 mL of whole blood is collected in a lavender-top (ethylenediaminetetraacetic acid [EDTA]) tube.
TECHNIQUE: Hemoglobin high-salt solubility
NORMAL VALUE: Negative.
EXPLAINATION:

The sickle cell test is one of a few screening tests for a group of inherited hemoglobinopathies. The test is positive in the case of rare sickle hemoglobin (Hgb) forms such as Hgb S and Hgb C Harlem. Hgb S is the result of an amino acid substitution during Hgb synthesis by which amino acid valine replaces glutamic acid. Hemoglobin C Harlem is the result of lysine substitution for glutamic acid. Persons with sickle cell disease have chronic anemia because abnormal Hgb cannot carry oxygen. The red blood cells of the affected people are also abnormally shaped, resembling a crescent or sickle rather than a typical disk shape. This abnormality, combined with the stiffness of the cell wall, prevents cells from passing through smaller blood vessels. Blockages in the blood vessels cause hypoxia, damage, and pain. Individuals with a sickle cell trait do not have clinical manifestations of the condition. Still, they can transfer the disorder on to children if the other person has a phenotype (or disease) as well.

INDICATIONS:

- Identify sickled red blood cells.
- Assess hemolytic anemias.

RESULT:

Positive findings in:
• Hgb C Harlem anemia
• Sickle cell anemia
• Sickle cell trait
• Thalassemias
• Combination of Hgb S with other hemoglobinopathies
Negative findings in N/A

IMPEDING FACTORS:

- Medications that may increase the number of sickle cells in vitro include prostaglandins.
- A positive test does not differentiate between sickle and sickle cell anemia; a follow-up a test using Hgb electrophoresis should be done to make this determination.
- False-negative results can occur in children < 3 months of age.
- False-negative findings may occur in patients who have received a previous blood transfusion before the collection of specimens due to dilution.
- False-positive results may occur in patients without a trait or illness who have undergone a blood transfusion from a sickle cell-positive donor; this effect may last for four months after the transfusion.
- The test results will not be accurate if the patient has pernicious anemia or polycythemia.

TRANSFERRIN (Siderophilin, TRF)

SAMPLING: 1 mL of serum is collected in a red- or tiger-top tube.
TECHNIQUE: Nephelometry
NORMAL VALUE:

Age	Conventional Units	SI Units (Conversion Factor 0.01)
Newborn	130–275 mg/dL	1.3–2.75 g/L
Adults		
Male	215–365 mg/dL	2.2–3.6 g/L
Female	250–380 mg/dL	2.5–3.8 g/L

EXPLAINATION:

Transferrin is a glycoprotein by nature that is formed in the liver. This contains circulating iron derived from dietary intake and the degradation of red blood cells. Transferrin contains 50 to 70 percent of the body's iron; it is normally about one-third saturated. Insufficient transferrin levels can lead to impaired hemoglobin synthesis and anemia. Transferrin is susceptible to diurnal variation and is responsible for changes in serum iron levels throughout the day.

INDICATIONS:

- Help to determine the iron-binding capacity of the blood.
- Evaluate the absorption of iron in iron deficiency anemia.
- Evaluate the dietary status.
- Hemochromatosis test.

RESULT:

Increased in:	
Iron-deficiency anemia	
Decreased in:	
Acute or chronic infection	
Cancer (especially of the gastrointestinal tract)	
Hereditary atransferrinemia	
Excessive protein loss from renal disease	
Hepatic damage	
Malnutrition	

IMPEDING FACTORS:

- Drugs that may raise transferrin levels include carbamazepine, danazole, mestranol, and oral contraceptives.

- Medications that may reduce transferrin levels include cortisone and dextran.

- Transferrin levels are dependent on diurnal variation and should be measured in the morning when the level is greatest.

WHITE BLOOD CELL COUNT & CELL DIFFERENTIAL
(WBC with diff, white cell count, leukocyte count)

SAMPLING: Whole blood in one full lavender-top tube with ethylenediaminetetraacetic acid [EDTA].

TECHNIQUE: Automated, computer-based, multichannel analyzers.

NORMAL VALUES:

The WBC count and differential specifies and identifies granulocytes, eosinophils, lymphocytes, monocytes, basophils, and platelets.

Age	SI Units (Conversion Factor X10 cells/L)*	Neutrophils Total (Absolute) and %	Neutrophils Bands (Absolute) and %	Neutrophils Segments (Absolute) and %
Birth	9.0–30.0	(6.0–26.0) 61%	(1.65) 9.1%	(9.4) 52%
1 d	9.4–34.0	(5.0–21.0) 61%	(1.75) 9.2%	(9.8) 52%
2 wk	5.0–20.0	(1.0–9.5) 40%	(0.63) 5.5%	(3.9) 34%
1 mo	5.0–19.5	(1.0–9.0) 35%	(0.49) 4.5%	(3.3) 30%
6 mo	6.0–17.5	(1.0–8.5) 32%	(0.45) 3.8%	(3.3) 28%
1 y	6.0–17.5	(1.5–8.5) 31%	(0.35) 3.1%	(3.2) 28%
10 y	4.5–13.5	(1.8–8.0) 54%	(0–1.0) 3.0%	(1.8–7.0) 51%
Adult	4.5–11.0	(1.8–7.7) 59%	(0–0.7) 3.0%	(1.8–7.0) 56%

Lymphocytes(Absolute) and %	Monocytes(Absolute) and %	Eosinophils(Absolute) and %	Basophils(Absolute) and %
(2.0–11) 31%	(0.4–3.1) 5.8%	(0.02–0.85) 2.2%	(0–0.64) 0.6%
(2.0–11.5) 31%	(0.2–3.1) 5.8%	(0.02–0.95) 2.0%	(0–0.30) 0.5%
(2.0–17.0) 48%	(0.2–2.4) 8.8%	(0.07–1.0) 3.1%	(0–0.23) 0.4%
(2.5–16.5) 56%	(0.15–2.0) 6.5%	(0.07–0.90) 2.8%	(0–0.20) 0.5%
(4.0–13.5) 61%	(0.1–1.3) 4.8%	(0.07–0.75) 2.5%	(0–0.20) 0.4%
(4.0–10.5) 61%	(0.05–1.1) 4.8%	(0.05–0.70) 2.6%	(0–0.20) 0.4%
(1.5–6.5) 38%	(0–0.8) 4.3%	(0–0.60) 2.4%	(0–0.20) 0.5%
(1.0–4.8) 34%	(0–0.8) 4.0%	(0–0.45) 2.7%	(0–0.20) 0.5%

EXPLAINATION:

White blood cells (WBCs) are the body's primary defense system against foreign tissues, organisms, and other compounds. The life of a healthy WBC is between 13 and 20 days. New WBCs have been eliminated by the lymphatic system and evacuated in the feces. The main types of WBCs are neutrophils, monocytes, eosinophils, basophils, and lymphocytes. These are yielded by the bone marrow, while lymphocytes can also be produced in other areas. The WBC count can be conducted on its own with the differential cell count or as part of the complete blood count (CBC). Increasing WBC count is termed leukocytosis, and reduced WBC count is called leukopenia. An overall WBC count indicates the degree of reaction to a pathological process, but the differential count gives a complete assessment of the specific diagnosis of any condition.

The WBCs in the count and the variance are stated as an absolute value and as a percentage.

The relative percentages of cell types are obtained by basing the classification of each cell type on a 100-cell count. The absolute count is acquired by multiplying the relative percentage of each cell type by the total WBC count.

Neutrophils are usually found to be the predominant type of WBC in circulating blood. Often called polymorphonuclear cells, they are the body's first line of defense through the phagocytosis process. They often contain enzymes and pyrogens that battle foreign invaders. Lymphocytes are agranular, mononuclear blood cells smaller than granulocytes. These are found in the next highest percentage of normal circulation. Lymphocytes are known as B and T cells.

All forms are produced in the bone marrow, while B cells get matured in the bone marrow, T cells mature in the thymus. Lymphocytes play a main role in the body's natural defense mechanism. B cells differentiate into plasma cell-synthesizing immunoglobulin cells. T cells serve as cellular immune mediators and include helper/inducer (CD4) lymphocytes, cytotoxic (CD8 or CD4) lymphocytes, and suppressor (CD8) lymphocytes, delayed hypersensitivity lymphocytes. Monocytes are mononuclear cells like lymphocytes but are more closely related to granulocytes in terms of their function. They are made from the same cells in the bone marrow as those that generate neutrophils.

Phagocytosis is the main function of monocytes. Monocytes remain in peripheral blood for about 70 hours, after which they migrate to the tissues and become macrophages. Eosinophils have the feature of phagocytosis of antigen-antibody complexes. During later stages of inflammation, they become aggressive.

Eosinophils come into action against allergic and parasitic diseases: they have specific granules of histamine used to destroy foreign cells in the body and specialized proteolytic enzymes that injure parasitic worms. Basophils are present in the circulating blood in small numbers. They have a phagocytic feature and contain several different granules, like eosinophils. Basophilic granules contain heparin, histamine, and serotonin. Basophils can also be found in tissues and are known as mast cells. Basophilia is seen in diseases such as asthma, polycythemia vera, ulcerative colitis, Hodgkin's disease, nephrosis, and chronic hypersensitivity.

INDICATIONS:
- Assist in verifying presumed bone marrow dysfunction.
- Assist in determining the cause of decreased WBC count (e.g., cancer, inflammatory process).
- Detecting hematological disease, neoplasm, or immunological abnormality.
- Determining the existence of inherited hematological abnormality.
- Monitor the effects of physical or emotional distress.
- Monitor the progression of non-hematological disorders, such as chronic obstructive pulmonary disease (COPD), malabsorption syndrome, cancer, and kidney disease.
- Monitor drug response or chemotherapy and assess undesired reactions to medications that may cause blood dyscrasias.
- Provide screening as part of the CBC for general physical examination, particularly upon entry to the health care facility.

RESULT:

WBC Abnormalities	Associated Condition
Alder-Reilly cytoplasmic granulations	A hereditary condition, ucopolysaccharidosis
Auer bodies or Auer rods	Acute myelocytic leukemia, yelomonocytic leukemia

Chédiak-Higashi lysosomal granulations	A hereditary condition, albinism, leukopenia, thrombocytopenia
Döhle bodies	Infections, inflammatory conditions, burns, myelocytic leukemia
Hypersegmented neutrophils	Megaloblastic anemia
Systemic lupus erythematosus (SLE) cells	SLE and other collagen diseases, drug reactions, chronic hepatitis
Left shift	Infections, intoxication, tissue necrosis, leukemia, pernicious anemia
Leukemic cells (immature blast forms)	Leukemia, leukemoid reaction, severe infection, myeloproliferative disorders, intoxication, malignancy, recovery from bone marrow suppression
May-Hegglin anomaly	The hereditary condition with thrombocytopenia and giant platelets
Smudge cells	Leukemias
Pelger-Huët cells	A hereditary condition, myelocytic leukemia, myeloproliferative disorders
Tart cell	Drug reactions
Toxic Granulation	Infections, inflammatory conditions

cells Left shift
- Leukemic cells (immature blast forms)
- May-Hegglin anomaly
- Smudge cells
- Pelger-Huët cells
- Tart cell
- Toxic granulation
- A hereditary condition, mucopolysaccharidosis
- Acute myelocytic leukemia, myelomonocytic leukemia
- A hereditary condition, albinism, leukopenia,
- thrombocytopenia
- SLE and other collagen diseases, drug
- reactions, chronic hepatitis
- Infections, intoxication, tissue necrosis,
- leukemia, pernicious anemia
- Leukemia, leukemoid reaction, severe
- infection, myeloproliferative disorders,
- intoxication, malignancy, recovery from bone marrow suppression
- Infections, inflammatory conditions, burns,
- myelocytic leukemia

- Megaloblastic anemia
- The hereditary condition with thrombocytopenia and giant platelets
  Leukemias
- A hereditary condition, myelocytic leukemia,
- myeloproliferative disorders
- Drug reactions
- Infections, inflammatory conditions

Increased in (leukocytosis):

Normal physiologic and environmental conditions:
- Increased epinephrine secretion
- Menstruation
- Pregnancy and labor
- Strenuous exercise
- Ultraviolet light
- Early infancy
- Emotional stress
- Exposure to cold

Pathologic conditions:
- Acute hemolysis, transfusion
- reactions
- All types of infections
- Anemias
- Appendicitis
- Collagen disorders
- Parasitic infestations
- Polycythemia vera
- Cushing's disease
- Inflammatory disorders
- Leukemias and other malignancies

Decreased in (leukopenia):

Normal physiologic conditions:
- Diurnal rhythms

Pathologic conditions:
- Alcoholism
- Anemias
- Bone marrow depression
- SLE and other autoimmune
- disorders
- Malaria
- Malnutrition
- Radiation
- Rheumatoid arthritis
- Toxic and antineoplastic drugs
- Viral infections

Neutrophils increased (neutrophilia):
- Extremes in temperature
- Inflammatory conditions (i.e., rheumatic fever, gout, rheumatoid arthritis, vasculitis, myositis)
- Acute hemolysis
- Infectious diseases
- Acute hemorrhage
- Malignancies
- Metabolic disorders (uremia, thyroid storm, eclampsia, diabetic ketoacidosis, Cushing's syndrome)
- Myelocytic leukemia
- Physiologic stress (e.g., allergies, asthma, exercise, childbirth, surgery)

Neutrophils decreased (neutropenia):
- Acromegaly
- Addison's disease
- Anaphylaxis
- Anorexia nervosa, starvation, malnutrition
- Vitamin B12 or folate deficiency
- Disseminated SLE
- Thyrotoxicosis
- Viral infection (mononucleosis, hepatitis, influenza)
- Bone marrow depression (viruses, radiation, toxic chemicals, overwhelming infection, Gaucher's disease)

Lymphocytes increased (lymphocytosis):
- Infections
- Lymphocytic leukemia
- Lymphomas
- Lymphosarcoma
- Malnutrition
- Myeloma
- Rickets
- Thyrotoxicosis
- Ulcerative colitis
- Waldenström's macroglobulinemia
- Addison's disease
- Felty's syndrome

Lymphocytes decreased (lymphopenia):
- Bone marrow failure
- Burns
- Gaucher's disease
- Hemolytic disease of the newborn
- High doses of adrenocorticosteroids
- Hodgkin's disease
- Hypersplenism

- Immunodeficiency diseases
- Antineoplastic drugs
- Aplastic anemia
- Pernicious anemia
- Pneumonia
- Radiation
- Rheumatic fever
- Septicemia
- Thrombocytopenic purpura
- Toxic chemical exposure
- Transfusion reaction

Monocytes increased (monocytosis):
- Carcinomas
- Cirrhosis
- Gaucher's disease
- Hemolytic anemias
- Hodgkin's disease
- Infections
- Radiation
- Sarcoidosis
- SLE
- Thrombocytopenic purpura
- Ulcerative colitis
- Lymphomas
- Monocytic leukemia
- Polycythemia vera
- Collagen diseases

CRITICAL VALUES:

< 2500 WBC/mm3 (on admission)

>30,000 WBC/mm3 (on admission)

The presence of abnormal cells, other morphologic features, or cellular inclusions may signify a potentially life-threatening or serious health condition.

IMPEDING FACTORS:

- drugs that may lower the overall WBC count include acetyldigitoxin, aminosalicylic acid, ampicillin, amsacrine, antazoline, acetylsalicylic acid, aminoglutethimide, aminopyrine, anticonvulsants, antineoplastic agents (therapeutic intent), antipyrine, cisplatin, colchicine, colistimethate, cycloheximide, cyclophosphamide, cytarabine, dacarbazine, dactinomycin, chloramphenicol, chlordane, chlorophenothane, chlortetracycline, barbiturates, busulfan, carbutamide, carmustine, chlorambucil, chlorthalidone,diaprim, diazepam, diethylpropion, digitalis, dipyridamole, dipyrone, fumagillin, glaucarubin, glucosulfone,
- hexachlorobenzene, hydroflumethiazide, hydroxychloroquine, thiouracil, iproniazid, lincomycin, local anesthetics, mercaptopurine, paramethadione, parathion, penicillin, phenacemide, mefenamic acid, mepazine, meprobamate, methotrexate, methylpromazine, mitomycin, phenindione, phenothiazine, pipamazine, prednisone, prochlorperazine, quinacrine, quinines, radioactive compounds, razoxane, ristocetin, primaquine, procainamide, procarbazine, sulfa drugs, promazine, promethazine, pyrazolones, tamoxifen, tetracycline, thenalidine, thioridazine, tolazamide, tolazoline, tolbutamide, trimethadione, and urethan.
- A noteworthy decrease in basophilic count occurs quickly following intravenous injection of propane and thiopental.
- A significant reduction in lymphocyte count happens quickly following administration of corticotropin, mechlorethamine, methysergide, and x-ray therapy; and megadoses of niacin, pyridoxine, and thiamine.
- Medications that may increase the overall WBC count include amphetamine, amphotericin B, chloramphenicol, chloroform (normal response to anesthesia), colchicine (leukocytosis causes leukopenia), erythromycin, corticotropin, ether (normal response to anesthesia), fluroxene (normal response to anesthesia), isoflurane (normal response to anesthesia), phenylbutazone, niacinamide, prednisone, and quinine.
- Drug allergies may have a considerable effect on the eosinophilic count and may affect the overall WBC count. Please refer to the specific monograph for a detailed list of intervention medicines.
- The WBC count may vary dependent on the position of the patient, decreasing when the patient is recumbent due to hemodilution and increasing when the patient rises due to hemoconcentration.
- Venous stasis may wrongly increase the results; the tourniquet should not be left on the arm for more than 60 seconds.
- Failure to fill the tube adequately (i.e., tube <three-quarters full) may result in insufficient sample volume for automated analyzers. It may be the cause of the rejection of the specimen.
- Hemolyzed or clotted specimens should be refused for analysis.
- The existence of nucleated red blood cells or giant or clustered platelets impacts the automated WBC, causing manual adjustment of the WBC count.

- Care should be taken to test the CBC during the first few hours after the transfusion.
- Persons/Patients with cold agglutinins or monoclonal gammopathies might have an incorrectly reduced WBC count due to cell clumping.

TUMOR MARKERS:

CARCINOEMBRYONIC ANTIGEN (CEA)

SAMPLING: 1 mL of serum is collected in a red-top tube. 1 mL of plasma collected in a lavender-top (ethylenediaminetetra-acetic acid [EDTA]) tube is also acceptable. Care should be taken to use the same type of collection container if serial measurements are to be made.

TECHNIQUE: Enzyme immunoassay

NORMAL VALUE:

Smoking Status	Conventional Units	SI Units (Conversion Factor X1)
Smoker	< 5.0 ng/mL	< 5.0 µg/L
Nonsmoker	< 2.5 ng/mL	< 2.5 µg/L

EXPLAINATION:

Carcinoembryonic antigen (CEA) is a glycoprotein mainly produced during the fetal period and the rapid division of epithelial cells, particularly in the digestive system. CEA is also present in chronic smokers' blood. Though this test is not useful in diagnosing any disease and is not beneficial as a screening test for carcinomas, it is useful in monitoring the responsiveness to antineoplastic therapy for breast and gastrointestinal cancer.

INDICATIONS:

- Determination of stage of colorectal cancer and recurrence tests.
- Monitor response to breast and gastrointestinal cancer treatment.

RESULT:

Increased in:
• Benign tumors, including benign breast disease
• Colorectal, gastric, pancreatic, pulmonary, breast, head, or neck, oesophageal, ovarian or prostate cancer
• Chronic tobacco smoking
• Radiation therapy (transient)
Decreased in: N/A

CA 125 (Carbohydrate antigen 125, cancer antigen 125)

SAMPLING: 1 mL of serum is collected in a red-top tube.

TECHNIQUE: Enzyme immunoassay

NORMAL VALUE:

Conventional Units	SI Units (Conversion Factor X1)
< 35 U/mL	< 35 kU/L

EXPLAINATION:

CA 125, a glycoprotein found in normal endometrial tissue, occurs in the blood when existing endometrial protective barriers are broken, as is the case in cancer or endometriosis. Persistently rising levels suggest poor prognosis, but the lack of a tumor marker does not rule out the existence of a tumor. Rates of the pancreatic, liver, colon, breast, and lung cancer may also raise. It is not as effective as a screening test.

INDICATIONS:

- Assist in the diagnosis of cervical and endometrial carcinoma.
- Assist in the detection of ovarian cancer.
- Monitor response to ovarian cancer treatment.

RESULT:

Increased in:
• **Endometriosis**
• **First-trimester pregnancy**
• **Menses**
• **Ovarian abscess**
• **Pelvic inflammatory disease**
• **Breast, colon, liver, lung, endometrial, ovarian, and pancreatic cancer**
• **Peritonitis**
Decreased in:
Effective therapy or removal of the tumor

CA 15-3 (cancer antigen 15-3, Carbohydrate antigen 15-3)

SAMPLING: 1 mL of serum is collected in a red-top tube.

TECHNIQUE: Immunoradiometric

NORMAL VALUE:

Conventional Units	SI Units (Conversion Factor 1)
< 30 U/mL	< 30 kU/L

EXPLAINATION:

CA 15-3 tracks the relapse of breast carcinoma in patients.

CA 27.29 (normal range < 38 U / mL), a more approved protein marker, replaces CA 15-3 in some normal laboratories.

INDICATIONS: Monitor Recurring Breast carcinoma.

RESULT:

Increased in: **Recurrent breast cancer**
Decreased in: **Effective treatment or removal of the tumor**

IMPEDING FACTORS: Recent radioactive scans or radiation exposure within the last seven days of the test that conflict with the test results while radioimmunoassay is a test method.

CA 19-9 (cancer antigen 19-9, Carbohydrate antigen 19-9)

SAMPLING: 1 mL of serum is collected in a red-top tube.

TECHNIQUE: Immunoradiometric

NORMAL VALUE:

Conventional Units	SI Units (Conversion Factor X1)
< 37 U/mL	< 37 kU/L

EXPLAINATION: CA 19-9 is used to manage patients with various types of cancer.

INDICATIONS:
- Monitoring efficacy of the treatment.
- Monitoring head and neck, gastrointestinal, and gynecological cancers.
- Predicting relapse of cholangiocarcinoma.
- Predicting recurrence of stomach pancreatic, gallbladder, liver, colorectal and urothelial carcinomas.

RESULT:

Increased in:
• **Gastrointestinal, head and neck, and gynecological carcinomas**
• **Relapse of gallbladder, stomach, pancreatic, liver colorectal, and urothelial carcinomas**
• **Relapse of cholangiocarcinoma**

Decreased in:
Effective treatment or removal of the tumor

IMPEDING FACTORS:
Fresh radioactive scans or radiation exposure within seven days of the test can intrude with the test results when radioimmunoassay is the method of choice.

5-HYDROXYINDOLEACETIC ACID (5-HIAA)

SAMPLING: 10 mL of urine from a timed specimen is collected in a clean plastic collection container with boric acid as a preservative.
TECHNIQUE: High-pressure liquid chromatography
NORMAL VALUE:

Conventional Units	SI Units (Conversion Factor5.23)
2–7 mg/24 h	10.5–36.6 µmol/24 h

EXPLAINATION:
Since 5-hydroxyindoleacetic acid (5-HIAA) is a serotonin metabolite, 5-HIAA levels reflect plasma serotonin concentrations. 5-HIAA is excreted in the urine. Increased urinary excretion happens when carcinoid tumors are present. This test, which removes serotonin, is most effective when obtained from a 24-hour urine specimen.
INDICATIONS: Detect early, small, or sporadic carcinoid tumors
RESULT:

Increased in:
• Celiac and tropical sprue
• Cystic fibrosis
• Ovarian carcinoid tumors
• Whipple's disease
• Foregut and midgut carcinoid tumors
• Oat cell carcinoma of the bronchus
Decreased in:
• Depressive illnesses
• Hartnup disease
• Mastocytosis
• Phenylketonuria
• Renal disease
• Small intestinal resection

IMPEDING FACTORS:

- Drugs that may raise 5-HIAA levels include acetaminophen, cisplatin, ephedrine, fluorouracil, glyceryl guaiacolate cough syrups, melphalan, naproxen, phenacetin, pindolol, and rauwolfia alkaloids.
- Medications that may decrease 5-HIAA levels include corticotropin, insulin, imipramine, isoniazid, levodopa, monoamine oxidase inhibitors, methenamine, methyldopa, mephenesin, methocarbamol, and phenothiazine.
- Serotonin-containing foods such as avocados, bananas, chocolates, aubergines, pineapples, plantains, red plums, tomatoes, and walnuts can falsely increase levels if consumed within four days of the collection of specimens.
- Severe gastrointestinal disturbance or diarrhea may interfere with the test results.
- Failure to gather all the semen and safely store the specimen during the 24-hour test period invalidates the findings.

PAPANICOLAOU SMEAR (Pap smear, cervical smear)

SAMPLING: Cervical and endocervical cells.
TECHNIQUE: Microscopic examination of a fixed and stained smear
NORMAL VALUE:

Reporting of pap smear results may be in one of several ways and may differ from laboratory to laboratory. Simplified content of the two most common interpretive formats is presented.

Traditional Method	Description
Class I	Normal cells only
Class II	Atypical cells but not malignant or inflammatory
Class III	Atypical cells suspicious of malignancy OR mild cervical dysplasia
Class IV	Atypical cells suggestive of malignancy OR severe cervical dysplasia
Class V	Cancerous cells definite for malignancy

Bethesda System	Explanation
Competence of the specimen	Satisfactory
	Satisfactory but limited by lack of required patient information, contamination, or poor technique, which prevents evaluation of 50–70% of the cells
	Unsatisfactory—should be rejected and recollected

General interpretation	Within normal limits Benign cellular changes Cellular abnormality
Descriptive diagnoses	
Benign cellular changes	Infection or reactive changes
Epithelial cell abnormalities	Graded squamous and glandular cell description
	Description of other malignant neoplasms
	Hormonal evaluation (vaginal smears only)

EXPLAINATION:
Papanicolaou (Pap) is mainly used for the early detection of cervical cancer. The analysis of pap smears is as dependent on the collection and fixation procedure as it is on the completeness and precision of the medical information provided with the specimen. Patient age, date of last menstrual period, parity surgical condition, postmenopausal status, hormone therapy (including oral contraceptive use), history of radiation or chemotherapy, irregular vaginal bleeding, and history of previous pap smears are essential for proper understanding.

INDICATIONS:
- Assist in the detection of cervical dysplasia.
- Assist in the evaluation of endometriosis, condylomas, and vaginal adenosis.
- Support in the diagnosis of genital infections (herpes, Candida spp., Trichomonas vaginalis, Chlamydia, lymphogranuloma venereum, human papillomavirus, cytomegalovirus, and Actinomyces spp.).
- Assist in the detection of primary and metastatic neoplasms.
- Evaluate hormonal function.

IMPEDING FACTORS:
- Before fixation, it should not be allowed to air dry.
- No lubricating gel should be applied to the speculum.
- Improper collection site can contribute to the rejection of the sample.
Specimens for cancer screening are taken from the posterior fornix of the vagina and the cervix. Samples are taken from the vagina for the hormone evaluation.
- Blood contamination from samples collected during a patient's menstrual period may cause the specimen to be rejected.

VANILLYLMANDELIC ACID, URINE (VMA)

SAMPLING: 25 mL of urine from a timed specimen collected in a clean plastic collection container with 6N hydrochloric acid as a preservative.

TECHNIQUE: High-pressure liquid chromatography

NORMAL VALUE:

Age	Conventional Units	SI Units (Conversion Factor X5.05)
3–6 y	1.0–2.6 mg/24 h	5–13 µmol/24 h
6–10 y	2.0–3.2 mg/24 h	10–16 µmol/24 h
10–16 y	2.3–5.2 mg/24 h	12–26 µmol/24 h
16–83 y	1.4–6.5 mg/24 h	7–33 µmol/24 h

EXPLAINATION:

Vanilylmandelic acid (VMA) is a major metabolite of epinephrine and norepinephrine. It is elevated in conditions that are also demonstrated by the overproduction of catecholamines. Creatinine is usually measured simultaneously to ensure sufficient accumulation and to determine the metabolite-creatinine excretion ratio.

INDICATIONS:

- Assist in the treatment of neuroblastoma, ganglioneuroma, or pheochromocytoma.
- Evaluate hypertension with unknown cause.

RESULT:

Increased in:
• **Ganglioneuroma**
• **Hypertension**
• **Neuroblastoma**
• **Pheochromocytoma**
Decreased in:
Not any specific disease

IMPEDING FACTORS:

- Drugs that may raise VMA levels include ajmaline, chlorpromazine, phenolsulfonphthalein, prochlorperazine, rauwolfia, reserpine, sulfobromophthalein, isoproterenol, methyldopa, nitroglycerin, glucagon, guaifenesin, guanethidine, oxytetracycline, phenazopyridine, and syrosingopine.
- Drugs that may lower VMA levels include brofaromine, guanethidine, methyldopa, morphine, nialamide (in people with schizophrenia), monoamine oxidase inhibitors, and reserpine.

- Stress, hypoglycemia, strenuous exercise, smoking, hyperthyroidism, and drugs can produce elevated catecholamines.
- Failure to save all urine and store 24- hour specimen appropriately will result in a falsely low result.

HER-2/NEU ONCOPROTEIN
c-erb-B2
SAMPLING: Breast tissue or cells.
TECHNIQUE: Immunocytochemical
NORMAL VALUE: Negative.
The presence of inappropriate amounts of a protein termed human epidermal growth factor receptor 2 (HER-2 / neu oncoprotein) is beneficial in the detection of histological proof of metastatic breast cancer. The specimen is obtained by a fine needle or by an open biopsy. The tissue sample is treated with a substance that binds to HER-2 / neu oncoprotein.
EXPLAINATION:
Breast cancer is the most diagnosed cancer among American women. It is the second chief cause of death related to cancer. The existence of excessive amounts of protein labeled human epidermal growth factor receptor 2 (HER-2 / neu oncoprotein) is helpful in the development of histological proof of metastatic breast cancer. Overexpression of this enzyme is the product of an inherited genetic mutation and occurs in 25 to 30% of patients with metastatic breast cancer.
Metastatic breast cancer patients with high rates of HER-2 / neu oncoprotein have a poor prognosis: accelerated tumor growth, higher recurrence rate, poor response to standard therapies, and reduced survival rate.
The specimen is obtained by a fine needle or by a transparent biopsy. The tissue sample is treated with a medium that binds to HER-2 / neu oncoproteins. The pigment is applied to the tissue sample; tissue areas with large amounts of HER-2 / neu oncoprotein are marked by a high-intensity stain on the tissue sample.
INDICATIONS:
Indication of breast lesion by palpation, mammography, or ultrasound.
RESULT:
Positive findings in Breast cancer
IMPEDING FACTORS: N/A

IMMUNOLOGY

Immunology is a subject of the immune system of the body and its roles and disorders. Serology is a blood serum analysis.

Immunology and serology laboratories concentrate on the following:

- Identification of antibodies. These are proteins formed by a type of white blood cell in response to foreign material (antigen).
- The investigation into issues in the immune system. This covers when the body's immune system destroys its own tissues (autoimmune diseases) and whether its immune system is underactive (immunodeficiency disorders).
- Determination of liver, tissue, and fluid viability for transplantation

Notes

ALLERGEN-SPECIFIC IMMUNOGLOBULIN E
[radioallergosorbent test (RAST), Allergen profile]
SAMPLING:2 mL of serum per group of six allergens, 0.5 mL for each additional an individual allergen is collected in a red- or tiger-top tube.
TECHNIQUE: Radioimmunoassay
NORMAL VALUE:

RAST Scoring METHOD		METHOD (ASM): Increasing Levels of Allergy Sensitivity	
Specific IgE Antibody Level	kIU/L	ASM Class	ASM % NORMAL
Absent or undetectable	< 0.35	0	< 70
Low	0.35–0.70	1	70–109
Moderate	0.71–3.50	2	110–219
High	3.51–17.50	3	220–599
Extremely high	>17.50	4	600–1999
		5	2000–5999
		6	>5999

EXPLAINATION:
Allergen-specific immunoglobulin E (IgE) or RAST is usually required for groups of allergens typically known to cause allergic reactions in the affected individual. The assessment is based on the use of a radiolabelled anti-IgE reagent to detect IgE in the patient's serum developed in response to specific allergens. The panels contain allergens such as animal dander, antibiotics, dust, food, grass, insects, trees mites, molds, poison, and weeds. Allergen monitoring is useful for assessing the cause of hay fever, extrinsic asthma, atopic eczema, nasal allergies, and potentially fatal reactions to insect venoms, penicillins, and other medications or chemicals. RAST replaced skin tests and provocation procedures that were inconvenient, painful, and hazardous to patients.
INDICATIONS:
- Test for specific allergic sensitivity before starting immunotherapy or desensitization shots.
- Check for precise allergic susceptibility where skin tests are not accurate.
- Monitor for allergens when there is a known history of severe allergic reactions to skin tests.

- Evaluate individuals who refuse to perform skin tests or who have systemic dermatitis or other dermatopathic disorders.
- Testing allergens where skin tests are not acceptable, such as in infants.
- Monitor responsiveness to desensitization procedures.

RESULT:
Different scoring systems are applied in the analysis of RAST results.
Increased in:
• **Allergic rhinitis**
• **Anaphylaxis**
• **Eczema**
• **Hay fever**
• **Hookworm infection**
• **Asthma (exogenous)**
• **Atopic dermatitis**
• **Echinococcus infection**
• **Schistosomiasis**
• **Visceral larva migrans**
Decreased in:
• **Asthma (endogenous)**
• **Pregnancy**
• **Radiation therapy**

IMPEDING FACTORS:
Fresh radioactive scans or radiation within one week of the test can affect test results when radioimmunoassay is the test method.

ANTIBODIES, ANTICYTOPLASMIC NEUTROPHILIC

Perinuclear antineutrophil cytoplasmic antibody (p-ANCA), Cytoplasmic antineutrophil cytoplasmic antibody (c-ANCA).
SAMPLING: 1 ml of serum is collected in a red-top tube.
TECHNIQUE: Indirect immunofluorescence
NORMAL value: Negative(-VE)
EXPLAINATION:

There are two forms of cytoplasmic neutrophil antibodies known by their cellular staining properties. C-ANCA (cytoplasmic) is unique to proteinase 3 in neutrophils and monocytes and is present in the sera of Wegener granulomatosis patients. Wegener's disease involves granulomatous swelling of the upper and lower respiratory tract, and vasculitis. P-ANCA (perinuclear) is specific to myeloperoxidase, elastase, and lactoferrin, as well as other neutrophil enzymes. P-ANCA is found in the sera of patients with glomerulonephritis necrotizing pauciimmune.

INDICATIONS:
- Differentiate between vasculitic disease and the effects of therapy.
- Help in establishing the diagnosis of Wegener's granulomatosis and its variants.
- Make a distinction between biliary cirrhosis and sclerosing cholangitis.
- Making a differential diagnosis of Inflammatory bowel disease (ulcerative Colitis).

RESULT

Increased in:
• c-ANCA
Wegener's granulomatosis and its variants
• p-ANCA
Alveolar hemorrhage
Angiitis and polyangiitis
Autoimmune liver disease
Capillaritis
Churg-Strauss syndrome
Felty's syndrome
Inflammatory bowel disease
Leukocytoclastic skin vasculitis
Necrotizing-crescentic
Glomerulonephritis
Rheumatoid arthritis
Vasculitis
Decreased in:
Not any specific condition

ANTIBODIES, ANTI–GLOMERULAR BASEMENT MEMBRANE

Goodpasture's antibody, anti-GBM.

SAMPLING:1ml serum is collected in a red- or tiger-top tube. Lung or kidney tissue can also be submitted for testing.

TECHNIQUE: Direct or indirect immunofluorescence

NORMAL VALUE: Negative.

EXPLAINATION: Autoimmune kidney disease can arise from the presence of antibodies to the renal glomerular basement membrane (GBM). 10 to 20 percent of patients with anti-GBM had false-negative results.

INDICATIONS:

Identify the presence of anti-GBM antibodies to distinguish glomerulonephritis caused by anti-GBM from other causes of glomerulonephritis.

RESULT

	Increased in:
•	Glomerulonephritis
•	Goodpasture's disease
•	Idiopathic pulmonary hemosiderosis
	Decreased in:
	Not any specific disease

ANTIBODIES, ANTINUCLEAR, ANTI-DNA, AND ANTICENTROMERE

[ANA, Anti-DNA (Anti-ds DNA)]

SAMPLING:2ml serum is collected in a red-top tube.

TECHNIQUE: Enzyme-linked immunosorbent assay [ELISA] for Anti- DNA and Indirect fluorescent antibody for ANA and anticentromere.

NORMAL VALUE:

- Anti-DNA: titer of < 1:1
- ANA & anticentromere: titer of 1:40 or less

EXPLAINATION:

Antinuclear antibodies (ANAs) are autoantibodies primarily located in the nucleus of the affected cells. The involvement of ANA suggests systemic lupus erythematosus (SLE), associated collagen vascular disorders, and complex immune diseases. Cellular DNA antibodies are strongly associated with SLE. Anticentromere antibodies are an ANA type.

Their presence is strongly related with CREST syndrome (calcinosis, Raynaud's disease, esophageal dysfunction, sclerodactyly, telangiectasia).

ANA and anticentromere antibodies are detected with Hep-2 (human epithelial cultured cells).

Anti-DNA antibodies may be observed using the Crithidia luciliae substrate.

Females are much more likely than males to have an SLE diagnosis.

INDICATIONS:
- Aid in the diagnosis and evaluation of SLE.
- Assess suspected immune disorders, e.g., rheumatoid arthritis, Sjögren's syndrome, systemic sclerosis, polymyositis, and mixed connective tissue disease.

Results:

ANA Pattern	Associated Antibody
Rim and/or homogeneous	Double-stranded DNA
	Single- or double-
	stranded DNA
ANA Pattern	Associated Antibody
Homogeneous	Histones
Speckled	Sm (Smith) antibody
	RNP
	SS-B/La, SS-A/Ro
Diffuse speckled with positive mitotic figures	Centromere
Nucleolar	Nucleolar, RNP

Increased in:
• Drug-induced lupus erythematosus
• Lupoid hepatitis
• Mixed connective tissue disorder
• Polymyositis
• Progressive systemic sclerosis
• Rheumatoid arthritis
• Sjögren's disease
• SLE
Decreased in:
Not any specific condition

IMPEDING FACTORS:
- Medications that may induce positive outcomes include carbamazepine, chlorpromazine, ethosuximide, hydralazine, isoniazid, mephenytoin, methyldopa, penicillin, phenytoin, primidone, procainamide, and quinidine.
- A patient may have clinical signs for lupus and ANA negative.

ANTIBODIES, ANTISCLERODERMA

Progressive systemic sclerosis antibody, Scl-70 antibody.

SAMPLING: 1 ml of serum is collected in a red-top tube.

TECHNIQUE: Indirect fluorescent antibody

NORMAL VALUE: Negative

EXPLAINATION: Antisclerodermic antibodies are associated with progressive systemic sclerosis, a condition that affects multiple systems, including the skin, lungs, blood vessels, gastrointestinal tract, heart, and kidneys. These antibodies are present in sera patients with CREST syndrome (calcinosis, Raynaud's phenomenon, esophageal dysfunction, sclerodactyly, telangiectasia).

INDICATIONS:

Aid in the diagnosis of scleroderma

RESULT

Increased in:
• CREST syndrome
• Progressive diffuse scleroderma
Decreased in:
No specific disease

IMPEDING FACTORS: Not any

ANTIBODIES, ANTISTREPTOLYSIN O

Streptozyme, ASO.

SAMPLING: 1 ml serum is collected in a red-top tube.

TECHNIQUE: Nephelometry

NORMAL VALUE: < 200 IU/mL.

EXPLAINATION:

Group A- β-hemolytic streptococci secretes the enzyme streptolysin O, which can destroy red blood cells. The enzyme acts as a receptor, which stimulates the immune system to develop antibodies to streptolysin O. Such antibodies will develop within one month of the initiation of streptococcal infection. Antibody detection for several weeks strongly suggests susceptibility to group A-β - hemolytic streptococci

INDICATIONS:

- Assist in the detection of streptococcal infection.

- Evaluate the risk of acute rheumatic fever or nephritis in patients with streptococcal infection.

- Monitor susceptibility to treatment in streptococcal disease.

RESULT

Increased in:	
• Rheumatic fever	
• Endocarditis	
• Glomerulonephritis	
• Scarlet fever	
Decreased in:	
Not any specific disease	

CRITICAL VALUES: Not any
IMPEDING FACTORS:
Medicines that may decrease ASO titer include antibiotics and corticosteroid because treatment suppresses antibody response.

ANTIBODIES, ANTITHYROGLOBULIN, AND ANTITHYROID PEROXIDASE
Thyroid antibodies, antithyroid peroxidase antibodies
(TPO antibodies were previously called thyroid anti microsomal antibodies).
SAMPLING:1 mL serum is collected in a red-top tube.
TECHNIQUE: Radioimmunoassay
NORMAL VALUE:

Antibody	Conventional Units	SI Units (Conversion Factor 1)
Antithyroglobulin antibody	< 0.3 U/mL	< 0.3 kU/L
Antiperoxidase antibody	< 0.3 U/mL	< 0.3 kU/L

EXPLAINATION:
Thyroid antibodies are mainly G-type immunoglobulin antibodies. Antithyroid peroxidase antibodies bind to microsomal antigens in cells that line the microsomal membrane. Thyroid tissue is believed to be damaged because of invasion by lymphocytic killer cells. Such antibodies are found in hypothyroid and hyperthyroid conditions. Antithyroglobulin antibodies are anti-thyroglobulin antibodies. The role of this antibody is not clear. The two tests are normally demanded together.
INDICATIONS:
- Assist in the diagnosis of possible thyroid inflammation.
- Aid in the diagnosis of suspected hypothyroidism caused by the destruction of thyroid tissue. -
Assist in the diagnosis of potential thyroid autoimmunity in patients with other autoimmune disorders.

RESULT

Increased in:
• Goiter
• Autoimmune disorders
• Graves' disease
• Hashimoto's thyroiditis
• Thyroid carcinoma
• Idiopathic myxedema
• Pernicious anemia
Decreased in:
Not any specific disease

IMPEDING FACTORS:
- Lithium can increase the levels of thyroid antibodies.
- Recent radioactive scans or contamination within one week of the test that conflict with the test results while radioimmunoassay is the test method.

ANTIBODIES, CARDIOLIPIN, IMMUNOGLOBULIN G, AND IMMUNOGLOBULIN M

The antiphospholipid antibody, lupus anticoagulant, LA, ACA.

SAMPLING: 1 ml serum is collected in a red-top tube.
TECHNIQUE: Immunoassay, enzyme-linked immunosorbent assay [ELISA]
NORMAL VALUE: Negative.
EXPLAINATION:
Cardiolipin antibody is one of several antiphospholipid antibodies known. Antiphospholipid antibody syndrome is characterized by non-inflammatory thrombosis of the blood vessels. Such receptors are found in people with lupus erythematosus, lupus-related conditions, infectious diseases, drug reactions, and sometimes fetal failure. Cardiolipin antibodies are often found in combination with lupus anticoagulant.
INDICATIONS:
Aid in the establishing diagnosis of antiphospholipid antibody syndrome.
RESULT

Increased in:
• Drug reactions

• Epilepsy
• Infectious diseases
• Chorea
• Mitral valve endocarditis
• Patients with lupus-like symptoms (often ANA negative)
• Placental infarction
• Recurrent fetal loss (strong link with two or more occurrences)
• Recurrent venous and arterial thromboses
Decreased in:
Not any specific

IMPEDING FACTORS:
- Cardiolipin antibody is partly cross-reactive with syphilis reagent antibody and lupus anticoagulant.
- False-positive, rapid plasma reagent tests can occur.

ANTIBODIES, GLIADIN
(IMMUNOGLOBULIN G AND IMMUNOGLOBULIN A)
Endomysial antibodies, EMA, gliadin (IgG and IgA) antibodies.
SAMPLING: 1 ml of serum collected in a red-top tube.
TECHNIQUE: Immunoassay
NORMAL VALUE:

Gliadin Antibody	Conventional Units
IgA	< 5 U
IgG	< 57 U

EXPLAINATION: Gliadin is a water-soluble protein found in wheat, rye, oats, and barley gluten. The digestive mucosa of some people does not absorb gluten, which results in a toxic build-up of gliadin. Gliadin antibodies develop and cause damage to the intestinal mucosa. For severe cases, intestinal mucosa may be lost; the disease is exacerbated by lactose intolerance. Immunoglobulin G (IgG) & immunoglobulin A (IgA) gliadin antibodies are detected in serum patients with gluten-sensitive enteropathy.
INDICATIONS:
- Help in the diagnosis of asymptomatic gluten-sensitive enteropathy in some cases of dermatitis herpetiformis.
- Aid in the diagnosis of gluten-sensitive enteropathies.

- Help in the diagnosis of nontropical sprue.
- Monitor food adherence in patients with gluten-sensitive enteropathies.

RESULT

Increased in:
• **Asymptomatic gluten-sensitive enteropathy**
• **Celiac disease**
• **Dermatitis herpetiformis**
• **Nontropical sprue**
Decreased in:
Not any specific disease

IMPEDING FACTORS:

- Factors other than gluten-sensitive enteropathy can result in higher levels of antibodies without accompanying histological evidence. Such factors include Crohn's disease, post-infection malabsorption, and food protein sensitivity.
- A negative IgA gliadin result, particularly with positive IgG gliadin, results in an untreated condition, and does not exclude active gluten-sensitive enteropathy.

ANTIBODY, ANTIMITOCHONDRIAL (AMA)

SAMPLING: 1 ml of serum is collected in a red-top tube.
TECHNIQUE: Indirect fluorescent antibody
NORMAL VALUE -ve (Negative) or titer < 1:20.
EXPLAINATION: Antimitochondrial antibodies are observed in 90 % of patients with primary biliary cirrhosis (PBC). PBC is most identified in women between 35 and 60 years of age.

INDICATIONS:

- Assist in the diagnosis of PBC.
- Aid in the differential diagnosis of chronic liver disease.

RESULT

Increased in:
• **PBC**
• **Hepatitis (alcoholic, viral)**
• **Rheumatoid arthritis (occasionally)**
• **Systemic lupus erythematosus (occasionally)**
• **Thyroid disease (occasionally)**
Decreased in:
Not any

CRITICAL VALUES: Not any
IMPEDING FACTORS: Not any

ANTIBODY, ANTI–SMOOTH MUSCLE (ASMA)

SAMPLING: 1 mL of serum is collected in a red-top tube.
TECHNIQUE: Indirect fluorescent antibody
NORMAL VALUE: Negative.
EXPLANATION: Anti-smooth muscle antibodies are autoantibodies found in high titers in sera patients with autoimmune liver and bile duct disorders.
INDICATIONS:
Differential diagnosis of liver disease.
RESULT

Increased in:
• **Autoimmune hepatitis**
• **Chronic active viral hepatitis**
• **Infectious mononucleosis**
Decreased in:
Not any specific disease

ANTIBODY, Jo-1

Antihistidyl transfer tRNA synthase.
SAMPLING: 1 mL of serum collected in a red-top tube.
TECHNIQUE: Immunoassay
NORMAL VALUE: Negative.
EXPLAINATION: Jo-1 is an autoantibody found in the sera of some antinuclear antibody-positive patients. Relative to the presence of other autoantibodies, the presence of Jo-1 suggests a more violent course of the disease and a greater risk of mortality. The clinical effects of this autoantibody include acute onset fever, dry cracking skin on the hands, Raynaud's phenomenon, and arthritis.
INDICATIONS:
Test for idiopathic inflammatory myopathies.
RESULT

Increased in:
Dermatomyositis

Polymyositis
Decreased in:
No specific disease

ANTIDEOXYRIBONUCLEASE-B, STREPTOCOCCAL

ADNase-B, AntiDNase-B titer, antistreptococcal DNase-B titer, streptodornase.

SAMPLING: 1 mL of serum is collected in a red-top tube.

TECHNIQUE: Spectrophotometry

NORMAL VALUE:

Age	Normal Results
Preschoolers	< 61 U
School-age children	< 171 U
Adults	< 86 U

EXPLAINATION:

The presence in streptococcal DNase antibodies is an indicator of recent infection, especially if antibody titer increases. The test is more sensitive than the antistreptolysin-O test. Clinically significant signs are the rise in the titer of two or more dilution intervals between acute and convalescent specimens:

RESULT

Increased in:
Streptococcal infections (systemic)
Decreased in:
Not any specific disease

ANTIGENS/ANTIBODIES, ANTI–EXTRACTABLE NUCLEAR

(La antibodies, SS-B antibodies, Ro antibodies, SS-A antibodies, ENA)

SAMPLING: 1 mL of serum is collected in a red-top tube.

TECHNIQUE: Immunoassay

NORMAL VALUE: Negative.

EXPLAINATION:

Extractive nuclear antigens (ENAs) include ribonucleoprotein (RNP), Smith (Sm), SSA/Ro, and SS-B/La antigens. ENAs and antibodies to them are observed in different concentrations of people with variations of concurrent rheumatologic symptoms.

INDICATIONS:

- Help in the diagnosis of mixed connective tissue disease.
- Assist in the diagnosis of Sjögren's syndrome.

- Aid in establishing the diagnosis of systemic lupus erythematosus (SLE).

RESULT

Increased in:
• Anti-SS-A/Ro-positive patients with photosensitivity.
• Anti-RNP has been linked with mixed connective tissue disorder.
• Anti-SS-A and anti-SS-B are useful in diagnosing antinuclear antibody (ANA)-negative cases of SLE.
• Anti-SS-A/La is associated with primary Sjögren syndrome.
• Anti-SS-A/anti-SS-B-positive sera are noticed in patients with neonatal lupus.
• Anti-SS-A-positive patients may also have antibodies consistent with antiphospholipid syndrome.
• Anti-SS-A/ANA-positive, anti-SSB-negative patients, are likely to suffer from nephritis.
• Anti-SS-A/Ro is a marker of congenital heart block in neonates born to SLE mothers.
Decreased in: N/A

CD4/CD8 ENUMERATION (T cell profile)

SAMPLING: 1ml of whole blood is collected in a green-top (heparin) tube.

TECHNIQUE: Flow cytometry

NORMAL VALUE:

Total lymphocytes	1500–4000/mm3
CD3	876–1900/mm3
CD4	450–1400/mm3
CD8	190–725/mm3
CD20	64–475/mm3
CD4/CD8	ratio 1.0–3.5

EXPLAINATION:

Enumeration of lymphocytes, cell lineage recognition, and cell stage development identification are used to identify and classify malignant myeloproliferative ailment and to plan treatment. T cell enumeration is also helpful in the assessment and treatment of immunodeficiency and autoimmune disease. Severely depressed CD4 counts are an excellent predictor of impending opportunistic infection.

INDICATIONS:

- Help in Hiv diagnosis and treatment plan.
- Evaluate malignant myeloproliferative disorders and treatment plan.
- Evaluate thymus-dependent or cell-dependent immunity.

RESULT:

Increased in case of:
Malignant myeloproliferative diseases (like acute and chronic lymphocytic leukemia, lymphoma)
Decreased in:
• **AIDS**
• **Aplastic anemia**
• **Hodgkin's disease**

IMPEDING FACTORS:

- Medications that can improve the T cell count include interferon-δ.
- Medications that may reduce T cell count include chlorpromazine and prednisone.
- Specimens should be kept at room temperature.
- Recent nuclear or radiation scans can reduce the number of T cells.
- Values may be atypical in patients with severe chronic disease or after recent surgery involving general anesthesia.

CHLAMYDIA GROUP ANTIBODY

SAMPLING: 1 mL of serum is collected in a red-top tube.

TECHNIQUE: Indirect fluorescent antibody, the polymerase chain reaction

NORMAL VALUE:

Negative or < fourfold increase in titer.

EXPLAINATION: Chlamydia is one of the quite common sexually transmitted infections caused by Chlamydia trachomatis. Such gram-negative bacteria are considered compulsive cell parasites because they allow living cells to grow. There are three C serotypes. Trachomatis: One group origins lymphogranuloma venereum, with symptoms of the first phase of the disease occurring 2 to 6 weeks after infection; the other group causes genital infections other than lymphogranuloma venereum, with symptoms appearing in men 7 to 28 days after intercourse (women are generally asymptomatic); and the third group causes ocular trachoma disease (incubation period, 7 to 1). Chlamydia psittaci is the source of psittacosis in both birds and humans. It is rising in prevalence as a pathogen responsible for other major respiratory system diseases. The period of incubation for C. psittaci in humans' infections is 7 to 15 days, accompanied by chills, fever, and recurrent non-productive cough.

Chlamydia is difficult to cultivate and grow, so antibody testing has become the technology of choice. The antigen used in several screening kits is not detailed to organisms and can only confirm the presence of Chlamydia spp. The organisms can be identified by newer technology using DNA probes. Tests that can specifically identify C. Trachomatis require special collection and transport kits. We also have specific instructions on the collection, and the specimens are gathered on the swabs. The laboratory performing this test should be consulted before the collection of specimens.

INDICATIONS:

- Identify Chlamydia as the cause of atypical pneumonia.
- Establish the prevalence of chlamydia infection.

RESULT:

Positive findings in:
• **Chlamydial infection**
• **Infantile pneumonia**
• **Infertility**
• **Ophthalmia neonatorum**
• **Pelvic inflammatory disease**
• **Urethritis**
• **Lymphogranuloma venereum**

COLD AGGLUTININ TITER (Mycoplasma serology)

SAMPLING:2 mL of serum is collected in a red-top tube. The tube should be placed in a water bath or heat block at 37°C for 1 hour and permitted to clot before the serum is separated from the red blood cells (RBCs).

TECHNIQUE: Patient sera containing autoantibodies titrated against RBCs of type O at 2°C to 8°C. Type O cells are used as they have no antigens on the surface of the cell membrane. Patient sera agglutination would not arise due to reactions between RBC blood type antigens and patients with blood type antibodies.

NORMAL VALUE:

Negative: Single titer < 1:32 or < a fourfold increase in titer over serial samples.

EXPLAINATION:

Cold agglutinins are antibodies that allow RBCs to clump or agglutinate at cold temperatures in people with certain diseases or who are attacked by specific organisms. Cold agglutinins are associated with infection with Mycoplasma pneumoniae. M. Pneumoniae has an antigen specificity to RBC human membranes. Fetal cells contain the most antigens, but most cells bear the I antigen for 18 months. Agglutinins are generally immunoglobulin M (IgM) antibodies and cause cell agglutination at temperatures between 0 °C and 10°C. The temperature of circulating blood in the limbs may be lower than the temperature of the heart. RBCs of affected individuals may agglutinate and block blood vessels in their fingers, toes, and ears, or may cause a complementary cascade. The affected cells may be lysed immediately within the capillaries and blood vessels because of the action of the complement on the cell wall or may return to the circulation and be destroyed by the spleen via macrophages.

The endpoint of titer is the maximum serum dilution that indicates a particular antigen-antibody reaction. Single titers >1:64, or a fourfold change in titer between specimens collected 5 days apart or more, are clinically significant. Patients with primary atypical viral pneumonia show an increase in titer 8 to 10 days after the onset of illness. IgM antibodies plateau in 12 to 25 days and begin to decrease 30 days after onset.

INDICATIONS:

- Assist in the diagnosis of primary atypical pneumonia, influenza, or pulmonary embolus.

- Provide additional diagnostic assistance for cold agglutinin disease associated with viral or lymphoreticular cancer.

RESULT:

Increased in:
• **Infectious mononucleosis**
• **Malaria**
• **Multiple myeloma**

• Raynaud's syndrome (severe)	
• Systemic lupus erythematosus	
• Trypanosomiasis	
• *M. pneumoniae* (primary atypical pneumonia)	
Decreased in: **N/A**	

IMPEDING FACTORS:
- Antibiotic use may interfere with or reduce the production of antibodies.
- High antibody titer can interfere with blood typing and cross-matching procedures.
- Raised titers may appear spontaneously in elderly patients and may continue for many years.
- Prompt and proper processing, storage, and analysis of specimens are important for the achievement of accurate results. Samples should always be transported to the laboratory as soon as possible after selection. The specimen must be clotted in a 37°C water bath for 1 hour before separation. The refrigeration of the sample before the serum separates from the RBCs may falsely reduce the titer.

COMPLEMENT C3 AND COMPLEMENT C4 (C3 and C4)
SAMPLING: 1 mL of serum is collected in a red-top tube.
TECHNIQUE: Nephelometry
NORMAL VALUE:
C3

Age	Conventional Units	SI Units (Conversion Factor X 10)
Newborn	57–116 mg/dL	570–1160 mg/L
6 mo–adult	74–166 mg/dL	740–1660 mg/L
Adult	83–177 mg/dL	830–1770 mg/L

C4

Age	Conventional Units	SI Units (Conversion Factor X10)
Newborn	10–31 mg/dL	100–310 mg/L
6 mo–6 y	15–52 mg/dL	150–520 mg/L

7–12 y	19–40 mg/dL	190–400 mg/L
13–15 y	19–57 mg/dL	190–570 mg/L
16–18 y	19–42 mg/dL	190–420 mg/L
Adult	12–36 mg/dL	120–360 mg/L

EXPLAINATION:

Complementary proteins act as enzymes that aid in the immunological and inflammatory response. The Complementary System is an important mechanism for the destruction and removal of foreign materials. Serum replacement levels are used to diagnose autoimmune diseases. C3 and C4 are the most frequently tested complement proteins along with the total compliment. Circulating C3 is produced in the liver and accounts for 70% of the complement system, but other tissues can also yield C3. C3 is an essential activating protein in classical and alternative complement cascades. It is reduced in patients with immunological diseases, in which it is ingested at a higher rate. C4 is produced mainly in the liver but may also be produced by monocytes, fibroblasts, and macrophages. C4 is part of the classic complementary pathway.

INDICATIONS:

- Detect genetic deficiencies.
- Evaluate immunologic diseases.

RESULTS:

Increased in:
• **C3 and C4**
• **Acute-phase reactions**
• **C3**
• **Amyloidosis**
• **Cancer**
• **Diabetes**
• **Myocardial infarction**
• **Pneumococcal pneumonia**
• **Pregnancy**
• **Rheumatic disease**
• **Thyroiditis**
• **Viral hepatitis**

• C4
• Certain malignancies
Decreased in:
• C3 and C4
• Hereditary deficiency
• Liver disease
• SLE
• C3
• Chronic infection (bacterial, parasitic, viral)
• Post–membranoproliferative
• glomerulonephritis
• Post–streptococcal infection
• Rheumatic arthritis
• C4
• Angioedema (hereditary and acquired)
• Autoimmune hemolytic anemia
• Autoimmune thyroiditis
• Cryoglobulinemia
• Glomerulonephritis
• Juvenile dermatomyositis
• Meningitis (bacterial, viral)
• Pneumonia
• Streptococcal or staphylococcal
• sepsis

IMPEDING FACTORS:
- Medications that may increase C3 levels include cimetidine and cyclophosphamide.
- Medications that may reduce C3 levels include phenytoin and danazol.
- Drugs that may raise C4 levels to include cimetidine, cyclophosphamide, and danazol.
- Drugs that may reduce C4 levels include dextran and penicillamine.

COMPLEMENT, TOTAL
(Total hemolytic complement, CH50, CH100)
SAMPLING:1 ml of serum is collected in a red-top tube.
TECHNIQUE: Quantitative hemolysis
NORMAL VALUE:

Conventional Units	SI Units (Conversion Factor (1000)
40–100 CH50 U/mL	40–100 CH50 kU/L

EXPLAINATION:
The complement system comprises of proteins that are activated and interact in a successive cascade. The complement system is a crucial part of the body's natural defense against allergic and immune reactions. It is activated by plasmin and interlinked with coagulation and fibrinolytic systems. Triggering of the complement system results in cell lysis, the release of histamine, white blood cell chemotaxis, increased vascular permeability, and smooth muscle contraction. The triggering of this mechanism may sometimes occur with unregulated self-destructive effects on the body. In the serum complement assay, the plasma of the patient is combined with the red blood cells of the animal coated with antibodies. If the complement is present in enough quantities, 50% of the red blood cells are destroyed. Lower amounts of lysed cells are related to lower complement levels.
INDICATIONS:
- Evaluate complement activity in autoimmune disorders.
- Assist in the treatment of inherited angioedema.
- Evaluate and monitor systemic lupus erythematosus therapy.
- Complementary dysfunction screening.
RESULT:

Increased in:
Acute-phase immune response
Decreased in:
Autoimmune diseases
Autoimmune hemolytic anemia
Burns
Cryoglobulinemia
Hereditary deficiency
Infections (bacterial, parasitic, viral)
Liver disease
Malignancy

• Rheumatoid arthritis
• Systemic lupus erythematosus
• Trauma
• Vasculitis
• Membranous glomerulonephritis

IMPEDING FACTORS:
- Medications that may increase total complement amounts include cyclophosphamide and danazole.
- Specimen should not stay at room temperature for more than 1 hour.

CYTOMEGALOVIRUS, IMMUNOGLOBULIN G & IMMUNOGLOBULIN M (CMV)
SAMPLING:1 mL of serum is collected in a plain red-top tube.
TECHNIQUE: Indirect fluorescent antibody
NORMAL VALUE: Negative or < a fourfold increase in titer.
EXPLAINATION:
Cytomegalovirus (CMV) is a double-stranded DNA herpes virus. The incubation period for the main infections ranges from 4 to 8 weeks. Transmission could still occur by close contact with others and excretion of nasal, digestive, or venereal fluids. CMV infection is a top consideration in pregnant or immunocompromised patient populations or in patients who had recently acquired organ transplants. Blood units are sometimes screened for CMV because patients in these high-risk groups are transfusion users. CMV serologic testing is part of the TORCH (toxoplasmosis, other [congenital syphilis and viruses], rubella, CMV, and herpesvirus type 2) panel used to monitor pregnant women. CMV, as well as other infectious agents, can cross the placenta and result in congenital malformations, miscarriage, or stillbirth. The presence of antibodies to immunoglobulin M (IgM) suggests acute infection. The presence of antibodies to IgG indicates current or previous infections.
INDICATIONS:
- Assist in the detection of congenital CMV infection in newborns.
- Determine susceptibility, especially in pregnant women, immunocompromised patients, and patients who have recently received organ transplantation.
- Screen blood for high-risk transfusion recipients.

RESULT

Positive findings in CMV infection
Negative findings in N/A

IMPEDING FACTORS:
- False-positive results can take place in the presence of a rheumatoid factor.
- False-negative results that occur if treatment has been begun before antibodies have been produced or if the test has been done < 6 days after exposure to the virus.

D-DIMER (Dimer, fibrin degradation fragment)

SAMPLING: 1 mL of plasma is collected in a filled blue-top (sodium citrate) tube.
TECHNIQUE: quantitative enzyme-linked immunosorbent assay [ELISA] or Latex semiquantitative screen.

NORMAL VALUE:
Semiquantitative: No fragments detected
Quantitative: < 250 ng/mL

EXPLAINATION:
The D-dimer is an asymmetric carbon compound founded by a cross-link between two similar fibrin molecules. The test is specific for secondary fibrinolysis as crosslinking happens with fibrin and not with fibrinogen. Positive testing is conclusive evidence of disseminated intravascular coagulation (DIC).

INDICATIONS:
- Assist in the diagnosis of DIC and deep venous thrombosis (DVT).
- Assist in the assessment of myocardial infarction and unstable angina.
- Assist in the evaluation of potential Veno-occlusive disease associated with bone marrow transplant sequelae.
- Assist in the assessment of pulmonary embolism.

RESULT:
The sensitivity and specificity of the sample vary between the test kits and the test methods (e.g., latex vs. ELISA).

Increased in:
• **Arterial or venous thrombosis**
• **DVT**
• **DIC**
• **Neoplastic disease**
• **Pre-eclampsia**
• **Pulmonary embolism**
• **Recent surgery (within 2 days)**
• **Secondary fibrinolysis**
• **Pregnancy (late and postpartum)**
Decreased in: N/A

IMPEDING FACTORS:
- High rheumatoid factor titers can induce a false-positive result.
- Increased CA 125 levels can result in a false-positive test.
- Medications that may cause an increase in plasma D-dimer include drugs that are used for antiplatelet therapy.
- Medications that may cause a decrease in D-dimer plasma include pravastatin and warfarin.
- Keeping the tourniquet in place for more than 1 minute may result in venous stasis and changes in the amount of plasma proteins to be measured. Activation of the platelet may also occur under these conditions, resulting in incorrect results.
- Vascular injury during phlebotomy can trigger platelets and coagulation factors, resulting in incorrect outcomes.
- Hemolyzed specimens must be refused as hemolysis is a sign of platelet activation and coagulation factor activation.
- Incompletely filled tubes mixed with heparin or clotted specimens shall be refused.
- Icteric or lipemic specimens' conflict with optical test methods and yield incorrect results.

INSULIN ANTIBODIES

SAMPLING: 1 mL of serum is collected in a red-top tube.
TECHNIQUE: Radioimmunoassay
NORMAL VALUE: < 3 percent; includes binding of human, beef, and pork insulin to antibodies in the patient's serum.
EXPLAINATION: Immunoglobulin G (IgG) is the most common anti-insulin antibody, but IgA, IgM, IgD, and IgE antibodies also have anti-insulin properties. These antibodies typically do not cause clinical problems but may hinder the testing of insulin assay. IgM is thought to be involved in insulin resistance and IgE in insulin allergy. Improvements in the safety of animal insulin and increased use of human insulin have led to a significant decrease in the rate of insulin antibody formation.
INDICATIONS:
- Assist in verifying insulin resistance.
- Assist in deciding whether hypoglycemia is caused by insulin misuse.
- Assist in evaluating insulin allergy.
RESULT:

Increased in:
• **Steroid-induced diabetes (a side effect of therapy for systemic lupus erythematosus)**
• **Insulin allergy or resistance**

• Factitious hypoglycemia
• Polyendocrine autoimmune syndromes
Decreased in: **N/A**

IMPEDING FACTORS:

- Recent radioactive scans or radiation exposure can interfere with test results when radioimmunoassay is the test method.

INTRINSIC FACTOR ANTIBODIES

IF-antibodies

SAMPLING: 1 mL of serum collected in a red-top tube. 1 mL of plasma collected in a lavender-top (ethylenediaminetetra-acetic acid) tube is also acceptable.

TECHNIQUE: Radioimmunoassay

NORMAL VALUE: None detected.

EXPLAINATION:

Intrinsic factor (IF) is released by gastric mucosa parietal cells and is required for normal absorption of vitamin B12.

In some disorders, antibodies have produced that bind the cobalamin-IF complex, prevent the complex from binding to ileum receptors, and inhibit the absorption of vitamin B12.

There are two forms of antibodies: type 1, the most widely employed blocking antibody, and type 2, the binding antibody. The blocking antibody blocks the absorption of vitamin B12 at the binding site of IF. Binding antibody blends with either a free or complex IF

INDICATIONS:

- Aid in the diagnosis of pernicious anemia.

- Access patients with decreased vitamin B12 levels.

RESULT:

Increased in:
• Megaloblastic anemia
• Pernicious anemia
• Some patients with hyperthyroidism
• Some patients with insulin-dependent (type 1) diabetes
Decreased in: **N/A**

IMPEDING FACTORS:

- Previous treatment with methotrexate or another folic acid antagonist can interfere with the test results.

- Vitamin B12 injected or consumed within 48 hours of the test results was invalidated.

- Recent radioactive scans or radiation exposure can interfere with the test results when the radioimmunoassay is a test method.

INFECTIOUS MONONUCLEOSIS SCREEN
Monospot, heterophil antibody test, IM serology
SAMPLING: 1 mL of serum is collected in a red-top tube.
TECHNIQUE: Agglutination
NORMAL VALUE: Negative
EXPLAINATION:
Infectious mononucleosis is produced by the Epstein-Barr (EBV) virus. The incubation period is around 10 to 50 days, and the symptoms begin 1 to 4 weeks after the full development of the infection. EBV infection is characterized by the presence of heterophilic antibodies, also known as Paul-Bunnell-Davidsohn antibodies, that are immunoglobulin M (IgM) antibodies, which can agglutinate sheep or horse red blood cells. The disorder causes the development of dysfunctional lymphocytes in the lymph nodes, stimulates the formation of heterophilic antibodies, and is characterized by fatigue, cervical lymphadenopathy, tonsillopharyngitis, and hepatosplenomegaly. EBV is also believed to have a role to play in Burkitt's lymphoma, nasopharyngeal carcinoma, and chronic fatigue syndrome. If the findings of the heterophilic antibody screening test are negative and infectious mononucleosis is highly suspected, an EBV-specific serology should be ordered.
INDICATIONS:
Aid in confirming infectious mononucleosis
RESULT:
Positive findings in Infectious mononucleosis
IMPEDING FACTORS:
- False-positive results may take place in the presence of narcotic addiction, serum sickness, lymphomas, hepatitis, leukemia, pancreatic cancer, and phenytoin treatment.
- False-negative findings that occur if therapy has been initiated before antibodies have been produced or if the test has been done < six days after exposure to the virus.

IMMUNOFIXATION ELECTROPHORESIS, SERUM, AND URINE (IFE)
SAMPLING: 1 mL of serum is collected in a red-top tube. 10 mL of urine from a random collection in a clean plastic container.
TECHNIQUE: Immunoprecipitation combined with electrophoresis
NORMAL VALUE:
A pathologist interprets test results. Normal placement and intensity of staining give information regarding the immunoglobulin bands.

EXPLAINATION: Immunofixation electrophoresis (IFE) is a qualitative procedure that provides a thorough classification of individual immunoglobulins according to their electrical loads. Abnormalities are identified by changes in the individual units, such as movement, brightness, or absence of color. Urine IFE replaced the Bence Jones Light Chain Screening Test. IFE substituted immunoelectrophoresis because it is more flexible and easier to interpret.

INDICATIONS:
- Assist in the cure of multiple myeloma and amyloidosis.
- Aid in the detection of presumed immunodeficiency.
- Assist in the diagnosis of possible immunoproliferative diseases such as multiple myeloma and Waldenström macroglobulinemia.
- Identify biclonal or monoclonal gammopathies.
- Identify cryoglobulinemia.
- Monitor the efficacy of chemotherapy or radiation therapy.

RESULT: Immunoglobulins A, D, G, and M

IMPEDING FACTORS:
- Drugs that may increase the levels of immunoglobulin include asparaginase, cimetidine, and narcotics.
- Medications that may decrease immunoglobulin levels include dextran, oral contraceptives, phenytoin, and methylprednisolone (high doses).
- Chemotherapy and radiation therapy can modify the bandwidth and make interpretation difficult.

IMMUNOGLOBULIN E (IgE)

SAMPLING: 1 mL of serum is collected in a red- or tiger-top tube.
TECHNIQUE: Immunoassay
NORMAL VALUE:

Age	Conventional Units	SI Unit (Conversion Factor X1)
Newborn	< 12 IU/mL	< 12 kIU/mL
< 1 y	< 50 IU/mL	< 50 kIU/mL
2–4 y	< 100 IU/mL	< 100 kIU/mL
5 y and older	< 300 IU/m	< 300 kIU/mL

EXPLAINATION:

Immunoglobulin E (IgE) is an antibody whose main responsibility is to allergic reactions and parasite infections. Many IgE cells in the body are bound to specific tissue cells; little is available in circulating blood. IgE attaches to the membrane of special granulocytes known as basophils in circulating blood and mast cells in tissues. Basophilic and mast cell membranes have IgE receptors. Mast cells are located within the skin and the tissues of the respiratory and digestive tract. When the IgE antibody is cross-linked to the antigen/allergen, heparin, the release of histamine and other chemical substances from the granules in the cells are activated. A sequence of events accompanies IgE activation, which affects vascular permeability, smooth muscle contraction, and inflammatory reactions. The inflammatory response permits proteins from the bloodstream to reach the tissues. Helminths (worm parasites) are particularly susceptible to immunoglobulin-mediated cytotoxic chemicals. Inflammatory response proteins recruit macrophages from the circulatory system and granulocytes, such as eosinophils, inflammation, and bone marrow. Eosinophils also contain enzymes that are effective against parasitic invaders.

INDICATIONS:

Helps in the evaluation of allergy and parasitic infection.

RESULT:

Increased in:
• **Bronchopulmonary aspergillosis**
• **Asthma**
• **Alcoholism**
• **Allergy**
• **Dermatitis**
• **Sinusitis**
• **Wiskott-Aldrich syndrome**
• **Eczema**
• **Hay fever**
• **IgE myeloma**
• **Parasitic infestation**
• **Rhinitis**
Decreased in:
• **IgE deficiency**
• **Advanced carcinoma**
• **Agammaglobulinemia**
• **Ataxia-telangiectasia**

IMPEDING FACTORS:
- Medications that may cause IgE levels to decrease include phenytoin and tryptophan.
- Penicillin G has been related to increased IgE levels in some patients with acute interstitial nephritis induced by drugs.
- Normal levels of IgE do not exclude allergic conditions as a possible diagnosis.

IMMUNOGLOBULINS A, D, G, & M (IgA, IgD, IgG, and IgM)

SAMPLING: 1 mL of serum is collected in a red-top tube.
TECHNIQUE: Nephelometry
NORMAL VALUE:
Immunoglobulin A

Age	Conventional Units	SI Units *Conversion Factor X10)*
Newborn	1–4 mg/Dl	10–40 mg/L
1–9 mo	2–80 mg/dL	20–800 mg/L
10–12 mo	15–90 mg/dL	150–900 mg/L
2–3 y	18–150 mg/dL	180–1500 mg/L
4–5 y	25–160 mg/dL	250–1600 mg/L
6–8 y	35–200 mg/dL	350–2000 mg/L
9–12 y	45–250 mg/dL	450–2500 mg/L
Older than 12 y	40–350 mg/dL	400–3500 mg/L

Immunoglobulin D

AGE	Conventional Units	SI Units (Conversion Factor X10)
Newborn	>2 mg/dL	>20 mg/L
Adult	< 15 mg/dL	< 150 mg/L

Immunoglobulin G

AGE	*Conventional Units*	*SI (Conversion Factor X0.01)*
Newborn	650–1600 mg/dL	6.5–16 g/L
1–9 mo	250–900 mg/dL	2.5–9 g/L
10–12 mo	290–1070 mg/dL	2.9–10.7 g/L
2–3 y	420–1200 mg/dL	4.2–12 g/L
4–6 y	460–1240 mg/dL	4.6–12.4 g/L
>6 y	650–1600 mg/dL	6.5–16 g/L

Immunoglobulin M

AGE	Conventional Units	SI Units (Conversion Factor X10)
Newborn	< 25 mg/dL	< 250 mg/L
1–9 mo	20–125 mg/dL	200–1250 mg/L
10–12 mo	40–150 mg/dL	400–1500 mg/L
2–8 y	45–200 mg/dL	450–2000 mg/L
9–12 y	50–250 mg/dL	500–2500 mg/L
>12 y	50–300 mg/dL	500–3000 mg/L

EXPLAINATION:
Most Immunoglobulins A, D, E, G, and M are formed by plasma cells in response to foreign particles.
Immunoglobulins neutralize toxic substances, facilitate phagocytosis, and kill invading microorganisms.
They are made up of heavy, light chains. Immunoglobulins produced by the expansion of a single plasma cell (clone) are called monoclonal cells.
Polyclonal improves the outcome as different cell lines produce antibodies. IgA is mainly observed in secretions such as saliva, tears, and breast milk. It is assumed to protect mucous membranes from viruses and bacteria. The IgD function is not well known. IgG is the leading serum immunoglobulin and is important for long-term disease protection. It is the only antigen that crosses the placenta. IgM is the largest immunoglobulin and the first antibody to respond to an antigenic stimulus. IgM also produces normal antibodies, such as ABO blood group antibodies.
The occurrence of IgM in cord blood is a symptom of congenital infection.

INDICATIONS:
- Assist in the evaluation of multiple myeloma.
- Test humoral immunity.
- Monitor treatment for multiple myeloma.
- IgA: assess anaphylaxis associated with blood transfusion and blood products (anti-IgA antibodies may build in patients with low levels of IgA, maybe resulting in anaphylaxis when blood is donated).

RESULT:
Increases in:
IgA:
Polyclonal:
- Chronic infections, particularly gastrointestinal (GI) and respiratory tracts

- Chronic liver disease
- Immunodeficiency states, such as Wiskott-Aldrich syndrome
- Inflammatory bowel disease
- Lower GI cancer
- Rheumatoid arthritis

Monoclonal:
- IgA-type multiple myeloma

IgD:

Polyclonal:
- Chronic infections
- Certain liver diseases
- Connective tissue disorders

Monoclonal:
- IgD-type multiple myeloma

IgG:

Polyclonal:
- Certain Autoimmune diseases, like systemic lupus erythematosus, rheumatoid arthritis, and Sjögren's syndrome
- Chronic liver disease
- Chronic or recurrent infections
- Intrauterine devices
- Sarcoidosis

Monoclonal:
- IgG-type multiple myeloma
- Leukemias
- Lymphomas

IgM:

Polyclonal:
- Active sarcoidosis
- Chronic hepatocellular disease
- Collagen vascular disease
- Early response to bacterial
- Parasitic infection
- Hyper-IgM dysgammaglobulinemia
- Rheumatoid arthritis
- Variable in nephrotic syndrome
- Viral infection (hepatitis or mononucleosis)

Monoclonal:
- Cold agglutinin hemolysis disease
- Malignant lymphoma
- Neoplasms (especially GI tract)
- Reticulosis
- Waldenström's macroglobulinemia

Decreases in:

IgA:
- Ataxia-telangiectasia
- Genetic IgA deficiency
- Chronic sinopulmonary disease

IgD:
- Genetic IgD deficiency
- Preeclampsia
- Malignant melanoma of the skin

IgG:
- Burns
- Nephrotic syndrome
- Pregnancy
- Genetic IgG deficiency

IgM:
- Burns
- Secondary IgM deficiency related to IgG or IgA gammopathies

IMPEDING FACTORS:
- Drugs that may enhance the level of immunoglobulin include asparaginase, cimetidine, and narcotics.
- Products that may reduce immunoglobulin levels include dextran, oral contraceptives, phenytoin, and methylprednisolone (high doses).
- Chemotherapy, immunosuppressive therapy, and radiation therapy, lower immunoglobulin levels.
- Samples with macroglobulins, cryoglobulins, or cold agglutinins tested at cold temperatures could give false low values.

LUPUS ANTICOAGULANT ANTIBODIES

Lupus antiphospholipid antibodies, Lupus inhibitor phospholipid type

SAMPLING: 1 mL of plasma is collected in the blue-top (sodium citrate) tube.

TECHNIQUE: Dilute Russell venom viper test time

NORMAL VALUE: Negative.

EXPLAINATION:

Lupus anticoagulant antibodies are immunoglobulins, typically in the IgG band. These are also referred to as lupus antiphospholipid antibodies because these interact with phospholipid-dependent coagulation tests such as active partial thromboplastin time (APTT) by interacting with phospholipids in the test system. They are not concerned with the bleeding disorder when thrombocytopenia or antiprothrombin antibodies are present. These are linked to an increased risk of thrombosis.

INDICATIONS:

- Evaluate extended activated partial thromboplastin time.
- Investigate the cause of fetal death.

RESULT:

Positive in:
• Fetal loss
• Raynaud's syndrome
• Rheumatoid arthritis
• Systemic lupus erythematosus
• Thromboembolism
Negative in: N/A

IMPEDING FACTORS:
- Drugs that can produce a positive lupus anticoagulant test result include chlorpromazine and heparin.
- Placing the tourniquet for more than 1 minute can result in venous stasis and changes in the concentration of plasma proteins to be tested. Activation of the platelet may also occur under these conditions, resulting in incorrect results.
- Vascular injury during phlebotomy can cause platelets and coagulation factors activation, resulting in incorrect outcomes.
- Hemolyzed specimens must be discarded as hemolysis is a sign of platelet activation and coagulation factor activation.
- Incompletely filled tubes mixed with heparin or clotted specimens should be declined.
- Icteric or lipemic specimens' conflict with optical test methods and yield incorrect results.

LATEX ALLERGY

SAMPLING:1 mL of serum is collected in a red-top tube.
TECHNIQUE: Immunoassay
NORMAL VALUE: Negative.
EXPLAINATION:
Latex is found in a wide range of medical supplies, such as gloves, catheters, and bandages. Many individuals who are routinely exposed to latex products, especially as part of their employment, have become highly allergic to latex. Health care workers are classified as high-risk, especially since the 1987 provision of standard / universal precautions resulting in increased use of latex gloves. It is calculated that 8 to 17 percent of health staff have become allergic to latex. There are two kinds of allergic reactions. Type IV allergic contact dermatitis is triggered by chemicals used in the latex manufacturing process. A delayed reaction occurs within 6 to 48 hours of direct skin or mucous membrane contact of latex products. The allergic reaction with the form I occurs in response to proteins in natural latex products by directly make contact of the skin or mucous membrane or by inhaling aerosolized material from the latex gloves. Other high-risk cases include those with spinal cord injury, spina bifida, myelodysplasia, eczema, atopic dermatitis, history of allergies (personal or family), history of chronic disease, or prolonged procedure.
INDICATIONS: Suspected latex allergy
RESULT:

Positive findings in Latex allergy
Negative findings in N/A

CRITICAL VALUES: N/A
IMPEDING FACTORS: N/A

LYME ANTIBODY

SAMPLING:1 mL of serum is collected in a red-top tube.
TECHNIQUE: Indirect immunofluorescence
NORMAL VALUE: Negative.
EXPLAINATION:
Borrelia burgdorferi, a deer tick-borne spirochete, that causes Lyme disease. Lyme disease is characterized by fever, arthralgia, and arthritis. Circular red rash characterizing erythema migrans can occur 3 to 30 days after the tick bite. Approximately one-half of those at an early stage with Lyme disease (stage 1) and nearly all those at an advanced stage (stage 2)—with neurological, cardiovascular, and rheumatoid manifestations—will have a positive test result. Those in remission will also have a positive response to the test. The presence of antibodies to immunoglobulin M (IgM) suggests acute infection. The existence of IgG antibodies indicates current or previous infections.

INDICATIONS:
Aid in the diagnosis of Lyme disease.

RESULT:

Positive findings in Lyme disease
Negative findings in Not any disease

IMPEDING FACTORS:
High titers of rheumatoid-factor, as well as cross-reactivity with Epstein-Barr virus and other spirochetes (e.g., Rickettsia, Treponema), can result in false-positive results.
Positive test results should be checked using the Western Blot process.

MUMPS SEROLOGY

SAMPLING: 1 mL of serum is collected in a red-top tube.
TECHNIQUE: Indirect immunofluorescence
NORMAL VALUE: Negative or < a fourfold increase in titer.
EXPLAINATION:
Mumps, also known as parotitis, is a viral disease of the parotid glands triggered by a myxovirus, which is transmitted by direct contact with or transmitted from the saliva of the infected person. The incubation period is typical of 3 weeks. The virus may be shed in saliva for two weeks after infection and in urine for two weeks after symptoms begin. Infection risks include aseptic meningitis, encephalitis, and infection of the testicles, ovaries, and pancreas. The presence of antibodies to immunoglobulin M (IgM) suggests acute infection.
INDICATIONS:
- Help to determine resistance or protection to mumps virus by a positive reaction or vulnerability to mumps by a negative reaction.
- Document immunity.
- Evaluate mumps viruses and differentiate between mumps and mumps-like conditions.
RESULT:

Positive findings in Previous or current mumps infection.

PARVOVIRUS B19 IMMUNOGLOBULIN G & IMMUNOGLOBULIN M ANTIBODIES

SAMPLING: 2 mL of serum is collected in a red- or tiger-top tube.

TECHNIQUE: Immunoassay

NORMAL VALUE:

Negative < 0.8

Equivocal 0.8–1.2

EXPLAINATION:

Parvovirus B19, a single-stranded DNA virus spread via respiratory secretions, is the only known parvovirus to infect humans. The main replication site is in red blood cell precursors in the bone marrow. It can cause a varied range of diseases ranging from self-limited erythema (fifth disease) to bone marrow malfunction or aplastic crisis in patients with sickle cell anemia, spherocytosis, or thalassemia. Fetal hydrops and spontaneous abortions may also occur because of infection during pregnancy.

The incubation period is about one week after exposure. B19-specific antibodies present in the serum approximately 3 days after symptoms have arisen. The presence of antibodies to immunoglobulin M (IgM) suggests acute infection. The presence of IgG antibodies suggests the previous infection and is believed to provide long-term immunity. Parvovirus may also be identified by DNA hybridization using a polymerase chain reaction.

INDICATIONS:

Aid in establishing a diagnosis of parvovirus B19 infection.

RESULT:

Positive findings in:
Arthritis
Erythrocyte aplasia
Hydrops fetalis
Erythema infectiosum (fifth disease)
Negative findings in N/A

IMPEDING FACTORS:

Immunocompromised patients may not develop adequate antibodies to be detected.

RUBEOLA ANTIBODIES (Measles serology)

SAMPLING: 1 mL of serum is collected in a red-top tube.
TECHNIQUE: Indirect immunofluorescence
NORMAL VALUE: Negative or < a fourfold increase in titer.
EXPLAINATION:
Measles is caused by a single-stranded paramyxovirus ribonucleic acid (RNA) that invades the respiratory tract and lymphoreticular tissues. It is transmitted via respiratory secretions and aerosolized secretion droplets. The incubation period is between 10 and 11 days. Signs often include conjunctivitis, cough, and fever. Koplik spots develop 4 to 5 days later, accompanied by papular eruptions, body rash, and lymphadenopathy. The presence of antibodies to immunoglobulin M (IgM) suggests acute infection. The presence of IgG antibodies suggests current or previous infections. A negative reaction demonstrates measles susceptibility. Most labs use a qualitative assay that detects the presence of both IgM and IgG antibodies. IgM- and IgG-specific immunoassays are also available to help distinguish acute infection from immune status. A rise in titer more than fourfold in paired specimens is a sign of current infection.
INDICATIONS:
- Determination of susceptibility to or protection against measles virus.
- Differential diagnosis of viral infection, especially in pregnant women with a history of exposure to measles.
RESULT:
Positive findings in Measles infection
CRITICAL VALUES: N/A
IMPEDING FACTORS: N/A

RUBELLA ANTIBODIES (German measles serology)

SAMPLING: 1 mL of serum is collected in a red-top tube.
TECHNIQUE: Indirect immunofluorescence
NORMAL VALUE: Immune or < a fourfold increase in titer.
EXPLAINATION:
Rubella, commonly referred to as German measles, is a communicable and contagious viral disease spread by contact with respiratory secretions and aerosolized secretion droplets. The incubation period is almost between 14 and 21 days. This disease causes a pink, macular rash that fades within 2 to 3 days. Rubella infection induces the production of immunoglobulin G (IgG) and IgM antibody. This test may determine the present infection or immunity from previous infections.

Serum rubella is part of the TORCH (toxoplasmosis, rubella, cytomegalovirus, herpes simplex type 2) panel routinely performed on pregnant women. Fetal infection during the first trimester will cause spontaneous abortion or congenital disabilities. Ideally, the immune state of women of childbearing age should be determined before birth, so vaccines can be provided to provide lifelong immunity. The presence of IgM antibodies suggests acute infection. The presence of IgG antibodies reveals current or past infections. Negative reactions indicate susceptibility to rubella. Often laboratories use a qualitative test to detect the presence of both IgM and IgG rubella antibodies. IgM- and IgG-specific immunoassays are also available to help differentiate acute infection from immune status. An increase in titer >fourfold in paired specimens is a sign of current infection.

INDICATIONS:
- Assist in the detection of rubella infection.
- Identify the presence of rubella antibodies.
- Determine the sensitivity to rubella, especially in pregnant women.
- Perform routine prenatal serological tests.

RESULT:

Positive findings in Rubella infection (past or present)
CRITICAL VALUES: N/A

IMPEDING FACTORS: N/A

RHEUMATOID FACTOR (RF, RA)

SAMPLING: 1 mL of the specimen is collected in a red-top tube.
TECHNIQUE: Nephelometry
NORMAL VALUE: 0 to 20 IU/mL.
EXPLAINATION:

Individuals with rheumatoid arthritis have a macroglobulin-type antibody called rheumatoid factor (RF) in their blood. Patients with other diseases (e.g., systemic lupus erythematosus [SLE] and sometimes tuberculosis, chronic hepatitis, infectious mononucleosis, and subacute bacterial endocarditis) might also have RF-positive tests. RF antibodies are normally M immunoglobulin (IgM) but may also be IgG or IgA.

INDICATIONS:
Assistance in the diagnosis of rheumatoid arthritis, particularly when the clinical diagnosis is difficult.

RESULT

Increased in:
Cirrhosis
Dermatomyositis
Infectious mononucleosis
Leishmaniasis
Leprosy
Malaria
Rheumatoid arthritis
Sarcoidosis
Scleroderma
Sjögren's syndrome
SLE
Syphilis
Tuberculosis
Chronic hepatitis
Chronic viral infections
Waldenström's macroglobulinemia
Decreased in: N/A

IMPEDING FACTORS:
- Older patients are likely to have higher values.
- Previous blood transfusions, multiple vaccinations or transfusions, or inadequately activated complements may have an impact on results.
- Serum with cryoglobulin or high lipid levels may cause a false-positive test and may allow a repeat test after a fat-restriction diet.

SYPHILIS SEROLOGY

Automated reagin testing (ART), microhemagglutination–Treponema pallidum (MHA-TP), fluorescent treponemal antibody testing (FTA-ABS), treponemal studies, Venereal Disease Research Laboratory (VDRL) testing, rapid plasma reagin (RPR)

SAMPLING: 1 mL of serum is collected in a red- or tiger-top tube.
TECHNIQUE: Darkfield microscopy, rapid plasma reagin, enzyme-linked immunosorbent assay [ELISA], microhemagglutination, fluorescence
NORMAL VALUE: Nonreactive or absence of treponemal organisms.

EXPLAINATION:

Numerous methods are used to detect Treponema pallidum, an agent known to cause syphilis. The serology of syphilis is regularly prescribed as part of a prenatal analysis and is required for the assessment of donated blood units before release for transfusion. It is crucial to select the right test method. Automated reagent processing (ART), rapid plasma reagent testing (RPR), and the Venereal Disease Research Laboratory (VDRL) testing should be used for screening purposes. Fluorescent Treponemal Antibody Testing (FTAABS) and Microhemagglutination–Treponema Pallidum (MHA-TP) are confirmatory methods for samples that are either positive or reactive. Cerebrospinal fluid should only be checked using the FTA-ABS method. The cord blood should not be tested using any of the above methods; rather, the serum of the mother should be tested to determine whether the baby should be treated.

INDICATIONS:

- Screening and verifying the existence of syphilis.
- Monitor the effectiveness of syphilis treatment.

RESULT:

Positive or reactive findings in:
Syphilis
False-positive or false-reactive findings in screening (RPR, VDRL) tests:
Infectious:
Chickenpox
Human immunodeficiency virus
Infectious mononucleosis
Leprosy
Leptospirosis
Lymphogranuloma venereum
Bacterial endocarditis
Chancroid
Malaria
Measles
Mumps
Psittacosis
Rickettsial disease
Relapsing fever
Scarlet fever
Trypanosomiasis
Tuberculosis
Vaccinia (live or attenuated)
Mycoplasma pneumoniae
Pneumococcal pneumonia
Viral hepatitis

Noninfectious:
Advanced cancer
Advancing age
Chronic liver disease
Connective tissue diseases
Intravenous drug use
Multiple blood transfusions
Narcotic addiction
Pregnancy
Multiple myeloma and other
Immunologic disorders
False-positive or false-reactive findings in confirmatory (FTA-ABS, MHA-TP) tests:
Infectious:
Infectious mononucleosis
Leprosy
Leptospirosis
Lyme disease
Malaria
Relapsing fever
Noninfectious:
Systemic lupus erythematosus
Negative or nonreactive findings in: N/A

TUBERCULIN SKIN TESTS

(TB tine test, PPD, Mantoux skin test)

SAMPLING: N/A

TECHNIQUE: Intradermal skin test

Prepare the PPD or old tuberculin in a tuberculin syringe with a short, 26-gauge needle. Prepare the correct dilution and quantity for the most widely used medium strength (5 tuberculin units in 0.1 mL) or the first strength normally found in infants (1 tuberculin unit in 0.1 mL). Inject the formulation intradermally at the prepared site if it is inserted into the syringe. When properly inserted, a blister or whale of 6 to 10 mm in diameter is formed within the skin layers. Mark the site and warn the patient to come back within 48 to 72 hours and get the result read. When reading, use a plastic ruler to determine the diameter of the largest indurated area, ensuring that space is adequately illuminated to do the reading. Palpate for thickening of the tissue; a favorable response of 5 mm or more with erythema and edema is suggestive.

NORMAL VALUE: Negative.

EXPLAINATION:

Tuberculin skin tests are performed to determine previous or current susceptibility to tuberculosis. Multipuncture or tine checking, a screening procedure, uses either tuberculin purified protein derivative (PPD) or old tuberculin. A positive reaction at the puncture site suggests cell-mediated immunity to the organism or impaired hypersensitivity caused by the interaction of sensitized T lymphocytes. Verification of the patient's positive response to multi puncture is performed with a more conclusive Mantoux test using Aplisol or Tubersol dispensed by intradermal injection. The Mantoux test is the investigation of choice for symptomatic patients. It is also used as a screening test in some settings. A negative result is concluded if there is no evidence of redness or induration at the injection site or if the redness and induration field is < 5 mm in diameter. A positive result is indicated by an area of more than 10 mm of erythema and induration at the injection site. A positive outcome does not distinguish between active and dormant infections. A positive reaction to the Mantoux test is accompanied by chest radiography and bacteriologic sputum tests to confirm the diagnosis.

INDICATIONS:

- Evaluate cough, weight loss, fatigue, hemoptysis, and suspicious x-rays to evaluate whether tuberculosis is the cause of symptoms.
- Evaluate known or suspected tuberculosis infection, with or without signs, to decide whether tuberculosis is present.
- Evaluate patients with medical problems that place them at risk for tuberculosis (e.g., acquired immunodeficiency syndrome [AIDS], lymphoma, diabetes).
- Screen children with a tine check at the time of first immunization to identify tuberculosis exposure.
- Screen individuals at risk of developing tuberculosis (e.g., health care professionals, nursing home patients, correctional staff, prisoners, and residents of the inner city living in poor hygienic conditions).

RESULT: Positive findings in Pulmonary tuberculosis
IMPEDING FACTORS:
- Medications such as immunosuppressive agents or steroids can influence the results.
- Diseases such as hematologic cancers or sarcoidosis can alter the results.
- Past or current bacterial, fungal, or viral infections can impact the result. False-positive results may be produced by the occurrence of non-tuberculous mycobacteria or by serial testing.
- False-negative results will occur if the sensitized T cells are temporarily depleted. False-negative outcomes may also occur in the presence of bacterial infections, immunological defects, immunosuppressive agents, live virus vaccinations (e.g., measles, mumps, polio, rubella), malnutrition, old age, significant tuberculosis, renal failure, and aggressive viral infections (e.g., chickenpox, measles, mumps).
- Inadequate storage of the tuberculin solution (e.g., concerning temperature, exposure to light, and stability at opening) can affect the results.
- Improper procedure during intradermal injection (e.g., injection into subcutaneous tissue) can lead to false-negative outcomes.
- Incorrect volume or dilution of the antigen injected, or delayed injection after the antigen has been applied to the syringe, can affect the results.
- Incorrect reading of the response measurement or timing of the reading can interfere with the tests.
- It is not understood whether the procedure has teratogenic or reproductive effects; the test should only be given to pregnant women as clearly indicated.
- The testing should not be applied to a patient with a previously successful tuberculin skin test due to the risk of serious reactions, including vesiculation, ulceration, and necrosis.
- The test does not differentiate between current and past infections.

TOXOPLASMA ANTIBODY (toxoplasmosis titer, Toxoplasmosis serology)

SAMPLING: 1 ml serum is collected in a red-top tube.

TECHNIQUE: Indirect fluorescent antibody

NORMAL VALUE: Negative or less than fourfold rise in titer.

EXPLAINATION:

Toxoplasmosis is a serious, systemic granulomatous central nervous system illness induced by the Toxoplasma gondii protozoan. Transmission among humans happens by consuming undercooked foods or the disposal of infected materials, such as cat litter. Immunoglobulin M (IgM) antibodies produce roughly five days after exposure and may remain high for three weeks to many months. IgG antibodies evolve 1 to 2 weeks after illness and may remain high for months or years. Toxoplasma serology is one of the TORCHES (toxoplasmosis, rubella, cytomegalovirus, herpes simplex type 2) group regularly conducted on pregnant women. Fetal illness during the first trimester can trigger spontaneous abortion or serious birth defects. Immunocompromised people are often at the risk of severe problems if they become exposed. IgM antibodies suggest acute or congenital disease; the presence of IgG antibodies implies present or previous infections.

INDICATIONS:

- Help in establishing a diagnosis of toxoplasmosis.
- Document previous exposure or immunity.
- Serologic screening during pregnancy.

RESULT:

Positive findings in Toxoplasma infection

CRITICAL VALUES: N/A

IMPEDING FACTORS: N/A

VARICELLA ANTIBODIES

Chickenpox, Varicella zoster antibodies, VZ

SAMPLING:1 mL of serum is collected in a red-top tube.

TECHNIQUE: Indirect fluorescent antibody

NORMAL VALUE: Negative or < a fourfold increase in titer.

EXPLAINATION:

Varicella-zoster is a herpes virus-carrying double-stranded DNA that is accountable for two clinical syndromes, i.e., chickenpox and shingles. The incubation period is almost 2 to 3 weeks and is highly contagious for about two weeks, beginning two days before the rash develops. Respiratory secretions spread it. The primary contact to the highly contagious virus typically occurs in susceptible school-aged children. Adults without previous exposure and who become infected may have serious complications, including pneumonia. A mother's neonatal infection is likely if exposure occurs within the last three weeks of gestation. Shingles occur when the potentially dormant virus is reactivated. The presence of antibodies to immunoglobulin M (IgM) indicates acute infection. The presence of IgG antibodies suggests current or past infections. The result of a reactive varicella antibody indicates immunity but does not protect an individual from shingles.

INDICATIONS:

Determine susceptibility or immunity to chickenpox.

RESULT:

Positive findings in Varicella infection
Negative findings in Not any disease

IMPEDING FACTORS: N/A

RENAL SYSTEM

The urinary system, also acknowledged as the renal or urinary tract system, consisting of the kidneys, urethra, bladder, and urethra. The urinary system is designed to eliminate waste from the body, manage blood flow and blood pressure, monitor the levels of electrolytes and metabolites, and manage the blood's pH.

The tests used in the renal screen can differ by laboratories, but the tests usually conducted include:

Electrolytes – electrically charged chemicals essential to natural body functions, such as nerve activity and muscle function, help control the body's volume, and preserve the acid-base balance. Electrolytes shall include:

- Sodium

- Potassium

- Sodium chloride

- Bicarbonate (total carbonate)

Minerals:

- Phosphorus – a mineral essential to energy output, muscle and nerve activity, and bone growth; it also plays an important role as a shield, helping to retain the body's acid-base balance.

- Calcium – one of the most important minerals in the body; it is necessary for the proper functioning of muscles, nerves, and the heart and is required for blood clotting and bone-forming.

Protein:

Albumin – a protein that makes up approximately 60 percent of the protein in the blood and serves various functions, such as preventing fluids from spilling out of blood vessels and moving nutrients, enzymes, medications, and ions like calcium throughout the body.

Other compounds:

- Urea / Blood Urea Nitrogen (BUN) – urea is a nitrogen-containing waste product produced by protein metabolism; it is absorbed into the blood by the liver and transferred to the kidneys, purified out of the blood, and passed in the urine.

- Creatinine – another waste product formed by the body; the kidneys excrete nearly all creatinine.

- Glucose – provides energy to the body; a consistent supply of glucose must be available for use, and a relatively stable volume of glucose must be retained in the blood.

Three values can also be calculated for the renal function:

- Urea (BUN)/Creatinine Ratio – a relation of urea (nitrogen) to creatinine in the blood
- Estimated Glomerular Filtration Rate (eGFR) – a measured approximation of the renal glomerular filtration rate (GFR, the volume of blood filtered by glomeruli in the kidneys per minute) derived from blood creatinine levels; the calculation takes into account the age, gender, race, and occasionally height and weight of the person.
- Anion Gap – anion gap (AG or AGAP) is a value determined from the electrolyte panel's effects. It measures the difference between measured and non-mediated electrical particles (ion or electrolyte) of the fluid's blood component.

NOTES

_____

_____

_____

_____

_____

_____

_____

_____

_____

_____

_____

CREATININE, SERUM

SAMPLING: 1 mL of serum is collected in a red- or tiger-top tube. 1 mL of plasma collected in a green-top (heparin) tube is also acceptable.

TECHNIQUE: Spectrophotometry

NORMAL VALUE:

Age	Conventional Units	SI Units (Conversion Factor X 88.4)
1–5 y	0.3–0.5 mg/dL	27–44 µ mol/L
6–10 y	0.5–0.8 mg/dL	44–71 µmol/L
Adult male	0.6–1.2 mg/dL	53–106 µ mol/L
Adult female	0.5–1.1 mg/dL	44–97 µmol/L

EXPLAINATION:

Creatinine is the final product of creatine breakdown. Creatine is located nearly entirely in the skeletal muscles, where it is active in energy-requiring biochemical reactions. Through these processes, a small volume of creatine is irreversibly transformed into creatinine and is then transferred to the kidneys and excreted in the urine. The quantity of creatinine formed in a person is related to the mass of his skeletal muscle. It remains relatively steady until major muscle damage is done by crushing or degenerative muscular disease. Creatinine also decreases with age gdue to reduced muscle mass.

Blood urea nitrogen (BUN) is very often recommended in comparative analysis with creatinine. The BUN/creatinine ratio is also a beneficial measure of disease. The usual ranges among 10:1 and 20:1. Creatinine is the ideal chemical for the estimation of renal clearance, as a nearly steady quantity is formed only within the body. The creatinine clearance test considers both the blood sample and the urine sample to calculate the rate at which creatinine is removed from the blood by the kidneys; this closely matches the GFR or glomerular filtration rate.

INDICATIONS:

- Evaluate known or suspected muscle disorder in the absence of renal disease.
- Evaluate known or suspected failure of renal function.

RESULT:

Increased in:
• **Acromegaly**
• **Congestive heart failure**
• **Dehydration**
• **Gigantism**
• **Hyperthyroidism**

• **Poliomyelitis**
• **Rhabdomyolysis**
• **Shock**
• **Renal disease, acute and chronic renal failure**
Decreased in:
• **Decreased muscle mass owing to debilitating disease or increasing age**
• **Inadequate protein intake**
• **Liver disease (severe)**
• **Muscular dystrophy**
• **Pregnancy**
• **Small stature**

CRITICAL VALUES:
Potential critical value is >15 mg / dL (non-dialysis patient). Possible interventions may involve renal or peritoneal dialysis and organ transplantation, but the early discovery of the cause of increased levels of creatinine may prevent such drastic interventions.

IMPEDING FACTORS:
- Medicines and substances that may increase the levels of creatinine include acebutolol, acetaminophen (overdose), aldatense, amikacin, amiodarone acid, barbiturates, capreomycin, captopril, carbutamide, carvedilol, doxycycline, enalapril, ethylene glycol, gentamicin, indomethacin, ipodate, kanamycin, levodopa, mannitol, amphotericin B, arginine, arsenicals, ascorbic acid, asparaginase, acetylsalicylic cephalothin, chlorthalidone, cimetidine, cisplatin, clofibrate, colistin, corn oil (Lipomul), cyclosporine, dextran, methicillin, methoxyflurane, mitomycin, neomycin, netilmycin, nitrofurantoin, nonsteroidal anti-inflammatory drugs, oxyphenbutazone, paromomycin, penicillin, tetracycline, thiazides, tobramycin, pentamidine, phosphorus, plicamycin, radiographic agents, semustine, streptokinase, streptozocin, triamterene, vancomycin, vasopressin, viomycin, and vitamin D.
- Medications that may decrease the levels of creatinine include citrate, dopamine, ibuprofen, and lisinopril.
- Bilirubin and glucose may cause false decreases in creatinine.
- A diet high in meat may cause increased levels of creatinine.
- Ketosis may cause a significant increase in creatinine.

CREATININE, URINE, & CREATININE CLEARANCE, URINE

SAMPLING: 5 mL of urine from an unpreserved random or timed specimen collected in a clean plastic collection container.

TECHNIQUE: Spectrophotometry

NORMAL VALUE:

Age	Conventional Units	SI Units
Urine Creatinine (Conversion Factor X 8.84)		
2–3 y	6–22 mg/kg/24 h	53–194 mol/kg/24 h
4–18 y	12–30 mg/kg/24 h	106–265 mol/kg/24 h
Adult male	14–26 mg/kg/24 h	124–230 mol/kg/24 h
Adult female	11–20 mg/kg/24 h	97–177 mol/kg/24 h
Creatinine Clearance (Conversion Factor X 0.0167)		
Infants and children	70–140 mL/min/1.73 m^2	1.17–2.33 mL/s/1.73 m^2
Male(adult)	85–125 mL/min/1.73 m^2	1.42–2.08 mL/s/1.73 m^2
Female (adult)	75–115 mL/min/1.73 m^2	1.25–1.92 mL/s/1.73 m^2
for every 10 yrs	Decrease by 6–7	Decrease by 0.06–0.07
after 40 y	**mL/min/1.73 m^2**	**mL/s/1.73 m^2**

EXPLAINATION:

Creatinine is the final product of the metabolism of creatine. Creatine occurs nearly entirely in the skeletal muscle, where it is active in energy-requiring metabolic reactions. In these phases, a small amount of creatine is irreversibly converted to creatinine, which is then transported to the kidneys and excreted. The amount of creatinine produced in a person is proportional to the mass of the skeletal muscle present. It remains constant until significant muscle damage is caused by crushing or degenerative muscle disease.

Creatinine levels decrease with the increasing age due to the reduced muscle mass. Although urine creatinine is a useful marker for renal function, the creatinine clearance test is much more accurate. The creatinine clearance test analyzes both the blood and the urine sample together to assess the rate at which the kidneys filter creatinine. This test specifically defines the glomerular filtration rate and is dependent on the body surface area estimation.

INDICATIONS:

- Determine the extent of nephrogenic damage in established renal disease (at least 50% of functional nephrons must be impaired before values are reduced).
- Determine renal function before nephrotic drugs are administered.
- Assess the validity of 24-hour urine collection based on the constant level of creatinine excretion.

- Evaluate glomerular function.
- Monitor the efficacy of treatment in renal disease.

RESULT:

	Increased in:
•	**Acromegaly**
•	**Acute tubular necrosis**
•	**Exposure to nephrotoxic drugs and chemicals**
•	**Carnivorous diets**
•	**Congestive heart failure**
•	**Dehydration**
•	**Diabetes**
•	**Exercise**
•	**Gigantism**
•	**Glomerulonephritis**
•	**Hypothyroidism**
•	**Infections**
•	**Neoplasms (bilateral renal)**
•	**Nephrosclerosis**
•	**Polycystic kidney disease**
•	**Pyelonephritis**
•	**Renal artery atherosclerosis**
•	**Renal artery obstruction**
•	**Renal disease**
•	**Renal vein thrombosis**
•	**Shock and hypovolemia**
•	**Tuberculosis**
	Decreased in:
•	**Chronic bilateral pyelonephritis**
•	**Hyperthyroidism**
•	**Leukemia**
•	**Muscle wasting diseases**
•	**Paralysis**
•	**Polycystic kidney disease**
•	**Shock**

• **Acute or chronic glomerulonephritis**
• **Anemia**
• **Urinary tract obstruction (e.g., from calculi)**
• **Vegetarian diets**

CRITICAL VALUES:
Degree of deficiency:
Borderline/only normal: 62.5–80 mL/min/ 1.73 m2
Insignificantly raised: 52–62.5 mL/min/1.73 m2
Mild: 42–52 mL/min/1.73 m2
Moderate: 28–42 mL/min/1.73 m2
Marked: < 28 mL/min/ 1.73 m2
IMPEDING FACTORS:
- Medications that may increase urinary creatinine levels include ascorbic acid, cefoxitin, cephalothin, corticosteroids, fluoxymesterone, levodopa, nitrofurans (including nitrofurazone), methandrostenolone, methotrexate, methyldopa, oxymetholone, phenolphthalein, and prednisone.
- Medications that may improve the clearance of creatinine in the urine include enalapril, oral contraceptives, prednisone, and ramipril.
- Medications that may decrease the levels of creatinine in urine include anabolic steroids, androgens, captopril, and thiazides.
- Drugs that may reduce the urine creatinine clearance include amphotericin B, ibuprofen, indomethacin, mitomycin, acetylsalicylic acid, carbenoxolone, chlorthalidone, cimetidine, cisplatin, cyclosporine, guancidine, oxyphenbutazone, paromomycin, probenecid (coadministered with digoxin), and thiazides.
- Excessive ketones in urine can cause false values to decrease.
- Failure to follow proper techniques in collecting a 24-hour specimen may invalidate the results of the test.
- Failure to refrigerate the specimen throughout the urine collection period allows the decomposition of creatinine, resulting in falsely decreased values.
- The consumption of large amounts of meat, excessive exercise, and stress should be avoided for 24 hours before the test.

OSMOLALITY, SERUM, AND URINE (Osmo)

SAMPLING:1 mL of serum is collected in a red- or tiger-top tube; 5 mL of urine from an unpreserved random specimen is collected in a clean, plastic collection container.

TECHNIQUE: Freezing point depression

NORMAL VALUE:

	Conventional Units	SI Units (Conversion Factor X1)
Serum	275–295 mOsm/kg	275–295 mmol/kg
Urine		
Newborn	75–300 mOsm/kg	75–300 mmol/kg
Children and adults	250–900 mOsm/kg	250–900 mmol/kg

EXPLAINATION:

Osmolality is used to help treat metabolic, renal, and endocrine diseases. Simultaneous determination of serum and urinary osmolality provides an opportunity to compare values between the two fluids. The typical ratio of urine to serum is about 0.2 to 4.7 for random samples and higher than 3.0 for first-morning samples (dehydration usually occurs overnight). Sodium, chloride, bicarbonate, urea, and glucose are the major dissolved particles that contribute to osmolality. Some of these chemicals are used in the following derived assessment:

The serum osmolality = {[2(Na+)] +[glucose/18] +[BUN/2.8]}

Original osmolality is higher than the estimated value. The osmolar gap is the difference between the observed and the calculated values and is usually between 5 and 10 mOsm / kg. If the discrepancy is >15 mOsm / kg, consider the toxicity of ethylene glycol, isopropanol, methanol, or ethanol. Such substances act as antifreeze, lower the freezing point in the body, and show misleadingly high results.

INDICATIONS:

Serum:
- Aid in the evaluation of antidiuretic hormone (ADH) activity.
- Assist in rapid screening of toxic substances such as ethylene glycol, ethanol, isopropanol, and methanol.
- Determine electrolyte and acid-base balance.
- Evaluate hydration state.

Urine:
- Renal Concentration Efficiency.
- Determine Diabetes Insipidus.
- Evaluate Neonatal Patients with Urinary Protein or Glucose.
- Sort out Kidney Disease.

RESULT:

Increased in:
Serum:
•   Hypernatremia
•   Azotemia
•   Dehydration
•   Diabetes insipidus
•   Diabetic ketoacidosis
•   Hypercalcemia
Urine:
•   Syndrome of inappropriate antidiuretic hormone production (SIADH)
•   Amyloidosis
•   Azotemia
•   Congestive heart failure
•   Dehydration
•   Hyponatremia
Decreased in:
Serum:
•   Water intoxication
•   Adrenocortical insufficiency
•   Hyponatremia
•   SIADH
Urine:
•   Hypokalemia
•   Hypernatremia
•   Primary polydipsia
•   Diabetes insipidus

CRITICAL VALUES:
Serum:
< 265 mOsm/kg
>320 mOsm/kg
Serious clinical situations may be associated with an elevated or reduced osmolality of the serum.
The following conditions are associated with an elevated osmolality of the serum:

- *Respiratory arrest:* 360 mOsm/kg
- *The stupor of hyperglycemia:* 385 mOsm/kg
- *Grand mal seizures:* 420 mOsm/kg
- *Death:* >420mOsm/kg

Symptoms with extremely high levels include poor skin turgor, listlessness, acidosis (lower pH), shock, seizures, coma, and cardiopulmonary arrest. Interventions can require close monitoring of electrolytes, administration of intravenous fluids with the appropriate composition to move water into or out of the intravascular space as required, monitoring of vital signals, continuing neurological tests, and taking seizure precautions.

IMPEDING FACTORS:

- Medications that may improve serum osmolality include citrate (as an anticoagulant), corticosteroids, ethylene glycol, glycerin, inulin, ioxithalamic acid, mannitol, and methoxyflurane.

- Medications that may reduce serum osmolality include bendroflumethiazide, carbamazepine, chlorpromazine, chlorthalidone, cyclophosphamide, cyclothiazide, hydrochlorothiazide, lorcainide, methyclothiazide, and polythiazide.

- Medications that may improve urinary osmolality include anesthetic agents, chlorpropamide, cyclophosphamide, furosemide, mannitol, metolazone, octreotide, phloridzin, and vincristine.

- Medications that may reduce the osmolality of urine include captopril, demeclocycline, glyburide, lithium, methoxyflurane, octreotide, tolazamide, and verapamil.

UREA NITROGEN, BLOOD (BUN)

SAMPLING:1 mL of serum is collected in a red- or tiger-top tube. 1 mL of plasma collected in a green-top (heparin) tube is also acceptable.

TECHNIQUE: Spectrophotometry

NORMAL VALUE:

Age	Conventional Units	SI UNITS (Conversion Factor _0.357)
Newborn–3 y	5–17 mg/dL	1.8–6.0 mmol/L
4–13 y	7–17 mg/dL	2.5–6.0 mmol/L
14 y–adult	8–21 mg/dL	2.9–7.5 mmol/L
Adult older than 90 y	10–31 mg/dL	3.6–11.1 mmol/L

EXPLAINATION:

Urea is a non-protein nitrogen compound formed in the liver by ammonia as the product of protein metabolism. Urea diffuses freely into extracellular and intracellular fluids and is eventually excreted by the kidneys. Blood urea nitrogen (BUN) levels indicate the balance between urea production and excretion. The levels of BUN and creatinine are commonly evaluated together.

The normal BUN/creatinine ratio is 15:1 to 24:1 (e.g., if a person has a BUN of 15 mg/dL, the creatinine should be roughly 0.6 to 1.0 mg/dL).

BUN is used in the subsequent calculation to approximate serum osmolality:
[(2[Na+]) + (glucose/18) + (BUN/2.8)]

INDICATIONS:
- Determining renal function.
- Evaluate liver function.
- Evaluate hydration.
- Scrutinize the effects of drugs known to be nephrotoxic or hepatotoxic.
- Evaluate hemodialysis therapy.
- Evaluate nutritional support.
- Evaluate patients with chemotherapy lymphoma (tumor lysis).

RESULT:

	Increased in:
•	**Acute renal failure**
•	**Chronic glomerulonephritis**
•	**Congestive heart failure**
•	**Decreased renal perfusion**
•	**Diabetes**
•	**Excessive protein ingestion**
•	**Gastrointestinal (GI) bleeding (too much blood protein in the GI tract)**
•	**Hyperalimentation**
•	**Hypovolemia**
•	**Ketoacidosis**
•	**Muscle wasting from starvation**
•	**Neoplasms**
•	**Nephrotoxic agents**
•	**Pyelonephritis**
•	**Shock**
•	**Urinary tract obstruction**

Decreased in:	
•	**Inadequate dietary protein**
•	**Low-protein/high-carbohydrate diet**
•	**Malabsorption syndromes**
•	**Pregnancy**
•	**Severe liver disease**

CRITICAL VALUES:
The potential critical value is >100 mg / dL (except in patients with renal dialysis). A patient with a grossly raised BUN may have signs and symptoms such as acidemia, agitation, fatigue, nausea, vomiting, confusion, and coma. Probable interventions include treatment of the cause, administration of intravenous bicarbonate, low protein diet, hemodialysis, and caution concerning prescribing and continuing nephrotoxic drugs.

IMPEDING FACTORS:
- Medicines, substances, and vitamins that may raise BUN levels include acetaminophen, alanine, aldatense, alkaline bismuth subsalicylate, capreomycin, antacids, amphotericin B, antimony compounds, arsenic, bacitracin, carbenoxolone, carbutamide, cephalosporins, chloral hydrate, chloramphenicol, chlorthalidone, colistimethate, guanethidine, ifosfamide, ipodate, kanamycin, guanoxan, ibuprofen, mephenesin, metolazone, mitomycin, neomycin, phosphorus, dexamethasone, dextran, diclofenac, doxycycline, ethylene glycol, gentamicin, colistin, cotrimoxazole, plicamycin, tertatolol, tetracycline, triamterene, triethylenemelamine, viomycin, and vitamin D.
- Medications that may decrease BUN rates include acetohydroxamic acid, chloramphenicol, iodine, paramethasone, phenothiazine, and streptomycin.

UREA NITROGEN, URINE

SAMPLING: 5 mL of urine from an unpreserved random or timed specimen collected in a clean plastic collection container.
TECHNIQUE: Spectrophotometry
NORMAL VALUE:

Conventional Units	SI Units (Conversion Factor X35.7)
12–20 g/24 h	428–714 mmol/24 h

EXPLAINATION:
Urea is a non-protein nitrogen complex formed in the liver by ammonia as the product of protein metabolism. Urea diffuses naturally into extracellular and intracellular fluids and is eventually excreted by the kidneys. Urine urea nitrogen levels reflect the equilibrium between urea production and excretion.

INDICATIONS:
- Evaluate renal disease.
- Predict the impact that other illnesses, such as diabetes and liver disease, will have on the kidneys.

RESULT:

Increased in:
• **Hyperthyroidism**
• **Increased dietary protein**
• **Postoperative period**
• **Diabetes**
Decreased in:
• **Liver disease**
• **Low-protein/high-carbohydrate diet**
• **Normal-growing pediatric patients**
• **Pregnancy**
• **Renal disease**
• **Toxemia**

IMPEDING FACTORS:
- Medications that may increase the level of urinary urea nitrogen include alanine and glycine.
- Drugs that may reduce urinary urea nitrogen levels include furosemide, growth hormone, insulin, and testosterone.
- All urine that has been emptied for the timed collection period must be included in the collection, or falsely decreased values may be obtained. Compare output records with the volume collected to verify that all voids have been included in the collection.

URIC ACID, URINE (Urine urate)

SAMPLING:5 mL of urine from a random or timed specimen collected in a clean plastic, unrefrigerated collection container. Sodium hydroxide preservative may be suggested to prevent precipitation of urates.

TECHNIQUE: Spectrophotometry

NORMAL VALUE:

Gender	Conventional Units*	SI Units (Conversion Factor X0.0059) *
Male	250–800 mg/24 h	1.48–4.72 mmol/24 h
Female	250–750 mg/24 h	1.48–4.43 mmol/24 h

INDICATIONS:

- Evaluate urine and serum uric acid levels to provide an indicator of renal function.
- Diagnose enzyme abnormalities and metabolic disorders that affect the body's production of uric acid.
- Monitor reaction to uricosuric medications.
- Monitor urinary symptoms of disorders that cause hyperuricemia.

RESULT:

Increased in:
• Disorders related to impaired renal tubular absorption, such as Wilson's Disease and Fanconi's syndrome
• Disorders of purine metabolism
• Excessive dietary intake of purines
• Gout
• Pernicious anemia
• Polycythemia vera
• Sickle cell anemia
• Neoplastic disorders, such as lymphosarcoma, leukemia, and multiple myeloma
Decreased in:
• Folic acid deficiency
• Lead toxicity
• Severe renal damage (possibly following chronic glomerulonephritis, lactic acidosis, ketoacidosis, collagen disorders, diabetic glomerulosclerosis, and alcohol abuse)

IMPEDING FACTORS:

Drugs that may raise urine uric acid levels include acetaminophen, acetohexamide, chlorprothixene, corticotropin, coumarin, cytotoxics, levodopa, mannose, merbarone, mercaptopurine, mersalyl, methotrexate, diatrizoic acid, dicumarol, ampicillin, ascorbic acid, azapropazone, benzbromarone, chlorpromazine, ethyl biscoumacetate, glycine, iodipamide, iodopyracet, iopanoic acid, ipodate, niacinamide, phenindione, phenolsulfonphthalein, phenylbutazone, phloridzin, probenecid, salicylates (long-term, large doses), seclazone, sulfinpyrazone, theophylline, verapamil, and xylitol.

Drugs that may reduce urine uric acid levels include acetylsalicylic acid (small doses), ethacrynic acid, ethambutol, ethoxzolamide, hydrochlorothiazide, levarterenol, ascorbic acid, azathioprine, benzbromaron, bumetanide, chlorothiazide, chlorthalidone, citrates, niacin, pyrazinoic acid, and thiazide diuretics.

All urine that has been voided for the timed collection period must be included in the collection or falsely decreased values may be obtained. Compare output records with the volume collected to verify that all voids have been included in the collection.

Notes

URINALYSIS (UA)

SAMPLING: 15 mL of urine from an unpreserved, random specimen is collected in a clean, plastic collection container.

TECHNIQUE: Macroscopic assessment by dipstick and microscopic examination

NORMAL VALUE: Urinalysis consists of a series of studies, including a description of the color and appearance of urine, a calculation of specific gravity and pH, and a semi-quantitative measurement of protein, glucose, ketones, urobilinogen, bilirubin, hemoglobin, nitrite, and leukocyte esterase. Urine deposits may also be examined for the presence of stones, casts, renal epithelial cells, temporary epithelial cells, white blood cells (WBCs), squamous epithelial cells, red blood cells (RBCs), bacteria, yeast, eggs, and any other compounds excreted in the urine that may have clinical worth. Examination of urine sediment is done microscopically under high power, and results are reported as the number seen per high power field (hpf). Normal urine color varies from light yellow to deep amber. Color depends on the patient's state of hydration (more concentrated samples are darker in color), diet, medications, and exposure to other substances that may contribute to unusual color or smell. The appearance of normal urine is noticeably clear. Cloudiness is sometimes due to the presence of amorphous phosphates or urates, as well as blood, WBCs, fat, or bacteria. Normal specific gravity is between 1,001 and 1,035.

Dipstick:

pH	5.0–9.0
Protein	< 20 mg/dL
Glucose	Negative
Ketones	Negative
Hemoglobin	Negative
Bilirubin	Negative
Urobilinogen	Up to 1 mg/dL
Nitrite	Negative
Leukocyte esterase	Negative

Microscopic examination:

Red blood cells	< 5/hpf
White blood cells	< 5/hpf
Renal cells	None has seen
Transitional cells	None has seen
Squamous cells	Rare; usually no clinical significance
Casts	Rare hyaline: otherwise, none has seen
Crystals in acid urine	Uric acid, calcium oxalate, amorphous urates
Bacteria, yeast, parasites	None has seen

EXPLAINATION:

Routine urinalysis, one of the most ordered laboratory procedures, is used for specific screening purposes. It is a group of tests that measure the capacity of the kidneys to excrete and reabsorb compounds while maintaining proper water balance selectively. The findings can provide useful information on the overall health of the patient and the patient's responsiveness to the disease and treatment. The urine dipstick has several pads on it to indicate different biochemical markers. Urine pH is an indicator of the ability of the kidneys to help maintain a balanced concentration of hydrogen ion in the blood. Specific gravity is a function of the coordination power of the kidneys. Urine protein is the most common indicator of renal disease, although there are disorders that may cause benign proteinuria. Glucose is used as a diabetes predictor.

The presence of ketones suggests abnormal metabolism of carbohydrates. Hemoglobin indicates the presence of blood associated with renal failure. Bilirubin is used to help detect liver disorders. Urobilinogen indicates liver or hematopoietic disorders. Nitrites and leukocytes are used to screen for bacteria and other causes of urinary tract infections (UTIs). Most laboratories have established criteria for microscopic examination of urine based on patient populations (e.g., pediatric, oncology, urology), unusual appearance, and biochemical reactions.

INDICATIONS:

- Determine the presence of genitourinary illness or abnormality.
- Observe the effects of physical or emotional stress.
- Monitor fluid imbalances or medical therapy for fluid imbalances.
- Monitor drug response and determine undesired reactions to medications that may impair renal function.
- Include monitoring as part of a general physical examination, particularly after entry to health care.

RESULT:

Unusual Color

Color	Presence of
Deep yellow	Riboflavin
Orange	Bilirubin, chrysophanic acid, Pyridium, santonin
Pink	Beet pigment, hemoglobin, myoglobin, porphyrin, rhubarb
Red	Beet pigment, hemoglobin, myoglobin, porphyrin, uroerythrin
Green	Oxidized bilirubin, Clorets (breath mint)
Blue	Diagnex, indican, methylene blue
Black	Homogentisic acid, melanin
Smokey	Red blood cells

Test	Increased in	Decreased in
pH	Ingestion of citrus fruits	**High-protein diets**
	Metabolic and respiratory alkalosis	**Ingestion of fruits (e.g., cranberries)**
	Vegetarian diets	**Metabolic or respiratory acidosis**
Protein	Benign proteinuria owing to stress, physical exercise, exposure to cold, or standing	N/A
	Diabetic nephropathy	
	Glomerulonephritis	
	Nephrosis	
	Toxemia of pregnancy	
	Diabetes	
	Diabetes	
Glucose	Fever	N/A
Ketones	Fasting	N/A
	Postanesthesia period	
	High-protein diets	
	Isopropanol intoxication	
	Starvation	
	Vomiting	
	Diseases of the bladder	
	Exercise (March hemoglobinuria)	
Hemoglobin	Glomerulonephritis	N/A
	Hemolytic anemia or other causes of hemolysis (e.g., drugs, parasites, transfusion reaction)	
	Malignancy	
	Menstruation	
	Paroxysmal cold hemoglobinuria	
	Paroxysmal nocturnal hemoglobinuria	
	Pyelonephritis	
	Snake or spider bites	
	Trauma	
	Tuberculosis	

	Urinary tract infections	
	Urolithiasis	
	Cirrhosis	
	Heart failure	
Urobilinogen	Hemolytic anemia	Antibiotic therapy (suppresses normal intestinal flora)
	Hepatitis	Obstruction of the bile duct
	Infectious mononucleosis	
	Malaria	
	Pernicious anemia	
Bilirubin	Cirrhosis	N/A
	Hepatic tumor	
	Hepatitis	
Nitrites	Bacterial infection Presence of nitrite-forming bacteria (e.g., Citrobacter, Enterobacter, Escherichia coli, Klebsiella, Proteus, Pseudomonas, Salmonella, and some species of Staphylococcus)	N/A
Leukocyte esterase	Fungal or parasitic infection	N/A
	Glomerulonephritis	
	Interstitial nephritis	
	Tumor	

Formed Elements in Urine:
Sediment
Cellular Elements:
- Clue cells (the bacterial membrane that induces epithelial cell adhesion) are present in non-specific vaginitis caused by Gardnerella vaginitis, Mobiluncus cortisii, and Mobiluncus mulieris.
- RBCs are present in glomerulonephritis, lupus nephritis, focal glomerulonephritis, calculus, malignancy, renal vein thrombosis, trauma, hydronephrosis, polycystic kidney, urinary tract disease, prostatitis, diverticulitis, gout, scurvy, subacute bacterial endocarditis, infectious mononucleosis, salpingitis, hemoglobinopathies, coagulation disorders, heart failure, infection, tuberculosis, infarction, pyelonephritis, appendicitis, and malaria.
- Renal cells that have absorbed cholesterol and triglycerides are also known as oval fat bodies.

- Renal cells originate from the lining of the collection ducts, and increased numbers indicate acute tubular damage as seen in acute tubular necrosis, pyelonephritis, malignant nephrosclerosis, acute glomerulonephritis, acute drug or substance (salicylate, lead, or ethylene glycol) intoxication, or chemotherapy resulting in desquamation, urolithiasis, and kidney transplant rejection.
- Squamous cells line the vagina and the distal part of the urethra. The presence of normal epithelial squamous cells in female urine is usually of no clinical significance. Abnormal cells with large nucleus show the need for cytological tests to rule out malignancy.
- Transitional cells line the renal pelvis, urethra, bladder, and proximal part of the urethra. Higher levels are seen with infection, trauma, and malignancy.
- WBCs are found in acute UTI, tubulointerstitial nephritis, lupus nephritis, pyelonephritis, renal transplant rejection, fever, and strenuous exercise.

Casts:
- Granular casts are formed by protein or by the decomposition of cellular elements. These can be seen in kidney disease, viral infection, or contribute to intoxication.
- Many hyaline casts can be seen in kidney disease, hypertension, congestive heart failure, nephrotic syndrome, and in more benign conditions such as fever, cold temperature use, exercise, or diuretic use.
- RBC castings can be found in acute glomerulonephritis, lupus nephritis, and subacute bacterial endocarditis.
- Waxy castings are seen in chronic renal failure or cases such as kidney transplant rejection, in which renal stasis occurs.
- WBC casts can be seen in lupus nephritis, acute glomerulonephritis, interstitial nephritis, and acute pyelonephritis.

Crystals:
- The crystals contained in recently passed urine have more clinical significance than the crystals seen in the urine sample that has been stored for more than 2 to 4 hours.
- Cystin crystals are seen in patients with cystinosis or cystinuria.
- Leucine or tyrosine crystals can be seen in patients with severe liver disease.
- Large numbers of uric acid crystals are seen in patients with urolithiasis, gout, high dietary intake of purine-rich foods, or chemotherapy.

CRITICAL VALUES:
Potential critical values are uric acid, cystine, leucine, or tyrosine crystals. The occurrence of highly elevated urinary glucose and ketones is also considered to be significant.

IMPEDING FACTORS:

- Other foods, such as onion, garlic, and asparagus, contain substances that may give urine an unpleasant smell. The presence of bacteria can emit an ammonia-like odor. Urine with a maple syrup-like odor can imply a congenital metabolic defect (maple syrup urine disease).
- The various biochemical strips are subject to interference, which may yield false-positive or false-negative results. Consult the laboratory for specific information on the limits of the method of use and the description of intervention medications.
- The dipstick protein detection method is most sensitive to albumin; light-chain or Bence Jones proteins may not be identified by this method. Alkaline pH can yield false-positive protein tests.
- Large amounts of ketones or ascorbic acid can cause false-negative or decreased color development on the glucose pad. Contamination of the collection container or specimen with chlorine, sodium hypochlorite, or peroxide can result in false-positive glucose.
- False-positive ketone findings may be obtained in the presence of ascorbic acid, levodopa metabolites, valproic acid, phenazopyridine, phenyl ketone, or phthalene.
- The hemoglobin pad can detect myoglobin, intact RBCs, and free hemoglobin. Contamination of the collection container or specimen with sodium hypochlorite or iodine may result in false-positive hemoglobin. Negative or decreased hemoglobin outcomes may occur in the presence of formalin, elevated protein, nitrite, ascorbic acid, or high specific gravity.
- False-negative results of nitrite are common. Weak or reduced effects can be seen in the presence of ascorbic acid and high specific gravity. Certain causes of false-negative values relate to the amount of time the urine was in the vagina before it was voided or the presence of pathogenic organisms that did not convert nitrates to nitrites.
- False-positive leukocyte esterase reactions are the result of specimens mixed with vaginal secretions. The presence of high concentrations of glucose, protein, or ascorbic acid may lead to false-negative results. Specimens with high specific gravity may also produce false-negative results. Patients with neutropenia (e.g., oncology patients) may also have false-negative results because they do not produce enough WBCs to exceed the biochemical reaction's sensitivity.
- Specimens that cannot be sent to the laboratory or checked within 1 hour should be refrigerated or added to the laboratory's preservative. Specimens obtained more than 2 hours before the collection may be rejected for analysis.
- Because changes in the urine specimen occur over time, prompt and proper processing, storage, and analysis of the specimen are important to achieve accurate results. Changes that may occur over time shall include:
- The development of a stronger odor and a rise in pH (the bacteria in the urine break down the urea to the ammonia).
- Decrease in clarity (as bacterial growth progresses or precipitates).

- Decrease in bilirubin and urobilinogen (oxidation of biliverdin and urobilin).
- Decreased ketone (lost by volatilization).
- Decreased glucose (consumed by bacteria).
- Increased bacteria (growth over time).
- Disintegration of castings, WBCs, and RBCs.
- Increased nitrite (overgrowth of bacteria).

MICROALBUMIN (Albumin, urine)

SAMPLING: 10 mL of urine from a random or timed specimen is collected in a clean plastic collection container.
TECHNIQUE: Nephelometry immunoassay
NORMAL VALUE:

Test	Conventional Units	SI Units (Conversion Factor X0.001)
Random		
microalbumin	0–30 µg/mL	0–0.03 g/L
24-h microalbumin	>40 µg/24 h	>0.04 g/24 h

Simultaneous assessment of urinary creatinine or creatinine clearance may be required.
EXPLAINATION:
The term microalbumin is used to identify amounts of albumin in urine that are >normal but not measurable by dipstick or by typical spectrophotometry methods. Microalbuminuria precedes diabetes-associated nephropathy and is often elevated for years until creatinine clearance reveals abnormal values. Research has shown that the median duration from the onset of microalbuminuria to nephropathy progression is between 5 and 7 years.
INDICATIONS:
- Assess renal disease.
- Scrutinize diabetic patients for early signs of nephropathy.

RESULT:

Increased in:
• Exercise
• Hypertension (uncontrolled)
• Preeclampsia
• Renal disease
• Urinary tract infections
• Cardiomyopathy
• Diabetic nephropathy
Decreased in: N/A

IMPEDING FACTORS:

- Medications that may decrease the rates of microalbumin include captopril, dipyridamole, enalapril, furosemide, indapamide, perindopril, quinapril, ramipril, tolrestat, and triflusal.
- Any urine sample that has been voided for the scheduled collection period must be included in the collection or mistakenly reduced values may be collected. Compare output records with the amount obtained to ensure that all voids have been included in the collection.

CALCULUS, KIDNEY STONE PANEL

(Kidney stone analysis, nephrolithiasis analysis)

SAMPLING: Kidney stones.
TECHNIQUE: Infrared spectrometry
NORMAL VALUE: None detected.
EXPLAINATION:

Renal stones are produced by the crystallization of calcium oxalate (most common), magnesium ammonium phosphate, calcium phosphate, uric acid, and cystine. The development of stones may be due to reduced urine flow and excessive amounts of the above-mentioned insoluble substances. The existence of stones is confirmed by diagnostic visualization or passage of stones in the urine. Qualitative proof of the chemical nature of the stones may be required.
INDICATIONS: Identify substances present in renal calculi
RESULT:

Positive findings in the **Presence of renal calculi**
Negative findings in **N/A**

IMPEDING FACTORS:

- Medications and substances that may enhance the production of urine calculi include probenecid and vitamin D.
- Adhesive tape should not be used to adhere stones to any transport or storage container, as the adhesive interferes with infrared spectrometry.

ENDOCRINE SYSTEM

The endocrine system is an interconnected network composed of numerous glands found in the body. Along with the nervous system, the endocrine system controls and manages many internal body functions. The endocrine system uses certain chemical messenger molecules called hormones produced, stored, and secreted by the gland network. When endocrine glands are released into the bloodstream, they hit cells, tissues, or organs with specific receptors. There are several parts of this network.

One, the hypothalamus, the other, the pituitary. Signals from the brain cause the hypothalamus to produce several hormones that stimulate or inhibit the pituitary gland. These signals allow the pituitary to increase or decrease the hormones that it produces and releases into the bloodstream. These hormones, released from the pituitary gland in varying amounts, travel through the bloodstream to endocrine glands such as thyroid glands, adrenal glands, testicles, and ovaries (gonads). Several other organs and tissues across the body are also hormone targets.

- A negative feedback mechanism controls some hormones.

- Some hormones, like cortisol, have a daily or monthly release pattern.

- Other hormones are usually present in exceedingly small amounts in the blood. They are released in specific situations, such as the release of epinephrine (adrenaline) from the adrenal glands in response to stress.

Anatomically endocrine system consists of
- Hypothalamus.
- Pineal body.
- Pituitary.
- Thyroid and parathyroid.
- Thymus.
- Adrenal gland.
- Pancreas.
- Ovary.
- Testis.

Important laboratory tests are,
- Adrenocorticotropic Hormone (ACTH)

- Antidiuretic Hormone (ADH)

- Androstenedione

- Cortisol

- Aldosterone and Renin

- Calcitonin

- Calcium
- Catecholamines
- DHEAS
- Electrolytes and Anion Gap
- Estrogens
- Follicle-stimulating Hormone (FSH)
- Growth Hormone
- hCG Tumor Marker
- Insulin-like Growth Factor-1 (IGF-1)
- Luteinizing Hormone (LH)
- Plasma Free Metanephrines
- Urine Metanephrines
- Progesterone
- Prolactin
- Parathyroid Hormone (PTH)
- Sex Hormone Binding Globulin (SHBG)
- T3 (Free and Total)
- T4, Free
- Testosterone
- Thyroid-stimulating Hormone (TSH)

ALDOSTERONE

SAMPLING: 1 ml of serum is collected in a red- or tiger-top tube. 1 ml of plasma collected in a green-top (heparin) or lavender-top (ethylenediaminetetraacetic Acid [EDTA]) tube is also acceptable.

TECHNIQUE: Radioimmunoassay

NORMAL value:

Age	Conventional Units	SI Units (Conversion Factor 0.0277)
Cord blood	40–200 ng/dL	1.11–5.54 nmol/L
3 d–1 wk	7–184 ng/dL	0.19–5.10 nmol/L
1 mo–1 y	5–90 ng/dL	0.14–2.49 nmol/L
13–23 mo	7–54 ng/dL	0.19–1.50 nmol/L
2–10 y		
Supine	3–35 ng/dL	0.08–0.97 nmol/L
Upright	5–80 ng/dL	0.14–2.22 nmol/L
11–15 y		
Supine	2–22 ng/dL	0.06–0.61 nmol/L
Upright	4–48 ng/dL	0.11–1.33 nmol/L
Adult		
Supine	3–16 ng/dL	0.08–0.44 nmol/L
Upright	7–30 ng/dL	0.19–0.83 nmol/L

EXPLAINATION:

Aldosterone is a mineralocorticoid produced by the adrenal cortex glomerulosa region in response to decreased serum sodium, decreased blood pressure, and increased serum potassium.

Aldosterone raises the reabsorption of sodium in the renal tubules, resulting in potassium excretion and increased water retention, blood volume, and blood pressure. Various factors influence serum aldosterone levels, certain medications, including sodium intake, and activity. This test is of not sufficiently diagnostic value unless plasma renin activity is calculated simultaneously. Patients with serum potassium < 3.6 mEq / L and 24-hour urine potassium >40 mEq / L meet the general aldosteronism test criteria.

Renin is low in primary aldosteronism and low in secondary aldosteronism. There is a significant ratio of plasma aldosterone to plasma renin activity >50.

INDICATIONS:

- Evaluate hypertension of unknown cause, particularly hypokalemia not caused by diuretics.
- Investigate alleged hyperaldosteronism as indicated by elevated levels.

- Perform tests for suspected hypoaldosteronism as indicated by decreased levels.

RESULT
Increased with Decreased Renin Levels
Primary hyperaldosteronism:
• Bilateral hyperplasia of the aldosterone-secreting cells of zona glomerulosa.
• Adenomas (Conn's syndrome)
Increased with Raised Renin Levels
Secondary hyperaldosteronism:
• Bartter's syndrome
• Hypovolemia secondary to hemorrhage and transudation
• Laxative abuse
• Nephrotic syndrome
• Starvation (after 10 days)
• Thermal stress
• Cardiac failure
• Chronic obstructive pulmonary disease
• Cirrhosis with ascites formation
• Diuretic abuse
• Toxemia of pregnancy
Decreased
Without hypertension:
• Addison's disease
• Hypoaldosteronism secondary to renin deficiency
• Isolated aldosterone deficiency
With hypertension:
• Excess secretion of deoxycorticosterone
• Turner's syndrome (25 percent of cases)
• Acute alcohol intoxication
• Diabetes

IMPEDING FACTORS:

- Drugs that may increase aldosterone concentrations include amiloride, ammonium chloride, angiotensin, angiotensin II, dobutamine, dopamine, endralazine, nifedipine, fenoldopam, hydralazine, hydrochlorothiazide, laxatives (abuse), metoclopramide, opiates, potassium, spironolactone, and zacopride.
- Drugs that may reduce aldosterone levels include atenolol, captopril, fadrozole, glycyrrhiza, ibopamine, indomethacin carvedilol, cilazapril, enalapril, lisinopril, nicardipine, NSAIDs (nonsteroidal anti-inflammatory drugs), perindopril, ranitidine, saline, sinorphan, and verapamil. Prolonged heparin therapy also decreases aldosterone levels.
- Upright body posture, stress, vigorous exercise, and late pregnancy may lead to increased levels.
- Current radioactive scans or radiation within one week of the test may interfere with the test results when radioimmunoassay is the test method.
- Food ingestion can have a significant impact on the results. Low sodium diets may increase serum aldosterone, while high sodium diets may decrease. Decreased sodium serum and increased serum potassium increase the secretion of aldosterone. Elevated serum sodium and decreased serum potassium stifle the secretion of aldosterone.

ANGIOTENSIN-CONVERTING ENZYME

The angiotensin-I-converting enzyme (ACE).
SAMPLING: 1 ml of serum is collected in a red- or tiger-top tube.
TECHNIQUE: Spectrophotometry

NORMAL VALUE:

Age	Conventional Units	SI Units (Conversion Factor 0.017)
0–2 y	5–83 U/L	0.09–1.41 Kat/L
3–7 y	8–76 U/L	0.14–1.29 Kat/L
8–14 y	6–89 U/L	0.10–1.51 Kat/L
>14 y	8–52 U/L	0.14–0.88 Kat/L

EXPLAINATION:

The production of angiotensin-converting enzyme (ACE) occurs primarily in the epithelial cells of the pulmonary bed. Smaller quantities are found in blood vessels and kidney tissue where ACE transforms angiotensin I to angiotensin II; this conversion helps to regulate blood pressure in the artery. Angiotensin II incites the adrenal cortex to produce aldosterone. Aldosterone is a hormone that helps the kidneys maintain water balance by retaining sodium and promoting potassium excretion. ACE levels are used mainly in the determination of hypertension and severe sarcoidosis, a granulomatous condition that can damage multiple organs, including the lungs. Serial rates are important in the analysis of the therapeutic response to corticosteroid therapy. Elevated ACE levels with positive gallium scans in sarcoidosis patients receiving steroids indicate poor response to therapy. Scrutinizing ACE levels may also have some utility in assessing the probability of pulmonary damage in patients receiving antineoplastic agents. Thyroid hormones may play a vital role in the regulation of ACE levels: decreased levels have been observed in patients with clinical hypothyroidism and anorexia nervosa, whereas increased levels have been observed in patients with hyperthyroidism.

Serum ACE elevations have been identified in 20 to 30 percent of patients with abnormal α-1 antitrypsin variants. ACE levels are sometimes prescribed on cerebrospinal fluid for the assessment of patients with neurosarcoidosis. Tests must be carefully interpreted due to the non-specificity between increased and reduced ACE levels. ACE is typically elevated in pediatric patients and is therefore not a useful marker for disease assessment in patients < 20 years of age.

INDICATIONS:

- Support in establishing a diagnosis of sarcoidosis.
- Assist in the assessment of Gaucher's disease.
- Aid in the treatment of sarcoidosis.
- Evaluate the cause of hypertension.
- Evaluate the seriousness and activity of sarcoidosis.

RESULT

Increased in:
• **Bronchitis (acute and chronic)**
• **Connective tissue disease**
• **Gaucher's disease**
• **Pulmonary fibrosis**
• **Rheumatoid arthritis**
• **Sarcoidosis**

•	Hansen's disease (leprosy)
•	Histoplasmosis and other fungal diseases
•	Hyperthyroidism (untreated)
	Decreased in:
•	Advanced pulmonary carcinoma
•	The period following corticosteroid therapy for sarcoidosis

IMPEDING FACTORS:
- Drugs that may raise serum ACE levels include triiodothyronine.
- Drugs that may lower serum ACE levels include captopril, cilazapril, perindopril, propranolol, quinapril, enalapril, fosinopril, lisinopril, nicardipine, pentopril, ramipril, and trandolapril.
- Quick and proper specimen processing, storage, and analysis are important to achieve accurate results. Failure to freeze samples if not tested instantly may cause falsely decreased values because ACE degrades rapidly.

RENIN (Plasma renin activity (PRA))

SAMPLING: 3 mL of plasma is collected in a lavender-top (ethylenediaminetetraacetic acid [EDTA]) tube.
TECHNIQUE: Radioimmunoassay
NORMAL VALUE:

Age and Position	Conventional Units	SI Units (Conversion Factor X1)
Newborn Supine, normal sodium diet	2.0–35.0 ng/mL per hour	2.0–35.0 µ g/L per hour
1–12 mo	2.4–37.0 ng/mL per hour	2.4–37.0 µg/L per hour
1–3 y	1.7–112 ng/mL per hour	1.7–112 µg/L per hour
3–5 y	1.0–6.5 ng/mL per hour	1.0–6.5 µg/L per hour
5–10 y	0.5–5.9 ng/mL per hour	0.5–5.9 µg/L per hour
10–15 y	0.5–3.3 ng/mL per hour	0.5–3.3 µg/L per hour
Adult Upright, normal sodium diet	0.2–1.6 ng/mL per hour	0.2–1.6 µg/L per hour
Adult	0.7–3.3 ng/mL per hour	0.7–3.3 µ g/L per hour

EXPLAINATION:

Renin is an enzyme that stimulates the mechanism of renin-angiotensin. The juxtaglomerular apparatus activates renal vessels in response to sodium deficiency and hypovolemia. Renin converts angiotensinogen into angiotensin I. Angiotensin I is converted to angiotensin II, a bioactive form. Angiotensin II is a strong vasoconstrictor that promotes the production of aldosterone in the adrenal cortex. Angiotensin II and aldosterone both increased blood pressure. Excessive amounts of angiotensin II cause renal hypertension. Renin checks for basic, renal, or renovascular hypertension. Plasma renin is expressed as angiotensin I formation rate per unit of time. The random collection of specimens without adequate dietary planning does not provide scientifically significant information. Values should also be measured along with aldosterone levels obtained at the same time.

INDICATIONS:

- Assist in the identification of primary hyperaldosteronism arising from aldosterone-secreting adrenal adenoma.
- Assist in monitoring patients with mineralocorticoid therapy.
- Assist in the assessment of the sources of essential renal or renovascular hypertension.

RESULT:

Increased in:
• **Gastrointestinal disorders with electrolyte loss**
• **Bartter's syndrome**
• **Cirrhosis**
• **Congestive heart failure**
• **Hepatitis**
• **Hypokalemia**
• **Malignant hypertension**
• **Nephritis**
• **Pheochromocytoma**
• **Pregnancy**
• **Renin-producing renal tumors**
• **Renovascular hypertension**
Decreased in:
• **Cushing's syndrome**
• **Essential hypertension**
• **Primary hyperaldosteronism**

IMPEDING FACTORS:

- Drugs that may increase renin levels include albuterol, amiloride, azosemide, benazepril, bendroflumethiazide, captopril, chlorthalidone, cilazapril, cromakalim, desmopressin, fenoldopam, fosinopril, furosemide, diazoxide, dihydralazine, doxazosin, hydralazine, hydrochlorothiazide, laxatives, lisinopril, lithium, methyclothiazide, enalapril, endralazine, felodipine, metolazone, muzolimine, nicardipine, nifedipine, opiates, oral contraceptives, perindopril, ramipril, spironolactone, triamterene, and xipamide.
- Medications and substances that may lower renin levels include angiotensin, angiotensin II, acetylsalicylic acid, atenolol, bopindolol, bucindolol, carbenoxolone, carvedilol, clonidine, cyclosporine A, dexfenfluramine, glycyrrhiza, ibuprofen, indomethacin, levodopa, metoprolol, naproxen, nicardipine, nonsteroidal anti-inflammatory drugs (NSAIDs), oral contraceptives, oxprenolol, propranolol, sulindac, and vasopressin.
- Upright body posture, tension, and strenuous exercise can increase renin levels.
- Recent radioactive scans or radiation exposure will interfere with the test results when the radioimmunoassay is a test method.
- Food can have a major impact on outcomes (e.g., low-sodium diets promote the production of renin).
- Hyperkalemia, an acute rise in blood pressure, and an increase in blood volume can inhibit renin secretion.

ANTIDIURETIC HORMONE

(Vasopressin, arginine vasopressin hormone, ADH.)
SAMPLING: 1 mL of plasma is collected in a lavender-top (ethylenediaminetetraacetic acid [EDTA]) tube.
TECHNIQUE: Radioimmunoassay
NORMAL VALUE:

Serum Osmolality	Antidiuretic hormone levels	SI Units (Conversion Factor X0.926)
270–280 mOsm/kg	< 1.5 pg/mL	< 1.4 pmol/L
280–285 mOsm/kg	< 2.5 pg/mL	< 2.3 pmol/L
285–290 mOsm/kg	1–5 pg/mL	0.9–4.6 pmol/L
290–295 mOsm/kg	2–7 pg/mL	1.9–6.5 pmol/L
295–300 mOsm/kg	4–12 pg/mL	3.7–11.1 pmol/L

RECOMMENDATION: This test should be ordered and clarified with the results of serum osmolality.

EXPLAINATION: The antidiuretic hormone (ADH) is produced by the hypothalamus and is stored in the posterior pituitary gland. ADH is released as a response to increased serum osmolality or reduced blood volume. When the hormone is functioning, small amounts of concentrated urine are released; in its absence, large amounts of dilute urine are produced. Although a 1% change in serum osmolality induces ADH secretion, the volume of blood must decrease by approximately 10% to induce ADH secretion. Psychogenic factors, such as stress, pain, and anxiety, may also stimulate the release of ADH, but the process is unknown.

INDICATIONS:
- Assess polyuria or altered serum osmolality to identify possible alterations in ADH secretion as the cause.
- Spot trauma, surgery, or disease of the central nervous system that may lead to impaired secretion of ADH.
- Distinguish neurogenic (central) diabetes insipidus from nephrogenic diabetes insipidus by reduced ADH rates in neurogenic diabetes insipidus, or increased levels of nephrogenic diabetes insipidus if normal feedback mechanisms are intact.
- Aid in the treatment of known or suspected malignancy associated with inadequate ADH secretion syndromes (SIADH), such as oat cell lung cancer, lymphoma, leukemia, pancreatic carcinoma, prostate gland carcinoma, and intestinal carcinoma; elevated ADH rates indicate the presence of this syndrome.
- Assist in the treatment of known or suspected pulmonary conditions related to SIADH, such as tuberculosis, pneumonia, and positive-pressure mechanical ventilation.

RESULT

Increased in:
• **Acute intermittent porphyria**
• **Brain tumor**
• **Ectopic production (systemic neoplasm)**
• **Guillain-Barré syndrome**
• **Nephrogenic diabetes insipidus**
• **Pain, stress, or exercise**
• **Pneumonia**
• **Pulmonary tuberculosis**
• **SIADH**
• **Tuberculosis meningitis**

•	**Disorders involving the thyroid gland, central nervous system, and adrenal gland**
	Decreased in:
•	**Nephrotic syndrome**
•	**Pituitary (central) diabetes insipidus**
•	**Psychogenic polydipsia**

CRITICAL VALUES:
Effective treatment of SIADH depends on the identification and resolution of the cause of increased ADH development. Signs and symptoms of SIADH are like hyponatremia, including irritability, tremor, muscle spasms, epilepsy, and neurological changes. The patient has enough sodium but is depleted more than the remaining volume.

IMPEDING FACTORS
- Medications that may raise ADH include barbiturates, carbamazepine, chlorpropamide, chlorthalidone, cisplatin, clofibrate, ether furosemide, haloperidol, hydrochlorothiazide, lithium methyclothiazide, narcotic analgesics, Phenothiazine, polythiazide, tolbutamide, tricyclic antidepressants, vidarabine, vinblastine, and vincristine.
- Drugs that may reduce ADH include clonidine, demeclocycline, ethanol, lithium carbonate, and phenytoin.
- Recent radioactive scans or radiation exposure within one week of the test can interfere with the test results when radioimmunoassay is the method of choice.
- ADH experiences diurnal variation, with the highest level of secretion occurring at night; the first-morning test is recommended.
- The secretion of ADH is also influenced by posture, with higher levels determined when upright.

CATECHOLAMINES (Epinephrine, norepinephrine, dopamine)

SAMPLING: 2 ml of plasma is collected in a green-top (heparin) tube.
TECHNIQUE: High-performance liquid chromatography
NORMAL VALUE:

	Conventional Units	SI Units
Epinephrine		(Conversion Factor 5.46)
Supine, 30 min	0–110 pg/mL	0–600 pmol/L
Standing, 30 min	0–140 pg/mL	0–764 pmol/L
Norepinephrine		(Conversion Factor 5.91)
Supine, 30 min	70–750 pg/mL	414–4432 pmol/L
Standing, 30 min	200–1700 pg/mL	1182–10,047 pmol/L
Dopamine (Conversion Factor 6.53)		
Supine or standing	0–30 pg/mL	0–196 pmol/L

EXPLAINATION:

Catecholamines are derived from the chromaffin tissue of the adrenal medulla. These are also located at the ends of the sympathetic nerves and the cortex. Epinephrine, norepinephrine, and dopamine are the main catecholamines. They prepare the body for a fight-or-flight stress response, help regulate metabolism, and excrete the kidneys from the body. Catecholamine levels are affected by diurnal variations, fluctuations in response to stress, changes in posture, nutrition, smoking drugs, and changes in temperature. As a result, blood tests are not as accurate as a 24-hour timed urine test. Results are most accurate if the specimen is obtained during a hypertensive period. Catecholamines are tested when there is a high level of suspicion of pheochromocytoma, but urine results are normal or borderline. The results should be compared with the derivatives of epinephrine and norepinephrine, metanephrine and vanillylmandelic acid and dopamine synthesis, homovanillic acid. The use of a clonidine suppression test to measure plasma catecholamines may be requested. Failure to inhibit the synthesis of catecholamines following the administration of clonidine confirms the diagnosis of pheochromocytoma.

INDICATIONS:

- Aid in the diagnostic testing of neuroblastoma, ganglioneuroma or dysautonomia.
- Help in the diagnosis of paraganglioma.
- Aid in the diagnosis of pheochromocytoma.
- Evaluate severe hypertensive episode.
- Evaluate hypertension with unknown origin.

- Pheochromocytoma screening for family members with an autosomal dominant pattern of inheritance for Lindau–von Hippel disease or multiple endocrine neoplasms.

RESULT:

Increased in:
• **Ganglioblastoma (epinephrine, slight increase; norepinephrine, large increase)**
• **Diabetic acidosis (epinephrine and norepinephrine)**
• **Ganglioneuroma (all are increased; norepinephrine, largest increase)**
• **Long-term manic-depressive disorders (epinephrine and norepinephrine)**
• **Hypothyroidism (epinephrine and norepinephrine)**
• **Myocardial infarction (epinephrine and norepinephrine)**
• **Neuroblastoma (all are raised; norepinephrine and dopamine, largest increase)**
• **Pheochromocytoma (a continuous or intermittent increase of epinephrine, a slight increase of norepinephrine)**
• **Shock (epinephrine and norepinephrine)**
• **Strenuous exercise (epinephrine and norepinephrine)**
Decreased in:
• **Orthostatic hypotension (norepinephrine)**
• **Parkinson's disease (dopamine)**
• **Autonomic nervous system dysfunction (norepinephrine)**

IMPEDING FACTORS:
- Medications that may raise catecholamine levels include ajmaline, chlorpromazine, cyclopropane, diazoxide, ether, monoamine oxidase inhibitors, nitroglycerine, pentazocine, perphenazine, phenothiazine, promethazine, and theophylline.
- Medications that may decrease catecholamine levels include clonidine, metyrosine, and reserpine.
- Anxiety and stress, hypoglycemia, smoking, and drugs can produce elevated plasma catecholamines.
- The release of catecholamines demonstrates diurnal variation, with the lowest levels happening at night.
- The release of catecholamines differs during the menstrual cycle, with higher levels excreted during the luteal phase and lower levels after ovulation.

- Diets rich in amines (e.g., bananas, avocados, beer, aged cheese, chocolate, cocoa, coffee, fava beans, grains, tea, vanilla, walnuts, Chianti wine) may contain elevated levels of plasma catecholamines. However, this effect is more likely to be seen concerning certain urinary metabolites.

CATECHOLAMINES, URINE

(Epinephrine, norepinephrine, dopamine)

SAMPLING: 25 mL of urine from a timed specimen collected in clean plastic, amber collection container with 6N hydrochloric acid as a preservative.
TECHNIQUE: High-performance liquid chromatography

NORMAL VALUE:

	Conventional Units	SI Units
Epinephrine (*Conversion Factor X5.46)*		
1–4 y	0–6.0 µg/24 h	0–32.8 nmol/24 h
4 – 10 y	0–10.0 µg/24 h	0–54.6 nmol/24 h
10–15 y	0.5–20 µg/24 h	2.7–109 nmol/24 h
Adult	0–20 µg/24 h	0–109 nmol/24 h
Norepinephrine (*Conversion Factor X5.91)*		
1–4 y	0–29 µg/24 h	0–171 nmol/24 h
4–10 y	8–65 µg/24 h	47–384 nmol/24 h
10 y–adult	15–80 µg/24 h	89–473 nmol/24 h
Dopamine (*Conversion Factor X6.53)*		
1–4 y	10–260 µg/24 h	65–1698 nmol/24 h
4 y–adult	65–400 µg/24 h	424–2612 nmol/24 h

EXPLAINATION: Catecholamines are formed from the chromaffin tissue of the adrenal medulla. These are also present in sympathetic nerve endings and the cortex. Epinephrine, norepinephrine, and dopamine are the main catecholamines. They prepare the body for a fight-or-flight stress response, help regulate metabolism, and excrete the kidneys from the blood. Diurnal variations, fluctuations in response to stress, changes in posture, diet, smoking, drugs, and changes in temperature are affected. As a result, blood tests are not as accurate as a 24-hour monitored urine test. For the test results to be accurate, all the environment variables listed above must be checked when the test is carried out. Elevated homovanillic acid levels preclude pheochromocytoma because this tumor secretes epinephrine mainly. Elevated catecholamine without hypertension indicates neuroblastoma or ganglioneuroma. Metanephrine and vanillylmandelic acid, which are epinephrine and norepinephrine derivatives, should be tested. The results should also be correlated with homovanillic acid, the product of dopamine metabolism.

INDICATIONS:
- Assists in the diagnosis of neuroblastoma, ganglioneuroma, or dysautonomia.
- Assist in the evaluation of pheochromocytoma.
- Assess acute hypertensive episode.
- Determine hypertension with unknown origin.
- Pheochromocytoma screening for family members with an autosomal dominant pattern of inheritance for Lindau–von Hippel disease or multiple endocrine neoplasms.

RESULT:

Increased in:
• **Diabetic acidosis (epinephrine and norepinephrine)**
• **Ganglioblastoma (epinephrine, slight increase; norepinephrine, large increase)**
• **Long-term manic-depressive disorders (epinephrine and norepinephrine)**
• **Ganglioneuroma (all are increased; norepinephrine, largest increase)**
• **Hypothyroidism (epinephrine and norepinephrine)**
• **Myocardial infarction (epinephrine and norepinephrine)**
• **Neuroblastoma (all are raised; norepinephrine and dopamine, largest increase)**
• **Strenuous exercise (epinephrine and norepinephrine)**
• **Pheochromocytoma (epinephrine, continuous or occasional increase; norepinephrine, slight increase)**
• **Shock (epinephrine and norepinephrine)**

	Decreased in:
•	Orthostatic hypotension (norepinephrine)
•	Parkinson's disease (dopamine)
•	Autonomic nervous system dysfunction (norepinephrine)

IMPEDING FACTORS:
- Medications that may increase urinary catecholamine levels include acetaminophen, atenolol, dopamine (intravenous), isoproterenol, methyldopa, niacin, nitroglycerin, prochlorperazine, rauwolfia, reserpine, syrosingopine, and theophylline.
- Medications that may decrease the level of catecholamine in the urine include clonidine, decaborane, guanethidine, guanfacine, methyldopa, ouabain, radiographs substances, reserpine, and bretyltosylate.
- Tension, hypoglycemia, smoking, and medications can produce elevated catecholamines.
- The release of catecholamines indicates diurnal variation, with the lowest levels happening at night.
- The release of catecholamines varies during the menstrual cycle, with higher levels excreted during the luteal phase and lower levels during ovulation.
- Foods rich in amines (e.g., bananas, avocados, beer, aged cheese, chocolate, cocoa, coffee, fava beans, grains, tea, almonds, walnuts, Chianti wine) can produce high levels of catecholamines.
- Failure to collect all urine and safely store a 24-hour test would result in a falsely low result.

CALCITONIN AND CALCITONIN STIMULATION TESTS

(Thyrocalcitonin, hCT)

SAMPLING: 3 mL of serum is collected in a red- or tiger-top tube.

TECHNIQUE: Radioimmunoassay

NORMAL VALUE:

	Conventional Units	SI Units (Conversion Factor X1)
Calcitonin		
Male	< 19 pg/mL	< 19 ng/L
Female	< 14 pg/mL	< 14 ng/L
	Maximum Response	
After Calcium and Pentagastrin Stimulation		
Male	< 350 pg/mL	< 350 ng/L
Female	< 94 pg/mL	< 94 ng/L
	Maximum Response	
After Pentagastrin Stimulation		
Male	< 110 pg/mL	< 110 ng/L
Female	< 30 pg/mL	< 30 ng/L

EXPLAINATION:

Calcitonin, also documented as thyrocalcitonin, is produced by the parafollicular or C cells of the thyroid gland concerning higher serum calcium levels. Calcitonin is acting opposite to the parathyroid hormone and vitamin D such that calcium remains in the bone instead of in the blood. Calcitonin also improves the renal excretion of magnesium and prevents the reuptake of phosphates by the renal tubular. The final effect is that calcitonin lowers the calcium content of the plasma. The Pentagastrin (Peptavlon) Provocation Test, as well as the Calcium Pentagastrin Provocation Test, are helpful in the diagnosis of medullary thyroid cancer.

INDICATIONS:

- Help in the diagnosis of hyperparathyroidism.
- Assist in the identification of medullary thyroid cancer in a patient.
- Evaluate changes in serum calcium levels.
- Monitor medullary thyroid carcinoma treatment.
- Predict relapse of medullary thyroid cancer.
- Investigate family members of patients with medullary thyroid carcinoma (20% of the family pattern).

RESULT:

Increased in:
• Alcoholic cirrhosis
• C-cell hyperplasia
• Carcinoid syndrome
• Pancreatitis
• Cancer of the breast, lung, and pancreas
• Hypercalcemia (any cause)
• Medullary thyroid cancer
• Chronic renal failure
• Pernicious anemia
• Pregnancy (late)
• Pseudohypoparathyroidism
• Zollinger-Ellison syndrome
• Thyroiditis
• Ectopic secretion (especially neuroendocrine origins)
Decreased in: N/A

IMPEDING FACTORS:
- Medications that may raise calcitonin rates include calcium, sincalide, epinephrine, estrogen, glucagon, pentagastrin, and oral contraceptives.
- Fresh radioactive scans or radiation exposure within seven days of the test could oppose the test results when radioimmunoassay method of choice.

C-PEPTIDE

(Connecting peptide insulin, proinsulin C-peptide, insulin C-peptide)

SAMPLING: 1 mL of serum is collected in a red-top tube.

TECHNIQUE: Radioimmunoassay

NORMAL VALUE:

Conventional Units	SI Units (Conversion Factor X0.333)
0.78–1.8 ng/mL	0.26–0.63 nmol/L

EXPLAINATION:

C-peptide is a bio-inactive peptide produced when pancreatic beta cells transform proinsulin to insulin. The kidneys secrete the majority of C-peptide. C-peptide levels are usually associated with insulin levels and provide a good measure of how well beta cells secrete insulin. C-peptide release is not impaired by exogenous insulin administration. C-peptide levels increase after glucose or glucagon activation. The insulin-C-peptide ratio of < 1.0 indicates an endogenous insulin secretion, while the ratio of more than 1.0 indicates an abundance of exogenous insulin.

INDICATIONS:

- Insulinoma diagnosis: Serum insulin and C-peptide levels are increased.
- Detecting the potential source of hypoglycemia (excessive insulin administration): C-peptide levels do not rise with serum insulin levels.
- Assess beta cell activity, as insulin antibodies prevent accurate measurement of serum insulin production.
- Differentiate between insulin-dependent (type 1) and non-insulin-dependent (type 2) diabetes (with C-peptide stimulation test): patients with diabetes whose C-peptide stimulation level is >18 ng / mL may be managed without insulin therapy.
- Assess hypoglycemia.

RESULT:

Increased in:
• **Endogenous hyperinsulinism**
• **Islet cell tumor**
• **Oral hypoglycemic medication**
• **Pancreas or beta cell transplants**
• **Renal failure**
• **Non–insulin-dependent (type 2) diabetes**
Decreased in:
• **Factitious hypoglycemia**
• **Insulin-dependent (type 1) diabetes**
• **Pancreatectomy**

IMPEDING FACTORS:

- Products that may raise C-peptide levels consist of danazol, betamethasone, chloroquine, deferoxamine, Ethinyl estradiol, prednisone, oral contraceptives, and rifampin.
- Drugs that might reduce C-peptide levels include atenolol and calcitonin.
- Recent radioactive scans or radiation exposure within seven days of the test may alter the test results when radioimmunoassay is the test method.
- C-peptide and endogenous insulin levels are not always related to obese patients.

CORTISOL AND CHALLENGE TESTS (Hydrocortisone, compound F)

SAMPLING:1 mL of serum is collected in a red- or tiger-top tube. 1 mL of plasma collected in a green-top tube (heparin tube) is also acceptable. Care must be engaged to use the same type of collection container if serial measurements are to be taken.

TECHNIQUE: Immunoassay

NORMAL VALUE:

Procedure	Medication Administered	Recommended Collection Times
ACTH stimulation	Synthetic ACTH (cosyntropin) IM or IV bolus	3 cortisol levels— baseline immediately before bolus, 30 min after bolus, and 60 min after bolus
CRH stimulation	CRH 1 µg/kg IV 9 a.m.	3 cortisol and ACTH levels—baseline before injection, 30 min after injection, and 60 min after injection
Dexamethasone suppression (overnight)	Oral dose dexamethasone at 11 p.m.	8 a.m. after morning collection of cortisol

Metyrapone stimulation (overnight)	An oral dose of metyrapone at midnight	8 a.m. after morning collection of cortisol and ACTH

	Conventional Units Cortisol (Conversion Factor X 27.6)	SI Units
8 a.m.	5–25 µg/dL	138–690 nmol/L
4 p.m.	3–16 µg/dL	83–442 nmol/L
ACTH Challenge Tests		
CRH stimulation	2–4-fold increase over baseline ACTH or cortisol level	2–4-fold increase over baseline values
Dexamethasone Suppressed		
		(Conversion Factor 27.6)
	Cortisol <3 µg/dL next day	< 83 nmol/L
ACTH (Cosyntropin) Stimulated		
		(Conversion Factor X 27.6)
	Cortisol greater than20 µg/dL	Greater than552 nmol/L

Conventional Units	SI Units
Metyrapone Stimulated	
ACTH greater than150 pg/mL	*(Conversion Factor X 0.22)* >33 pmol/L
Cortisol <3 g/dL next day	(Conversion Factor X 27.6) < 83 nmol/L

EXPLAINATION:

Cortisol (hydrocortisone) is the major glucocorticoid secreted in response to hypothalamus stimulation and pituitary adrenocorticotropic hormone (ACTH). Cortisol stimulates gluconeogenesis, mobilizes fats and proteins, inhibits insulin, and suppresses inflammation. Measuring cortisol levels in the blood is the best indicator of adrenal activity. Cortisol secretion varies daily, with the highest levels occurring at dawn and the lowest levels occurring late in the day. Bursts of cortisol excretion may occur at night. Cortisol and ACTH test results are done together because they control each other's concentrations (i.e., any change in one, triggers a change in the other). ACTH levels show diurnal variation, peaking between 6 a.m. and 8 a.m. Moreover, to reach the lowest point between 6 and 11 p.m. The evening standard is usually one-half to two-thirds lower than the morning level.

INDICATIONS:

- Detect adrenal hyperfunction (Cushing's syndrome).
- Detect adrenal hypofunction (Addison's disease).

RESULT:

The dexamethasone suppression test is useful for differentiating the causes of elevated cortisol levels. Dexamethasone is a synthetic steroid that suppresses ACTH secretion. The normal morning cortisol level is collected with this test, and a 1-mg dose of dexamethasone is given to the patient at bedtime. A second specimen shall be collected the following morning. An adrenal adenoma may be suspected when cortisol levels have not been suppressed. The dexamethasone suppression test also yields abnormal results in patients with psychiatric disorders. The stimulation test for corticotropin-releasing hormone (CRH) works as well as the suppression test for dexamethasone in distinguishing Cushing's disease from the ectopic secretion of ACTH. In this test, cortisol levels are measured following the injection of CRH. Cushing's disease reveals a fourfold increase in cortisol levels above baseline. No increase in cortisol is seen if the cause is ectopic ACTH secretion. The cosyntropin test is used if adrenal insufficiency is suspected. Cosyntropin is an ACTH synthetic form. The baseline level of cortisol is collected before the injection of cosyntropin. Specimens are then collected at 30- and 60-minute intervals. If the adrenal glands are functioning normally, the levels of cortisol will increase significantly following cosyntropin administration. The metyrapone stimulation test is used to differentiate corticotropin-dependent (pituitary Cushing's disease and ectopic Cushing's disease) from corticotropin-independent (pulmonary or thyroid carcinoma) causes of increased cortisol levels. Metyrapone inhibits the conversion of 11-deoxycortisol into cortisol. Cortisol levels should be >3 g / dL if regular pituitary stimulation with ACTH happens after an oral dose of metyrapone. The specimen collection and administration of the medication is performed as with the overnight dexamethasone test.

Increased in:
• **Adrenal adenoma**
• **Cushing's syndrome**
• **Ectopic ACTH production**
• **Hyperglycemia**
• **Pregnancy**
• **Stress**
Decreased in:
• **Addison's disease**
• **Adrenogenital syndrome**
• **Hypopituitarism**

IMPEDING FACTORS:

- Medications and compounds that may raise cortisol levels include amphetamine, anticonvulsants, clomipramine, corticotropin, cyclic AMP, ether fenfluramine, CRH, cortisone, hydrocortisone, insulin, lithium, methadone, metoclopramide, naloxone, opioids, oral contraceptives, prednisolone, tetracosactrin, ranitidine, spironolactone, and vasopressin.
- Medications and substances that may decrease cortisol levels include barbiturates, beclomethasone, betamethasone, clonidine, danazole, desoximetasone, ephedrine, etomidate, fluocinolone, ketoconazole, levodopa, lithium, methylprednisolone, desoxycorticosterone, dexamethasone metyrapone, midazolam, morphine, nitrous oxide, oxazepam, phenytoin, ranitidine, and trimipramine.
- The test results are affected by the time this test is performed because the levels of cortisol vary daily.
- Stress and excessive physical activity can lead to higher levels of stress.
- Normal values may be obtained in the presence of a partial pituitary deficiency.
- The stimulation test for metyrapone is contraindicated in patients with suspected adrenal insufficiency.
-Metyrapone can cause gastrointestinal distress and/or confusion.

DEHYDROEPIANDROSTERONE SULFATE (DHEAS)

SAMPLING:1 mL of serum is collected in a red- or tiger-top tube. 1 ml of plasma collected in a lavender-top (ethylenediaminetetra-acetic [EDTA]) tube is also acceptable.

TECHNIQUE: Radioimmunoassay

NORMAL VALUE:

Age	Conventional Units	SI Units (Conversion Factor X 0.027)
Newborn		
Male	108–406 µg/dL	2.9–10.9 µmol/L
Female	10–248 µg/dL	0.3–6.7 µ mol/L
6–9 y	25–145 µg/dL	0.07–3.9 µ mol/L
10–11 y		
Male	15–115 µ g/dL	0.4–3.1 µ mol/L
Female	15–260 µg/dL	0.4–7.0 µmol/L
12–17 y		
Male	20–555 µg/dL	0.5–15.0 µmol/L
Female	20–535 µg/dL	0.5–14.4 µmol/L
19–30 y		
Male	125–619 µg/dL	3.4–16.7 µ mol/L
Female	29–781 µ g/dL	0.8–21.1 µ mol/L
31–50 y		
Male	59–452 µ g/dL	1.6–12.2 µ mol/L
Female	12–379 µg/dL	0.8–10.2 µmol/L
51–60 y		
Male	20–413 µ g/dL	0.5–11.1 µmol/L
61–83 y		
Male	10–285 µg/dL	0.3–7.7 µmol/L
Postmenopausal woman	30–260 mg/dL	0.8–7.0 mmol/L

EXPLAINATION:

Dehydroepiandrosterone sulfate (DHEAS) is the main precursor of 17-ketosteroids.

DHEAS is a metabolite of DHEA, the main adrenal androgen, which is mainly synthesized in the adrenal gland and in a small amount by ovaries. It is secreted in combination with cortisol, under the influence of adrenocorticotropic hormone (ACTH) and prolactin. Excessive production induces masculinization in both women and children.

DHEAS replaced the calculation of urinary 17-ketosteroids in the estimate of the development of adrenal androgen.

INDICATIONS:
- Assist in the measurement of androgen excess, including congenital adrenal hyperplasia, adrenal tumor, and Stein-Leventhal syndrome.
- Evaluate people with fertility issues, amenorrhea, or hirsutism.

RESULT:

Increased in:
• **Anovulation**
• **Cushing's syndrome**
• **Ectopic ACTH-producing tumors**
• **Hirsutism**
• **Hyperprolactinemia**
• **Polycystic ovary**
• **Stein-Leventhal syndrome**
• **Virilizing adrenal tumors**
Decreased in:
• **Addison's disease**
• **Adrenal insufficiency (primary or secondary)**
• **Pregnancy**
• **Psoriasis**
• **Psychosis**
• **Aging adults**
• **Hyperlipidemia**

IMPEDING FACTORS:
- Drugs that may improve DHEAS include clomiphene, corticotropin, danazol, DHEA, mifepristone, and nitrendipine.
- Products that may decrease DHEAS include carbamazepine, dexamethasone, ketoconazole, oral contraceptives, and phenytoin.
- Recent radioactive scans or contamination within one week of the test can conflict with the test results when radioimmunoassay is the test method.

INSULIN AND INSULIN RESPONSE TO GLUCOSE

SAMPLING: 1 mL of serum is collected in a red-top tube.

TECHNIQUE: Radioimmunoassay

NORMAL VALUE:

	Insulin	Insulin 6.945 SI Units	Glucose (Tolerance for Hypoglycemia)
Fasting	< 2mIU/L	< 174pmol/L	65–115 mg/dL
30 min	30–230mIU/L	208–1597pmol/L	N/A
1 h	18–276mIU/L	125–191pmol/L	< 200 mg/dL
2 h	16–166mIU/L	111–1153pmol/L	< 140 mg/dL
3 h	< 25mIU/L	< 174pmol/L	65–120 mg/dL
4 h	< 25mIU/L	< 174pmol/L	65–120 mg/dL
5 h	< 25mIU/L	< 174pmol/L	65–115 mg/dL

EXPLAINATION:

Increased blood glucose levels lead to an increase in insulin secretion. Its overall effect is to facilitate glucose use and energy storage. The insulin reaction test measures the amount of insulin secreted by the beta cells of the islets of Langerhans in the pancreas; a 5-hour glucose tolerance test for hypoglycemia may be performed simultaneously.

INDICATIONS:

- Aid in the diagnosis of early or developing non-insulin-dependent (type 2) diabetes, as shown by elevated insulin production in comparison to blood glucose levels (best shown with glucose tolerance testing or 2-hour postprandial examinations).

- Assist in the diagnosis of insulinoma, as demonstrated by sustained high insulin levels and lack of blood glucose-related variations.

- Verify functional hypoglycemia, as indicated by circulating insulin levels that are sufficient for increasing blood glucose levels.

- Difference between insulin-resistant diabetes with elevated insulin levels and non-insulin-resistant diabetes with low insulin levels.

- Evaluate fasting hypoglycemia of unknown cause.

- Evaluate postprandial hypoglycemia of unknown cause.

- Analyze uncontrolled insulin-dependent (type 1) diabetes.

RESULT:

Increased in:
• **Insulin- and proinsulin-secreting tumors (insulinomas)**
• **Acromegaly**
• **Alcohol use**
• **Cushing's syndrome**
• **Diabetes**
• **Excessive administration of insulin**
• **Obesity**
• **Reactive hypoglycemia in developing diabetes**
• **Severe liver disease**
Decreased in:
• **Beta-cell failure**

CRITICAL VALUES:

>35 mIU/L

Symptoms with elevated insulin levels include dizziness, diaphoresis, fainting, pallor, fatigue, stupor, and seizures. Possible interventions include the administration of 50 percent dextrose in water (D5W) solution, the administration of glucagon, and hourly blood glucose monitoring.

IMPEDING FACTORS:

- Drugs and substances that may raise insulin levels include acetohexamide, alanine, albuterol, amino acids, calcium gluconate, cannabis, chlorpropamide, beclomethasone, betamethasone, broxaterol, cyclic AMP, glibornuride, glipizide, glisoxepide, glucagon, pancreozymins, prednisolone, prednisone, rifampin, salbutamol, glyburide, ibopamine, insulin, insulin-like growth factor–I, oral contraceptives, tolbutamide, terbutaline, tolazamide, trichlormethiazide, and verapamil.

- Medicines that may decrease insulin levels include acarbose, asparaginase, calcitonin, diltiazem, doxazosin, enalapril, enprostil, ether, hydroxypropyl methylcellulose, insulin-like growth factor–I, metformin, niacin, cimetidine, clofibrate, dexfenfluramine, nifedipine, nitrendipine, octreotide, phenytoin, propranolol, and psyllium.

- The dispensation of insulin or oral hypoglycemic agents within 8 hours of the test can lead to false elevations.

- Hemodialysis removes insulin and changes the test results.

- Recent radioactive scans or radiation exposure may conflict with the test results when the radioimmunoassay is a test method.

ADRENOCORTICOTROPIC HORMONE (AND CHALLENGE TESTS) (Corticotropin, ACTH)

SAMPLING:

2 ml of plasma in lavender-top (ethylenediamine tetra-acetic acid [EDTA]) tube of adrenocorticotropic hormone (ACTH) and serum (1 mL) of a red-top tube of cortisol. The specimens should be processed immediately. Plasma for ACTH processing is to be moved to a plastic container.

Procedure	Medication Administered, Adult Dosage	Recommended Collection Times
ACTH stimulation, rapid test	250 µg cosyntropin IM or IV bolus after overnight fast	Three cortisol levels: Baseline, immediately before bolus, 30 min after
Corticotropin-releasing hormone (CRH) stimulation	An IV dose of 1 µg/kg ovine CRH between 9 a.m. and 8 p.m.	Three cortisol and 3 ACTH levels: baseline before injection, 30 min after injection, and 60 min after Injection
Dexamethasone suppression (overnight)	The oral dose of 1 mg dexamethasone (Decadron) at 11 p.m.	Collect cortisol at 8 a.m. on the morning after the dexamethasone dose
Metyrapone stimulation (overnight)	The oral dose of 30 mg/kg metyrapone with snack at midnight	Collect cortisol and ACTH at 8 a.m. on the morning after the metyrapone dose

For ACTH

Age	Conventional Units	SI Units (Conversion Factor 0.22)
Cord blood	50–570 pg/mL	11–125 pmol/L
Newborn	10–185 pg/mL	2–41 pmol/L
Adult supine specimen collected in morning	9–52 pg/mL	2–11 pmol/L
Women on oral contraceptives	5–29 pg/mL	1–6 pmol/L

ACTH Challenge Tests

ACTH (Cosyntropin) Stimulated, Rapid Test	Conventional Units	SI Units (Conversion Factor 27.6)
Baseline	Cortisol greater than 5 µg/dL	>138 nmol/L
Peak response	Cortisol greater than 20 µg/dL	>552 nmol/L
Corticotropin-Releasing Hormone Stimulated	2–4-fold increase over baseline ACTH or cortisol level	2–4-fold increase over baseline values
Dexamethasone Suppressed, Overnight Test	Cortisol < 3 µg/dL next day	< 83 nmol/L
Metyrapone Stimulated, Overnight Test	ACTH greater than 150 pg/mL	>33 pmol/L
	Cortisol < 3 µg/dL next day	< 83 nmol/L

EXPLAINATION:

ACTH secretes the anterior pituitary gland. This hormone stimulates the adrenal cortex secretion of glucocorticoids, androgens, and, to a lesser degree, mineral corticosteroids. The hypothalamic-releasing factor stimulates the release of ACTH. The measurements of the Cortisol and ACTH test are analyzed together because any change in one causes a change in the other. ACTH levels show diurnal variation, peaking between 6 a.m. and 8 a.m.

Moreover, to reach the lowest point between 6 and 11 p.m. The evening level is generally one-half to two - thirds lower than the daytime level. Cortisol levels often differ daily, with the lowest values increasing during the morning hours and peak levels happening at night.

INDICATIONS:

- Establish adequacy of replacement therapy in congenital adrenal hyperplasia.

- Establish adrenocortical dysfunction.

- Make a distinction between increased ACTH release with decreased cortisol levels and decreased ACTH release with increased cortisol levels.

RESULT:

The ACTH secretion demonstrates diurnal variation with the highest values in the morning. The lack of change in values from morning to night is clinically significant.

Increased in:
Addison's disease (primary adrenocortical hypofunction)
Congenital adrenal hyperplasia
Cushing's disease (pituitary-dependent)
Ectopic ACTH-producing tumors
Menstruation
Nelson's syndrome
Pregnancy
Stress
Decreased in:
Adenoma
Adrenal Carcinoma
Hypopituitarism
Secondary adrenocortical insufficiency

IMPEDING FACTORS:

- Drugs that may increase ACTH rates include aminoglutethimide, amphetamines, insulin, levodopa, metoclopramide, metyrapone, pyrogens, mifepristone (RU 486), and vasopressin.

- Drugs that may decrease the levels of ACTH include adrenal corticosteroids and dexamethasone.
- The test results are influenced by the moment the test is performed because the ACTH levels vary regularly, with the highest values between 6 and 8 a.m. Moreover, the lowest values exist at night. Samples should be withdrawn at the same time of day, between 6 a.m. and 8 a.m.
- Excessive physical activity may yield elevated levels of activity.
- Recent radioactive scans or contamination within one week of the test may conflict with the test results if the immuno-radiometric assay is the test method.
- The relaxation test for metyrapone is contraindicated in patients with suspected adrenal insufficiency.
- Metyrapone can cause gastrointestinal pain and/or confusion.

OSTEOCALCIN

Bone GLA protein, BGP
SAMPLING: 1 mL of serum is collected in a red-top tube.
TECHNIQUE: Radioimmunoassay
NORMAL VALUE:

Age and Sex	Conventional Units	SI Units (Conversion Factor X1)
Newborn	20–40 ng/mL	20–40 µg/L
1–17 y	2.8–41 ng/mL	2.8–41 µg/L
Adult		
Male	3–13 ng/mL	3–13 µg/L
Female		
Premenopausal	0.4–8.2 ng/mL	0.4–8.2 µg/L
Postmenopausal	1.5–11 ng/mL	1.5–11 µg/L

EXPLAINATION:
Osteocalcin is an important protein in the bone cell-matrix and a critical marker for bone metabolism. It is delivered by osteoblasts during the matrix mineralization process of bone formation and is the most abundant protein in bone cells. The synthesis of osteocalcin relies on vitamin K. Osteocalcin has parallel alkaline phosphatase levels. Osteocalcin levels are affected by several causes, including hormone estrogen. The estimation of osteocalcin levels allows for indirect measurement of osteoblast activity and bone formation. Because osteocalcin is released into the bloodstream during bone resorption, there is some doubt about whether osteocalcin may also be considered a marker for bone matrix deterioration and turnover.

INDICATIONS:
- Assist with a bone cancer diagnosis.
- Evaluate bone disease.
- Evaluate bone metabolism.
- Monitor the effectiveness of estrogen replacement therapy.

RESULT:

Increased in:
Hyperthyroidism (primary and secondary)
Adolescents undergoing a growth spurt
Chronic renal failure
Metastatic skeletal disease
Paget's disease
Renal osteodystrophy
Some patients with osteoporosis
Decreased in:
Pregnancy
Primary biliary cirrhosis
Growth hormone deficiency

IMPEDING FACTORS:
- Medications that may increase calcitonin levels contain anticonvulsants, calcitriol, and estrogens.
- Drugs that may reduce calcitonin levels include glucocorticoids.
- Recent radioactive scans or contamination within one week of the serum osteocalcin test can interfere with the test results, while radioimmunoassay is the test method.

PARATHYROID HORMONE: INTACT, C-TERMINAL, AND N-TERMINAL (Parathormone, PTH)

SAMPLING:1 mL of serum collected in a red- or tiger-top tube is recommended for C-terminal and N-terminal. 1 mL of plasma collected in a lavender top (EDTA) tube is recommended for intact PTH. Specimens should be transported tightly capped and in an ice slurry.
TECHNIQUE: Immunoassay

NORMAL VALUE:

	Conventional Units	SI Units (Conversion Factor X1)
C-terminal		
1–16 y	51–217 pg/mL	51–217 ng/L
Adults	50–330 pg/mL	50–330 ng/L
N-terminal		
2–13 y	14–21 pg/mL	14–21 ng/L
Adult	8–24 pg/mL	8–24 ng/L
Intact		
Cord blood	< 3 pg/mL	< 3 ng/L
2–20 y	9–52 pg/mL	9–52 ng/L
Adult	10–65 pg/mL	10–65 ng/L

EXPLAINATION:

Parathyroid glands produce parathyroid hormone (PTH) in response to decreased levels of circulating calcium. PTH aids in retrieving calcium from the bone into the bloodstream, encouraging renal tubular reabsorption of calcium and phosphate reabsorption depression, thereby reducing calcium excretion, and increasing renal phosphate excretion. PTH also increases the renal release of hydrogen ions, which leads to increased renal excretion of bicarbonate and chloride. PTH increases the renal production of activated vitamin D metabolites, leading to increased absorption of calcium in the small intestine. The net result of PTH intervention is that sufficient serum calcium levels are maintained. For normal individuals, preserved PTH has a circulating half-life of approximately 5 minutes.

INDICATIONS:

- Aid in the diagnosis of hyperparathyroidism.

- Assist in the diagnosis of presumed secondary hyperparathyroidism due to malignant tumors that produce ectopic PTH, chronic renal failure, and malabsorption syndromes.

- Spot unintended or unintentional disruption of the parathyroid gland during thyroid or neck surgery.

- Differentiated parathyroid and non-parathyroid reasons for hypercalcemia.

- Determine the autoimmune destruction of parathyroid glands.

- Evaluate the response of parathyroids to altered serum calcium levels, particularly those resulting from malignant processes leading to decreased PTH production.

- Assess the source of altered calcium metabolism.

RESULT:

Increased in:
Fluorosis
Pseudogout
Pseudohypoparathyroidism
Spinal cord trauma
Zollinger-Ellison syndrome
Primary, secondary, or tertiary hyperparathyroidism
Decreased in:
DiGeorge syndrome
Hyperthyroidism
Hypomagnesemia
Nonparathyroid hypercalcemia (in the non-existence of renal failure)
Autoimmune destruction of the parathyroids
Sarcoidosis
Secondary hypoparathyroidism due to surgery

IMPEDING FACTORS:

- Drugs that may raise PTH levels include clodronate, dopamine, estrogen/progestin therapy, foscarnet, furosemide, hydrocortisone, isoniazid, lithium octreotide, pamidronate, phosphate, prednisone, tamoxifen, and verapamil.

- Medications and vitamins that may lower PTH levels include calcitriol, cimetidine (C-terminal only), diltiazem, magnesium sulfate, alfacalcidol, aluminum hydroxide, pindolol, prednisone (intact), and vitamin D.

- PTH levels are responsive to diurnal variation, with the highest level occurring in the morning.

- PTH levels should always be measured following calcium for proper interpretation.

THYROGLOBULIN (Tg)

SAMPLING: 1 mL of serum is collected in a red- or tiger-top tube.
TECHNIQUE: Radioimmunoassay
NORMAL VALUE:

Age	Conventional Units	SI Units (Conversion Factor 1)
Cord blood	20.7–28.1 ng/mL	20.7–28.1 g/L
1 h	25.5–33.9 ng/mL	25.5–33.9 g/L
48 h	36.1–47.7 ng/mL	36.1–47.7 g/L
Adult	3.0–42.0 ng/mL	3.0–42.0 g/L
Athyrotic patient	< 5 ng/mL	< 5 g/L

EXPLAINATION:

Thyroglobulin is an iodine glycoprotein secreted by the follicular epithelial cells of the thyroid gland. It is the processing component of thyroid hormones thyroxine (T4) and triiodothyronine (T3). Once thyroid hormones are released into the bloodstream, they are isolated from thyroglobulin in response to the thyroid-stimulating hormone. Values >50 ng / mL are predictive of recurrence of tumors in athyrotic patients.

INDICATIONS:

- Assist in the treatment of subacute thyroiditis.

- Help in the evaluation of potential diseases with excessive thyroid hormone.

- Regulation of differentiated or metastatic thyroid cancer.

- Monitor responsiveness to goiter therapy.

- Monitor T4 therapy in patients/individuals with solitary nodules.

RESULT:

Increased in:
Differentiated thyroid cancer
Graves' disease (untreated)
Neonates
Pregnancy
T4-binding globulin deficiency
Thyroiditis
Thyrotoxicosis
Surgery or irradiation of the thyroid (raised levels to indicate residual or disseminated carcinoma)
Decreased in:
Congenital arthrosis (neonates)
Thyrotoxicosis factitial
Administration of thyroid hormone

IMPEDING FACTORS:

- Drugs that may decrease the level of thyroglobulin include neomycin and T4.

- Thyroglobulin autoantibodies can cause decreased values.

- Recent radioactive scans or radiation can conflict with the test results when the radioimmunoassay is a test method.

- Recent thyroid surgery or needle biopsy can hinder with test results.

THYROID-BINDING INHIBITORY IMMUNOGLOBULIN

(thyrotropin binding inhibitory immunoglobulin, Thyrotropin-receptor antibodies, TBII)

SAMPLING:1 mL of serum is collected in a red-top tube.

TECHNIQUE: Radioreceptor

NORMAL VALUE: < 10 % inhibition.

(Note: In patients with Graves' disease, inhibition is anticipated to be 10 to 100 percent.)

EXPLAINATION: There are two functional forms of thyroid receptor immunoglobulins: thyroid-stimulating immunoglobulin (TSI) and thyroid-binding immunoglobulin (TBII). TSI interacts with receptors, stimulates intracellular enzymes, and facilitates epithelial cell function, which functions outside the TBII thyroid-stimulating hormone feedback regulation, inhibits the action of TSH, and is believed to cause some forms of hyperthyroidism. Such antibodies were formerly known as long-acting thyroid stimulants. High levels of pregnancy may have some predictive value for neonatal thyrotoxicosis: positive results suggest that the antibodies are stimulating (TSI); negative results indicate that the antibodies are blocking (TBII). The TBII test measures the level of thyroid-receptor immunoglobulin in the determination of thyroid disease.

INDICATIONS:

- Test possible acute toxic goiter.

- Investigate suspected neonatal thyroid disease due to maternal thyroid disease.

- Monitor hyperthyroid patients at risk of relapse or remission.

RESULT:

Increased in:
Toxic goiter
Maternal thyroid disease
Neonatal thyroid disease
Graves' disease
Hyperthyroidism (various forms)
Decreased in:
Not any specific disease

IMPEDING FACTORS:

- Lithium will produce false-positive results.

- Recent radioactive scans or radiation exposure within one week of the test conflict with the test results while radioimmunoassay is the test method.

THYROID-STIMULATING HORMONE (Thyrotropin, TSH)

SAMPLING: 1 mL of serum is collected in a red- or tiger-top tube; for a neonate, using filter paper.

TECHNIQUE: Immunoassay

NORMAL VALUE:

Age	Conventional Units	SI Units (Conversion Factor X 1)
Neonates–3 d	< 20 IU/mL	< 20 mIU/L
Adults	0.4–4.2 IU/mL	0.4–4.2 mIU/L

EXPLAINATION:

The pituitary gland produces Thyroid-stimulating hormone (TSH) in response to thyrotropin-releasing hormone (TRH) stimulation, a hypothalamic releasing factor. TRH regulates the release and circulation of thyroid hormones in response to variables such as cold, stress, and increased metabolic needs. Thyroid and pituitary function may be evaluated by TSH measurement. TSH shows diurnal variation, peaking between midnight and 4 a.m. Furthermore, snorkeling between 5 and 6 p.m., TSH levels are high at birth but extend to adult levels in the first week of life. Raised TSH levels combined with decreased thyroxine (T4) levels indicate hypothyroidism and thyroid dysfunction. Decreased TSH and T4 levels generally indicate residual congenital hypothyroidism and pituitary hypothalamic dysfunction. Normal TSH and depressed T4 levels may indicate (1) hypothyroidism due to congenital defect in T4-binding globulin, or (2) transient congenital hypothyroidism due to hypoxia or prematurity. Early diagnosis and neonate therapy are critical to the reduction of cretinism and mental retardation.

INDICATIONS:

- Assist in the treatment of congenital hypothyroidism.

- Assist in the detection of hypothyroidism or hyperthyroidism or possible pituitary or hypothalamic dysfunction.

- Differentiate actual euthyroidism from real hypothyroidism in vulnerable individuals.

RESULT:

Increased in:
Congenital hypothyroidism in the neonate (filter paper test)
Ectopic TSH-producing tumors (lung, breast)
Primary hypothyroidism
Secondary hyperthyroidism owing to pituitary hyperactivity
Thyroid hormone resistance
Thyroiditis (Hashimoto's autoimmune disease)
Decreased in:
Excessive thyroid hormone replacement
Graves' disease
Primary hyperthyroidism
Secondary hypothyroidism (pituitary involvement)
Tertiary hypothyroidism (hypothalamic involvement)

IMPEDING FACTORS:

- Drugs and hormones that may increase TSH include amiodarone, benserazide, erythrosine, flunarizine (males), iobenzamic acid, iodides, lithium, methimazole, metoclopramide, morphine, propranolol, radiographic agents, TRH, and valproic acid.

- Drugs and hormones that may decrease TSH levels include amiodarone, anabolic steroids, acetylsalicylic acid, carbamazepine, corticosteroids, dopamine, glucocorticoids, hydrocortisone, insulin-like growth factor I, interferon-alfa-2b, iodamide, josamycin, levodopa, levothyroxine, methergoline, nifedipine, pyridoxine, T4, and triiodothyronine (T3).

- If the filter paper sample did not dry, it might affect test results.

THYROID-STIMULATING IMMUNOGLOBULIN
Thyrotropin-receptor antibodies, TSI

SAMPLING: 1 mL of serum is collected in a red-top tube.
TECHNIQUE: Radioimmunoassay
NORMAL VALUE: < 130 percent of basal activity.
EXPLAINATION:
There are two functional forms of thyroid-receptor immunoglobulins: thyroid-stimulating immunoglobulin (TSI) and thyroid-binding immunoglobulin (TBII). TSI interacts with receptors, stimulates intracellular enzymes, and facilitates epithelial cell function, which functions outside the TBII thyroid-stimulating hormone feedback regulation, inhibits the action of TSH, and is believed to cause some forms of hyperthyroidism. Such antibodies were formerly known as long-acting thyroid stimulants. High levels of pregnancy may have some predictive value for neonatal thyrotoxicosis: positive results suggest that the antibodies are stimulating (TSI); negative results indicate that the antibodies are blocking (TBII). TSI research measures the level of thyroid-receptor immunoglobulin in the determination of thyroid disease.
INDICATIONS:
Follow-up with positive TBII test in differentiating antibody activation from neutral or suppressive activity.
Monitor hyperthyroid patients at risk of relapse or recovery.

RESULT:

Increased in: Graves' disease
Decreased in: No specific disease

IMPEDING FACTORS:
- Lithium may cause false-positive TBII results.
- Recent radioactive scans or exposure to radiation can intrude with test results when radioimmunoassay is the test method.

THYROTROPIN-RELEASING HORMONE STIMULATION TEST
TRH stimulation
SAMPLING: 1 mL of serum is collected in a red- or tiger-top tube.
TECHNIQUE: Immunoassay
NORMAL VALUE:
Minimal rise of 1 to 2 mIU/L above baseline.
the typical response is a 5- to 10-fold increase above baseline.

EXPLAINATION:

In the thyrotropin-releasing hormone (TRH) stimulation test, TRH is administered intravenously after a normal assessment of the thyroid-stimulating hormone (TSH) has been obtained. Subsequent specimens are collected for TSH measurements at 30- and 60-minute intervals. An exaggerated response is a sign of impaired thyroid function or hypothalamic-pituitary axis disorders. Third generation or "responsive" TSH assays are now favored over TRH stimulation.

INDICATIONS:

- Assistance in the diagnosis and treatment of hypothalamic and pituitary conditions.

- Distinguishing of mania from schizophrenia.

RESULT:

Increased in:
Pregnancy
Primary hypothyroidism
Decreased in:
Major depressive illnesses
Primary hyperthyroidism
Secondary hypothyroidism

IMPEDING FACTORS: Not any

THYROXINE-BINDING GLOBULIN (TBG)

SAMPLING: 1 mL of serum is collected in a red- or tiger-top tube.
TECHNIQUE: Radioimmunoassay
NORMAL VALUE:

Age	Conventional Units	SI Unit (Conversion Factor 10)
0–1 wk	3–8 mg/dL	30–80 mg/L
1–12 mo	1.6–3.6 mg/dL	16–36 mg/L
14 y–adult	1.2–2.5 mg/dL	12–25 mg/L
Adult		
Pregnancy, third trimester	4.7–5.9 mg/dL	47–59 mg/L
Oral contraceptives	1.5–5.5 mg/dL	15–55 mg/L

EXPLAINATION:

Thyroxine-binding globulin (TBG) is the prevalent carrier protein for circulating thyroxine (T4) and triiodothyronine (T3). The other transport proteins are T4-binding pre-albumin and T4-binding albumin. Conditions that affect the TBG level and binding ability also affect the free T3 and free T4 levels.

INDICATIONS:

- Helps to make a difference between elevated T4 due to hyperthyroidism and increased TBG binding in euthyroid patients.

- Assess hypothyroid patients.

- Detect deficiency or excess TBG due to hereditary abnormality.

RESULT:

Increased in:
Acute intermittent porphyria
Infectious hepatitis and other liver diseases
Genetically high TBG
Hypothyroidism
Neonates
Pregnancy
Decreased in:
Acromegaly
Major illness
Nephrotic syndrome
Ovarian hypofunction
Surgical stress
Testosterone-producing tumors
Chronic hepatic disease
Genetically low TBG
Marked hypoproteinemia, malnutrition

IMPEDING FACTORS:

- Drugs and hormones that may raise TBG levels include estrogens, oral contraceptives, tamoxifen, and perphenazine.

- Drugs that may reduce TBG levels include anabolic steroids, androgens, asparaginase, corticosteroids, corticotropin, danazole, phenytoin, and propranolol.

- Recent radioactive scans and radiation exposure within one week of the test, may interfere with the test results especially when radioimmunoassay is the test method.

THYROXINE, FREE (Free T4, FT4)

SAMPLING: 1 mL of serum is collected in a red- or tiger-top tube. 1 mL of plasma is collected in a green-top (heparin) tube is also acceptable.

TECHNIQUE: Immunoassay

NORMAL VALUE:

Age	Conventional Units	SI Units (Conversion Factor 12.9)
Newborn	0.8–2.8 ng/dL	10–36 pmol/L
1–12 mo	0.8–2.0 ng/dL	10–26 pmol/L
1–18 y	0.8–1.7 ng/dL	10–22 pmol/L
Adult	0.8–1.5 ng/dL	10–19 pmol/L

EXPLAINATION:

Thyroxine (T4) is a hormone produced and excreted by the thyroid gland. Newborns are commonly tested for reduced T4 rates using a filter paper system (see the monograph titled "Thyroxine, Total"). The bulk of T4 in serum (99.97%) is bound to globulin-binding thyroxine (TBG), pre-albumin, and albumin. The remainder (0.03%) circulates as unbound or free T4, a physiologically active form. The free T4 levels are proportional to the total T4 levels. The advantage of calculating free T4 instead of total T4 is that, unlike total T4 values, free T4 levels are not influenced by variations in TBG levels; thus, free T4 levels are thought to be the most precise indicator of T4 and its hypometabolic behavior. Free T4 measurements are useful in assessing thyroid disease, where thyroid-stimulating hormone (TSH) levels alone provide insufficient information. Free T4 and TSH are inversely proportional. Assessment of free T4 is also prescribed during hyperthyroidism therapy before symptoms have decreased, and levels have decreased to the normal range.

INDICATIONS:

- Evaluate signs of hypothyroidism as well as hyperthyroidism.

- Monitor response to drug therapy against hypothyroidism or hyperthyroidism.

RESULT:

Increased in:
Hyperthyroidism
Hypothyroidism treated with T4
Decreased in:
Hypothyroidism
Pregnancy (late)
Hypothyroidism treated with triiodothyronine (T3)

IMPEDING FACTORS:

- Medications that may raise the free T4 levels include amiodarone, acetylsalicylic acid, halofenate, heparin, iopanoic acid, levothyroxine, methimazole, and radiographic agents.

- Medications that may decrease T4-free levels include amiodarone, anabolic steroids, asparaginase, methadone, methimazole, oral contraceptives, and phenylbutazone.

THYROXINE, TOTAL (T4)

SAMPLING: 1 mL of serum is collected in a red- or tiger-top tube. 1ml of plasma is collected in a green-top (heparin) tube is also acceptable.

TECHNIQUE: Immunoassay

NORMAL VALUE:

Age	Conventional Units	SI Units (Conversion Factor 12.9)
1–3 d	11.8–22.6 g/dL	152–292 nmol/L
1–2 wk	9.8–16.6 g/dL	126–214 nmol/L
1–4 mo	7.2–14.4 g/dL	93–186 nmol/L
5–12 mo	7.8–16.5 g/dL	101–213 nmol/L
1–5 y	7.3–15.0 g/dL	94–194 nmol/L
5–10 y	6.4–13.3 g/dL	83–172 nmol/L
10–15 y	5.6–11.7 g/dL	72–151 nmol/L
Adult		
Man	4.6–10.5 g/dL	59–135 nmol/L
Woman	5.5–11.0 g/dL	71–142 nmol/L
Pregnant woman	5.5–16.0 g/dL	71–155 nmol/L
Over 60 y	5.0–10.7 g/dL	65–138 nmol/L

EXPLAINATION:

Thyroxine (T4) is a hormone produced and excreted by the thyroid gland. Newborns are commonly tested for reduced T4 rates using a filter paper form. The bulk of T4 in serum (99.97%) is bound to globulin-binding thyroxine (TBG), prealbumin, and albumin. The rest (0.03%) circulates as unbound or free T4, a physiologically active form. The free T4 levels are proportional to the total T4 levels. The advantage of calculating free T4 instead of total T4 is that, unlike total T4 values, free T4 levels are not influenced by variations in TBG levels; thus, free T4 levels are considered to be the most precise indicator of T4 and its hypometabolic behavior.

INDICATIONS:
- Assess signs of hypothyroidism or hyperthyroidism and neonatal screening for congenital hypothyroidism (required in many states).
- Evaluate the response of thyroid to protein deficiency associated with severe diseases.
- Monitor response to hypothyroidism or hyperthyroidism.

RESULT:

Increased in:
Acute psychiatric illnesses
Excessive intake of iodine
Hepatitis
Hyperemesis gravidarum
Hyperthyroidism
Obesity
Thyrotoxicosis factitia
Thyrotoxicosis due to Graves' disease
Decreased in:
Hypothyroidism
Panhypopituitarism
Strenuous exercise
Decreased TBG (liver disease, gastrointestinal protein loss, nephrotic syndrome, malnutrition)

CRITICAL VALUES:
Hypothyroidism:
< 2.0 µg/dL
Hyperthyroidism:
>20.0 µg/dL
At rates below 2.0 µg/dL, the patient is at risk for myxedema coma. Signs and symptoms of severe hypothyroidism include bradycardia, hypoventilation, hypothermia, hypotension, lethargy, and coma. Possible therapies include airway support, regular control of neurological activity and blood pressure, and intravenous thyroid hormone.

The patient is at risk for thyroid storms at levels >20.0 g / dL. Signs and symptoms of extreme hyperthyroidism include hyperthermia, diaphoresis, diarrhea, fatigue, and discomfort.

Possible interventions include shock therapy, sodium, electrolyte replacement for dehydration, and antithyroid medications (propylthiouracil and Lugol solution).

IMPEDING FACTORS:
- Medications that may raise T4 levels include amiodarone, amphetamines, corticosteroids, estrogen, fluorouracil, insulin, glucocorticoids, halofenate,

iobenzamic acid, levodopa, levothyroxine, opiates, oral contraceptives, iopanoic acid, ipodate, levarterenol phenothiazine, and prostaglandins.

- Medicines, drugs, substances, and treatments that may decrease T4 levels include aminoglutethimide, aminosalicylic acid, colestipol, corticotropin, cortisone, amiodarone, anabolic steroids, anticonvulsants, danazol, dehydroepiandrosterone, asparaginase, acetylsalicylic acid, barbiturates, carbimazole, dexamethasone, diazepam, diazo dyes, chlorpromazine, chlorpropamide, dinitrophenol, ethionamide, Evans blue, fenclofenac, halofenate, hydroxyphenylpyruvic acid, lithium, lovastatin, methimazole, methylthiouracil, mitotane, cholestyramine, clofibrate, cobalt, cotrimoxazole, cytostatic therapy, thiouracil, iron, isotretinoin, liothyronine, norethindrone, penicillamine, penicillin, propylthiouracil, reserpine, salicylate, sodium nitroprusside, stanozolol, interferon alfa-2b, phenylacetic acid derivatives, phenylbutazone, potassium iodide, sulfonylureas, tetrachloro-thyronine, tolbutamide, and triiodothyronine (T3).

TRIIODOTHYRONINE, FREE (Free T3, FT3)

SAMPLING: 1 mL of serum is collected in a red- or tiger-top tube.
TECHNIQUE: Immunoassay
NORMAL VALUE:

Age	Conventional Units	SI Units (Conversion Factor 0.0154)
Children and adults	260–480 pg/dL	4.0–7.4 pmol/L
Pregnant women (4–9 mo gestation)	196–338 pg/dL	3.0–5.2 pmol/L

EXPLAINATION:
Unlike the thyroid hormone thyroxine (T4), the bulk of T3 is enzymatically transformed from T4 of tissues rather than specifically formed by the thyroid gland. Approximately one-third of T4 is converted to T3. The bulk of T3 in serum (99.97%) is bound to globulin-binding thyroxine (TBG), prealbumin, and albumin. The rest (0.03%) circulates as unbound or free T3, a physiologically active form. The free T3 levels are proportional to the total T3 levels. The benefit of calculating T3 free instead of T3 total is that, like fixed T3 tests, free T3 levels are not influenced by variations in TBG levels. T3 is four to five times more biologically efficient than T4. This hormone, along with T4, is responsible for maintaining the status of the euthyroid.

Free T3 measurements are rarely required but are demonstrated in the diagnosis of T3 toxicity and when certain medications are administered that interact with the conversion of T4 to T3.

INDICATIONS:

- Adjunctive assistance for thyroid-stimulating hormone (TSH) and free T4 testing.

- Assist in the evaluation of T3 toxicosis.

RESULT:

Increased in:
High altitude
Hyperthyroidism
T3 toxicosis
Decreased in:
Hypothyroidism
Malnutrition
Pregnancy (late)
Nonthyroidal chronic diseases

IMPEDING FACTORS:

- Products that may increase T3 free include amiodarone, acetylsalicylic acid, and levothyroxine.

- Drugs that may reduce T3 free include amiodarone, methimazole, phenytoin, propranolol, and radiographic agents.

TRIIODOTHYRONINE, TOTAL (T 3)

SAMPLING: 1mL of serum is collected in a red- or tiger-top tube. 1 mL of plasma collected in a green-top (heparin) tube is also acceptable.

TECHNIQUE: Immunoassay

NORMAL VALUE:

Age	Conventional Units	SI Units (Conversion Factor X 0.0154)
1–3 d	100–740 ng/dL	1.54–11.40 nmol/L
1–12 mo	105–245 ng/dL	1.62–3.77 nmol/L
1–5 y	105–269 ng/dL	1.62–4.14 nmol/L
6–10 y	94–241 ng/dL	1.45–3.71 nmol/L
16–20 y	80–210 ng/dL	1.20–3.20 nmol/L
Adult	70–204 ng/dL	1.08–3.14 nmol/L
Pregnant woman (last 4 mo gestation)	116–247 ng/dL	1.79–3.80 nmol/L

EXPLAINATION:
Unlike the thyroid hormone thyroxine (T4), most T3 is enzymatically transferred from T4 to tissues rather than specifically produced by the thyroid gland. Approximately one-third of T4 is translated to T3. The majority of T3 in serum (99.97%) is bound to globulin-binding thyroxine (TBG), prealbumin, and albumin. The rest (0.03%) circulates as unbound or free T3, a physiologically active form. The free T3 levels are proportional to the total T3 levels. The benefit of calculating T3 free instead of T3 fixed is that, like total T3 values, free T3 levels are not influenced by variations in TBG levels. T3 is four to five times more biologically efficient than T4. This hormone, along with T4, is responsible for maintaining the state of the euthyroid.

INDICATIONS:
Adjunctive help for thyroid stimulation hormone (TSH) and unrestricted measurement of T4.

RESULT:

Increased in:
Hyperthyroidism
Iodine-deficiency goiter
Pregnancy
T3 toxicosis
Conditions with increased TBG
Early thyroid failure
Thyrotoxicosis factitial
Treat hyperthyroidism
Decreased in:
Conditions with decreased TBG
Hypothyroidism
Acute and subacute nonthyroidal disease

IMPEDING FACTORS:
- Drugs that may raise the total T3 levels include amiodarone, amphetamine, fluorouracil, halofenate, insulin, levothyroxine, methadone, opiates, benziodarone, clofibrate, fenoprofen, prostaglandins, T3, oral contraceptives, phenytoin, and valproic acid.

- Drugs that may reduce total T3 levels include amiodarone, anabolic steroids, cholestyramine, clomiphene, asparaginase, acetylsalicylic acid, carbamazepine, dexamethasone, fenclofenac, furosemide, colestipol, cotrimoxazole, interferon alfa-2b, glucocorticoids, hydrocortisone, iobenzamic acid, iodides, ipodate, isotretinoin, netilmicin, oral contraceptives, penicillamine, lithium, methimazole, neomycin, phenobarbital, phenylacetic acid derivatives, phenylbutazone, phenytoin, potassium iodide, prednisone, propranolol, propylthiouracil, radiographic agents, salicylate, sodium ipodate, sulfonylureas, and tyropanoic acid.

NOTES

REPRODUCTIVE SYSTEM

PROLACTIN
(Luteotropic hormone, lactogenic hormone, lactogen, HPRL, PRL)

SAMPLING: 1 mL of serum is collected in a red- or tiger-top tube. The sample should be transported tightly capped and in an ice slurry.

TECHNIQUE: Immunoassay

NORMAL VALUE:

Age	Conventional Units	SI Units (Conversion Factor X1)
Prepubertal males and females	3.2–20.0 ng/mL	3.2–20.0 µg/L
Men	2.4–13.8 ng/mL	2.4–13.8 µg/L
Women	3.3–26.7 ng/mL	3.3–26.7 µg/L
Pregnant	5.3–215.3 ng/mL	5.3–215.3 µ g/L
Postmenopausal	2.4–24.0 ng/mL	2.4–24.0 µg/L

EXPLAINATION:

Prolactin is secreted from the pituitary gland. It is peculiar among hormones in that it responds to hypothalamus suppression rather than activation. The only known purpose of prolactin is to promote the production of milk in female breasts that are already activated by elevated estrogen levels. Lactation can continue without elevated prolactin levels when milk production is achieved. Prolactin levels rise late in pregnancy, a peak with the initiation of lactation, and rise every time a woman breastfeeds. The function of prolactin in males is unknown.

INDICATIONS:

- Assist in the detection of primary hypothyroidism, as suggested by elevated levels.

- Assist in the diagnosis of possible lung or kidney tumors (high levels suggesting ectopic prolactin production).

- Evaluate postpartum lactation failure.

- Evaluate possible postpartum hypophyseal infarction (Sheehan's Syndrome), as demonstrated by decreased levels.

- Evaluate sexual dysfunction of unknown cause in both men and women.

RESULT:

Increased in:
Ectopic prolactin-secreting tumors (e.g., lung, kidney)
Adrenal insufficiency
Amenorrhea
Anorexia nervosa
Breastfeeding
Chiari-Frommel and Argonz–Del
Castillo syndromes
Chest wall injury
Chronic renal failure
Galactorrhea
Hypothyroidism (primary)
Insulin-induced hypoglycemia
Liver failure
Pituitary tumor
Polycystic ovary (Stein-Leventhal) syndrome
Hypothalamic and pituitary disorders
Pregnancy
Surgery (pituitary stalk section)
Decreased in:
Sheehan's syndrome

IMPEDING FACTORS:

- Drugs and hormones that may raise prolactin levels include amitriptyline, megestrol, mestranol, methyldopa, sultopride, thiethylperazine, thioridazine, thiothixene, thyrotropin-releasing hormone, trifluoperazine, metoclopramide, molindone, morphine, nitrous oxide, oral contraceptives, oxcarbazepine, parathyroid hormone, phenothiazines, phenytoin, pimozide, prochlorperazine, promazine, ranitidine, benserazide, butaperazine, butorphanol, carbidopa, chlorophenylpiperazine, pentagastrin, perphenazine, remoxipride, reserpine, sulpiride, β-endorphin, enflurane, fenfluramine, fenoldopam, flunarizine, amoxapine, arginine, azosemide, chlorpromazine, cimetidine, fluphenazine, growth hormone-releasing hormone, imipramine, insulin, clomipramine, desipramine, diethylstilbestrol, interferon-β, labetalol, loxapine, trimipramine, tumor necrosis factor, veralipride, verapamil, and zometapine.

- Drugs and hormones that may reduce prolactin levels include anticonvulsants, apomorphine, bromocriptine, D-Trp-6-LHRH, levodopa, metoclopramide, morphine, nifedipine, octreotide, cabergoline, calcitonin, cyclosporine, dexamethasone, dopamine, pergolide, ranitidine, rifampin, ritanserin, ropinirole, secretin, thyroid hormones, and terguride.

- Episodic peaks can occur in response to sleep, stress, exercise, hypoglycemia, and breastfeeding.

- Venipuncture can cause falsely elevated levels.

- The release of prolactin is subject to diurnal variation, with the highest levels occurring in the morning.

ANTIBODIES, ANTISPERM

SAMPLING: 1 ml serum is collected in a red-top tube.
TECHNIQUE: Immunoassay
NORMAL VALUE:

Result	Sperm Bound by Immunobead (%)
Negative	0–15
Weak positive	16–30
Moderate positive	31–50
Strong positive	51–100

EXPLAINATION: A major cause of male infertility is the obstruction of efferent testicular ducts. As a result of the reabsorption of sperm from blocked ducts, antibodies to sperm may be produced over time, which may minimize the fertility of the individual.

Semen and cervical mucus may also be screened for anti-sperm antibodies.

INDICATIONS:
Evaluation of infertility
RESULT

Increased in:
Blocked testicular efferent duct
Postvasectomy
Decreased in:
Not any specific disease

IMPEDING FACTORS:
- If semen is tested, the patient should not ejaculate until 3 to 4 days before the test is obtained.
- Sperm antibodies have been found in pregnant women and women with primary infertility.

SEMEN ANALYSIS

SAMPLING:

Ejaculate semen stored in a clean, dry, glass container considered to be free of detergent. The specimen container should be held at body temperature (37°C) during transport.

TECHNIQUE: Macroscopic and microscopic examination

NORMAL VALUE:

Volume	2–5 mL
Color	White or opaque
Appearance	Viscous (pours in droplets, not clumps or strings)
Clotting and liquefaction	Complete in 20–30 minutes
pH	7.5–8.5
Sperm count	20–200 million/mL
Motility	At least 60%
Morphology	At least 70% of normal oval-headed forms

EXPLAINATION:

Semen analysis is a reliable measure of overall male fertility. Semen contains a combination of elements produced by different parts of the male reproductive system. Spermatozoa are formed in the testicles and account for only a small volume of seminal fluid. Fructose and other nutrients are provided by the fluid produced in the seminal vesicles. The prostate gland provides the acid phosphatase and other enzymes needed for semen coagulation and liquefaction. The motility of the sperm depends on the presence of a sufficient level of ionized calcium. If the specimen has an abnormal appearance (e.g., red, unusually colored, turbid), the patient may have an infection. Specimens may be tested with a leukocyte esterase strip to detect the presence of white blood cells.

INDICATIONS:

- Assist in the evaluation of azoospermia and oligospermia.

- Infertility assessment.

- Vasectomy feasibility evaluation.

- Paternity suits help.

RESULT: There is a marked intraindividual difference in sperm count. Indications of suboptimal fertility should be confirmed through serial analysis of two to three samples collected over several months. When suspicious results are obtained, additional tests may be required.

Increased in: N/A
Decreased in:
Orchitis
Postvasectomy period

Primary and secondary testicular failure
Testicular atrophy (e.g., recovery from mumps)
Hyperpyrexia
Obstruction of the ejaculatory system
Varicocele

IMPEDING FACTORS:

- Medicines and substances that may decrease sperm count include arsenic, fluoxymesterone, ketoconazole, lead, methotrexate, methyltestosterone, nitrofurantoin, nitrogen mustard, procarbazine, azathioprine, cannabis, cimetidine, cocaine, cyclophosphamide, estrogens, sulfasalazine, and vincristine.

- Testicular radiation can reduce sperm counts.

- Cigarette smoking is associated with reduced semen production.

- Intake of caffeine is associated with increased sperm production and the number of unusual shapes.

- Delays in the transfer of the specimen and inability to keep the specimen warm during transportation are one of the most common reasons for the rejection of the specimen.

TESTOSTERONE, TOTAL

SAMPLING: 1ml of serum is collected in a red- or tiger-top tube. 1 ml of plasma collected in a green-top (heparin) tube is also acceptable.

TECHNIQUE: Radioimmunoassay

NORMAL VALUE:

Age	Conventional Units	SI Units (Conversion Factor 0.0347)
Cord blood		
Male	13–55 ng/dL	0.45–1.91 nmol/L
Female	5–45 ng/dL	0.17–1.56 nmol/L
Newborn		
Male	75–400 ng/dL	2.6–13.9 nmol/L
Female	20–64 ng/dL	0.69–2.22 nmol/L
1–5 mo		
Male	1–177 ng/dL	0.03–6.14 nmol/L
Female	1–5 ng/dL	0.03–0.17 nmol/L
6–11 mo		
Male	2–7 ng/dL	0.07–0.24 nmol/L
Female	2–5 ng/dL	0.07–0.17 nmol/L

	1–5 y	
Male	2–25 ng/dL	0.07–0.87 nmol/L
Female	2–10 ng/dL	0.07–0.35 nmol/L
	6–9 y	
Male	3–30 ng/dL	0.10–1.04 nmol/L
Female	2–20 ng/dL	0.07–0.35 nmol/L
	10–11 y	
Male	5–50 ng/dL	0.17–1.73 nmol/L
Female	5–25 ng/dL	0.17–0.87 nmol/L
	12–14 y	
Male	10–572 ng/dL	0.35–19.83 nmol/L
Female	10–40 ng/dL	0.35–1.39 nmol/L
	15–17 y	
Male	220–800 ng/dL	7.63–27.74 nmol/L
Female	5–40 ng/dL	0.17–1.39 nmol/L
	Adult	
Male	280–1100 ng/dL	9.71–38.14 nmol/L
Female	15–70 ng/dL	0.52–2.43 nmol/L

EXPLAINATION:

Testosterone is the primary androgen responsible for sexual differentiation. For males, testosterone is developed by the Leydig cells in the testicles and is responsible for spermatogenesis and the production of secondary sex characteristics. In females, the ovarian and adrenal gland secretes small amounts of this hormone; nevertheless, most of the testosterone in females is extracted from the metabolism of androstenedione. For males, testicular, adrenal, or pituitary tumors may induce an overabundance of testosterone, leading to premature puberty. In females, adrenal tumors, hyperplasia, and drugs can induce an overabundance of this hormone, resulting in masculinization or hirsutism.

INDICATIONS:

- Help in the treatment of hypergonadism.

- Help in the evaluation of male sexual precocity before the age of 10.

- Distinguishment of primary and secondary hypogonadism.

- Evaluate hirsutism.

- Evaluate the male infertility.

RESULT:

Increased in:
Hirsutism
Hyperthyroidism
Idiopathic sexual precocity

Polycystic ovaries
Syndrome of androgen resistance
Testicular or extragonadal tumors
Adrenal hyperplasia
Adrenocortical tumors
Trophoblastic tumors during pregnancy
Virilizing ovarian tumors
Decreased in:
Anovulation
Cryptorchidism
Delayed puberty
Down's syndrome
Impotence
Klinefelter's syndrome
Malnutrition
Myotonic dystrophy
Orchiectomy
Excessive alcohol intake
Hepatic insufficiency
Primary and secondary hypogonadism
Primary and secondary hypopituitarism
Uremia

IMPEDING FACTORS:

- Drugs that may lead to a rise in testosterone levels include levonorgestrel, barbiturates, bromocriptine, cimetidine, flutamide, gonadotropin, mifepristone, moclobemide, nafarelin (males), nilutamide, oral contraceptives, rifampin, and tamoxifen.

- Drugs that may decrease testosterone levels include cyclophosphamide, cyproterone, danazole, dexamethasone, diethylstilbestrol, digoxin, D-Trp-6-LHRH, fenoldopam, goserelin, ketoconazole, leuprolide, magnesium sulfate, medroxyprogesterone, methylprednisone, nandrolone, oral contraceptives, pravastatin, prednisone, pyridoglutethimide, spironolactone, stanozolol, tetracycline, and thioridazine.

- Recent radioactive scans or radiation exposure within one week of the test may interfere with the test results, while radioimmunoassay is the test method.

PROSTATE-SPECIFIC ANTIGEN (PSA)

SAMPLIG:1 mL of serum is collected in a red- or tiger-top tube.

TECHNIQUE: Immunoassay

NORMAL VALUE:

Sex	Conventional Units	SI Units (Conversion Factor X 1)
Male	< 4 ng/mL	< 4 g/L
Female	< 0.5 ng/mL	< 0.5 g/L

EXPLAINATION:

The prostate-specific antigen (PSA) is produced exclusively by the epithelial cells of the prostate, peri-urethral, and perirectal glands. Used in arrangement with a digital rectal examination, PSA is a useful test for the diagnosis of prostate adenocarcinoma. PSA circulates in a free and bound (complex) form. A less ratio of free to complexed PSA (i.e., < 10%) is predictive of prostate cancer; a ratio of more than 30% is rarely associated with prostate cancer. Serial measurements are often carried out before and after surgery. Important note: Use the same method of measurement continuously when performing serial testing in patients.

INDICATIONS:

- Evaluate prostate cancer treatment (prostatectomy): levels decrease if treatment is effective; can levels are associated with recurrence and poor prognosis.

- Investigate or examine an enlarged prostate gland, particularly if the cancer of the prostate is suspected.

- Stage cancer of the prostate.

RESULT:

Increased in:
Benign prostatic hypertrophy
Prostate cancer
Prostatic infarct
Urinary retention
Decreased in: N/A

IMPEDING FACTORS:

- Medications that reduce PSA levels include buserelin, finasteride, and flutamide.

- Specimens should not be obtained for at least four weeks after the digital rectal examination, biopsy, other prostate manipulation, or findings may be wrongly increased.

ACID PHOSPHATASE, PROSTATIC
(o-phosphoric monoester phosphohydrolase, PAP, Prostatic acid phosphatase)

SAMPLING:
Serum/Plasma (1 mL) stored in a bottle with lavender top (ethylenediaminetetraacetic acid [EDTA]). Serum (1 mL) in a red-top tube is also appropriate, but care must be taken to make use of the same type of collection container for serial measurements. Swab with vaginal secretions may be put forward in the appropriate transfer container. Other items, such as clothing, may be provided for review. Consult the Department of Hospital or Emergency Services for advice on collecting specimens and containers.

TECHNIQUE: Enzyme immunoassay

NORMAL value:

Conventional Units:	< 2.5 ng/mL
SI Units:	< 2.5 µg/L

EXPLAINATION:
Acid phosphatases are proteins present in many organs, including the prostate gland, bone, spleen, liver, and kidney, as well as RBCs and platelets. Seminal fluid also comprises high concentrations of acid phosphatase, and the presence of this enzyme in vaginal swabs or other physical evidence is used to prosecute abuse. The activity of acid phosphatase is highest in the prostate gland; however, prostatic acid phosphatase (PAP) are not significantly raised in the early stages of prostatic cancer, so this test is not utilized as a screening tool. A prostate-specific antigen substituted PAP for the treatment of prostate carcinoma and the diagnosis of metastatic prostate adenocarcinoma.

INDICATIONS:
- Support in the investigation of sexual assault and rape.

- Assist for differential diagnosis of other disorders associated with elevated PAP, red blood cell phosphatase, or platelet phosphatase, such as leukemia.

- Evaluate the efficacy of prostatic cancer therapy (prostatectomy, recurrence). Levels are lower with effective treatment. Rising levels are linked to poor prognosis.

- Investigate or assess an enlarged prostate gland, especially if prostatic Carcinoma is suspected.

RESULT

Increased in:
• Acute myelogenous leukemia
• Benign prostatic hypertrophy
• Gaucher's disease

• Liver disease
• Metastatic bone cancer
• Niemann-Pick disease
• Paget's disease
• After prostate surgery, biopsy, or manipulation
• Prostatic cancer
• Prostatic infarct
• Prostatitis
• Sickle cell crisis
• Thrombocytosis
Decreased in: Not any

IMPEDING FACTORS:

- Products that may raise PAP levels include alglucerase, androgens (female), buserelin, and clofibrate.

- Drugs that may decrease PAP levels include caffeine, fluoride, ketoconazole, oxalate, and phosphate.

- Prostatic massage, rectal, or urinary catheterization within 48 hours of the test can cause elevated PAP rates.

- Specimens should be taken in the morning because PAP has diurnal variation.

PROGESTERONE

SAMPLING:1 mL of serum is collected in a red- or tiger-top tube.
TECHNIQUE: Radioimmunoassay
NORMAL VALUE:

Hormonal State	Conventional Units	SI Units (Conversion Factor X 0.0318)
Prepubertal males and females	< 20 ng/dL	< 0.6 nmol/L
Men	10–50 ng/dL	0.3–1.6 nmol/L
Women		
Follicular phase	< 50 ng/dL	< 1.6 nmol/L
Luteal phase	300–2500 ng/dL	9.5–79.5 nmol/L
Pregnancy, first trimester	725–4400 ng/dL	23.0–139.9 nmol/L
Pregnancy, second trimester	1950–8250 ng/dL	62.0–262.3 nmol/L
Pregnancy, third trimester	6500–22,900 ng/dL	206.7–728.2 nmol/L
Postmenopausal period	< 40 ng/dL	< 1.3 nmol/L

EXPLAINATION:

Progesterone is a sex hormone for women. Its role is to prepare the uterus for conception and breasts for breast lactation. Progesterone monitoring may be used to ensure that ovulation has occurred and to determine the activity of the corpus luteum. Serial measurements may be done to help determine the day of ovulation.

INDICATIONS:

- Assist in the treatment of luteal phase defects (in combination with endometrial biopsy).
- Evaluate patients at risk of early or spontaneous abortion.
- Identify patients at risk of ectopic pregnancy and evaluation of corpus luteum function.
- Monitor ovulating patients during human chorionic gonadotropin (HCG), human menopausal gonadotropin, follicle-stimulating hormone / luteinizing hormone-releasing hormone, or clomiphene induction (serial measurements can help to determine the day of ovulation).
- Monitor patients receiving progesterone replacement therapy.

RESULT:

Increased in:
Congenital adrenal hyperplasia
Hydatidiform mole
Lipoid ovarian tumor
Theca lutein cyst
Chorioepithelioma of the ovary
Decreased in:
Primary or secondary hypogonadism
Short luteal phase syndrome
Threatened abortion
Galactorrhea-amenorrhea syndrome

IMPEDING FACTORS:

- Medicines that may increase the levels of progesterone include clomiphene, corticotropin, hydroxyprogesterone, ketoconazole, mifepristone, progesterone, tamoxifen, and valproic acid.
- Medications that may reduce progesterone levels include ampicillin, epostane, goserelin, leuprolide, and F2 prostaglandin.
- Recent radioactive scans or radiation exposure within one week of the test can conflict with the test results, while radioimmunoassay is the test method.

ESTRADIOL (E2)

SAMPLING:1 mL of serum is collected in a red- or tiger-top tube. 1 ml of Plasma collected in a green-top (heparin) tube is also acceptable.

TECHNIQUE: Immunoassay

NORMAL VALUE:

Age	Conventional Units	SI Units (Conversion Factor 3.67)
6 m–10 y	< 15 pg/mL	< 55 pmol/L
11–15 y		
Male	< 40 pg/mL	< 147 pmol/L
Female	10–300 pg/mL	37–1100 pmol/L
Adult male	10–50 pg/mL	37–184 pmol/L
Adult female		
Early follicular phase	20–150 pg/mL	73–551 pmol/L
Late follicular phase	40–350 pg/mL	147–1285 pmol/L
Midcycle peak	150–750 pg/mL	551–2753 pmol/L
Luteal phase	30–450 pg/mL	110–1652 pmol/L
Post menopause	< 20 pg/mL	< 73 pmol/L

EXPLAINATION:

Estrogens are hormones secreted in large amounts by the ovaries and the placenta during pregnancy. Estradiol is also secreted by the adrenal cortex and the testicles in minute amounts. Just three types of estrogen are present in the blood in quantifiable amounts: estrone, estradiol, and estriol.

Estradiol is the most active of all estrogens. Estron (E1) is the immediate precursor of estradiol (E2). Estriol (E3) is naturally produced in large amounts from the placenta during pregnancy by precursors produced by the fetal liver.

INDICATIONS:

- Help in establishing the prevalence of gonad dysfunction.
- Assess menstrual abnormalities, fertility problems, and estrogen-producing tumors in women and testicular or adrenal tumors and feminization defects in men.
- Monitoring of menotropin (Pergonal) therapy.

Menotropin is a mixture of follicle-stimulating hormone (FSH), and luteinizing hormone (LH) used to stimulate ovulation and increase the probability of conception.

RESULT:

Increased in:
Estrogen-producing tumors

Feminization in children	
Gynecomastia	
Hepatic cirrhosis	
Hyperthyroidism	
Adrenal tumors	
Decreased in:	
Primary and secondary hypogonadism	
Ovarian failure	
Turner's syndrome	

IMPEDING FACTORS:
- Medications that may raise estradiol concentrations include cimetidine, clomiphene, dehydroepiandrosterone, diazepam, estrogen/progestin therapy, ketoconazole, mifepristone (some patients with meningiomas and receiving no other medications), nafarelin, nilutamide, phenytoin, tamoxifen, and troleandomycin.
- Medications that may decrease estradiol levels include aminoglutethimide, chemotherapy drugs, cimetidine, danazol, fadrozole, goserelin, leuprolide, megestrol, mepartricin, mifepristone (pregnant women with pregnancy expulsion), nafarelin (women who are being treated for endometriosis), and oral contraceptives.
- Estradiol is secreted under a biphasic pattern during normal menstruation. Awareness of the menstrual cycle stage may aid in the analysis of estradiol levels.

ESTROGEN AND PROGESTERONE RECEPTOR ASSAYS
Estrogen receptor protein (ERP), progesterone receptor protein (PRP)
SAMPLING: h Breast tissue.
TECHNIQUE: Cytochemical or immunocytochemical
NORMAL VALUE:
The interpretation of the results is subjective, depending on the staining intensity and the number of cells classified as positive. More recently, immunoperoxidase methods using monoclonal antibodies have been introduced. These antibodies are more specific and do not interfere with exogenous hormones.

Cytochemical Findings	Values
Favorable	>20% of cell nuclei are stained
Borderline	11–20% of cell nuclei are stained
Unfavorable findings	<10% of cell nuclei are stained

EXPLAINATION:

Estrogen and progesterone receptor assays are used to classify patients with a form of breast cancer that may be more receptive to estrogen-deprivation (antiestrogen) treatment or ovarian removal than other tumor forms. Patients of these tumor types usually have a clearer diagnosis. Flow cytometry examination of DNA ploidy can also be conducted on malignant cells. Cancer cells contain an unnatural volume of DNA. The larger the tumor cells, the more likely the excessive DNA is to be detected. The number of chromosomes as a set in the nucleus or polidy shows the speed of cell division and the development of the tumor.

INDICATIONS:

- Recognize patients with breast or other varieties of cancer that may respond to hormone or antihormonal therapy.
- Monitor hormonal or antihormonal response for treatment.

RESULT:

Positive findings in:
• **Hormonal therapy**
• **Receptor-positive tumors**
Negative findings in:
Receptor-negative tumors

IMPEDING FACTORS:

- Antiestrogen preparations (e.g., tamoxifen) taken two months before tissue sampling will affect the test results.
- Tissue samples soiled with formalin or failure to properly freeze the specimen using liquid nitrogen or dry ice will deceptively reduce the results.
- Considerable necrosis of tumors or tumors with low cellular composition mistakenly decreases the results.
- Instantly, failure to transport specimens to the laboratory can cause degradation of the receptor sites. Prompt and proper processing, storage, and analysis of specimens are important for the achievement of accurate results.

LUTEINIZING HORMONE

LH, luteotropin, interstitial cell-stimulating hormone (ICSH)

SAMPLING:1 mL of serum is collected in a red- or tiger-top tube. 1 mL of plasma collected in a green-top (heparin) tube is also acceptable.

TECHNIQUE: Immunoassay

NORMAL VALUE:

Concentration by Sex and by Phase (in Women)	Conventional Units	SI (Conversion Factor X1)
Male		
< 2 y	0.5–1.9 mIU/mL	0.5–1.9 IU/L
2–10 y	< 0.5 mIU/mL	< 0.5 IU/L
11–20 y	0.5–5.3 mIU/mL	0.5–5.3 IU/L
Adult	1.2–7.8 mIU/mL	1.2–7.8 IU/L
Female		
< 2–10 y	< 0.5 mIU/mL	< 0.5 IU/L
11–20 y	0.5–9.0 mIU/mL	0.5–9.0 IU/L
Phase in Women		
Follicular	1.7–15.0 mIU/mL	1.7–15.0 IU/L
Ovulatory	21.9–56.6 mIU/mL	21.9–56.6 IU/L
Luteal	0.6–16.3 mIU/mL	0.6–16.3 IU/L
Postmenopausal	14.2–52.3 mIU/mL	14.2–52.3 IU/L

EXPLAINATION:

Luteinizing hormone (LH) is secreted from the anterior pituitary gland among response to a gonadotropin-releasing stimulus, the same hypothalamic release factor that activates follicle-stimulating hormone production. LH affects the gonadal function of both men and women. Among women, LH spikes usually occur at the midpoint of the menstrual cycle (ovulation phase) and are believed to be caused by elevated estrogen levels. LH induces the ovum to be released from the ovaries and stimulates the development of corpus luteum and progesterone output. As progesterone levels rise, LH output decreases. In males, LH accelerates the interstitial cells of Leydig, found in the testicles, to produce testosterone. For this function, LH is sometimes referred to as an interstitial cell-stimulating hormone in males. LH release is pulsatile and maintains circadian rhythm in response to the usual irregular secretion of gonadotropin-releasing hormone.

INDICATIONS:

- Distinguishment between primary and secondary causes of gonadal failure.
- Evaluate children with precocious puberty.
- Evaluate male and female infertility as shown by reduced LH rates.
- Evaluate reaction to ovulation-induced therapy.
- Support treatment of anovulation-induced infertility as shown by lack of LH in the midpoint of the menstrual cycle.

RESULT:

Increased in:
• **Anorchia**
• **Gonadal failure**
• **Menopause**
• **Primary gonadal dysfunction**
Decreased in:
• **Anorexia nervosa**
• **Kallmann's syndrome**
• **Malnutrition**
• **Pituitary or hypothalamic dysfunction**
• **Severe stress**

IMPEDING FACTORS:
- Medications and hormones that may improve LH include clomiphene, gonadotropin-releasing hormone, goserelin, ketoconazole, mestranol, nafarelin, naloxone, nilutamide, spironolactone, and tamoxifen.
- Drugs and hormones that may lower LH include anabolic steroids, anticonvulsants, conjugated estrogens, danazole, digoxin, D-Trp-6-LHRH, estrogen/progestin therapy, goserelin, octreotide, oral contraceptives, phenothiazine, megestrol, norethindrone, pimozide, pravastatin, progesterone, stanozolol, and tamoxifen.
- In menstruating women, values vary depending on the phase of the menstrual cycle.
- LH secretion follows the circadian rhythm, with higher levels increasing during the night.

FOLLICLE-STIMULATING HORMONE (Follitropin, FSH)

SAMPLING: 1 mL of serum is collected in a red- or tiger-top tube.

TECHNIQUE: Immunoassay

NORMAL VALUE:

Status	Conventional Units	SI Units (Conversion Factor X 1)
Prepuberty	< 10 mIU/mL	< 10 IU/L
Men	1.4–15.5 mIU/mL	1.4–15.5 IU/L
Women		
Follicular phase	1.4–9.9 mIU/mL	1.4–9.9 IU/L
Ovulatory peak	6.2–17.2 mIU/mL	6.2–17.2 IU/L
Luteal phase	1.1–9.2 mIU/mL	1.1–9.2 IU/L
Post menopause	19–100 mIU/mL	19–100 IU/L

EXPLAINATION:

Follicular-stimulating hormone (FSH) is produced and stored in the anterior portion of the pituitary gland. In women, FSH facilitates the maturation of the Graafian (germinal) follicle, inducing the production of the estrogen and enabling the ovum to develop. In men, FSH regulates spermatogenesis in part, but testosterone is also required. Gonadotropin-releasing hormone secretion induces a decline in estrogen and testosterone levels. Gonadotropin-releasing hormone release stimulates the secretion of FSH. The development of FSH is impaired by an increase in estrogen and testosterone levels. The development of FSH is pulsatile, episodic, cyclic, and is subject to diurnal variation. Serial measurements are often needed.

INDICATIONS:

- Assistance in deciding between primary and secondary (pituitary or hypothalamic) gonadal dysfunction or menstrual cycle phases as part of infertility study.
- Evaluate undefined (ambiguous) sexual differentiation in infants.
- Assess early sexual maturity of girls younger than nine years of age or boys younger than ten years of age (precocious puberty linked with elevated levels).
- Assess sexual maturation impairment in adolescents.
- Assess testicular dysfunction.
- Investigate impotence, gynecomastia, and menstrual disorders.

RESULT:

Increased in:
• Alcoholism
• Castration
• Gonadal failure
• Klinefelter's syndrome
• Menopause
• Orchitis
• Precocious puberty in children
• Gonadotropin-secreting pituitary tumors
• Primary hypogonadism
• Reifenstein's syndrome
• Turner's syndrome
Decreased in:
• Anorexia nervosa
• Hemochromatosis
• Hyperprolactinemia
• Hypothalamic disorders
• Polycystic ovary disease
• Pregnancy
• Sickle cell anemia
• Anterior pituitary hypofunction

IMPEDING FACTORS:

- Medications that may raise FSH include cimetidine, clomiphene, digitalis, gonadotropin-releasing hormone, ketoconazole, levodopa, nafarelin, naloxone, nilutamide, oxcarbazepine, and pravastatin.
- Medications that may lower FSH levels include anabolic steroids, anticonvulsants, goserelin, megestrol, buserelin, estrogens, corticotropin-releasing hormone, mestranol, oral contraceptives, phenothiazine, progesterone, stanozolol, pimozide, pravastatin, tamoxifen, toremifene, and valproic acid.
- In menstruating women, results vary depending on the phase of the menstrual cycle. Values are higher among postmenopausal women.

ANTI-MÜLLERIAN HORMONE TEST

AMH hormone test, müllerian-inhibiting hormone, MIH, müllerian inhibiting factor, MIF, müllerian-inhibiting substance, MIS

SPECIMEN: 2 ml blood in Red top (plain, no additive) or Gold top (serum separator-SST Gel)

TECHNIQUE: Electrochemiluminescence immunoassay (ECLIA)

NORMAL VALUES:

Higher AMH values (>1 ng/mL) usually signify that a woman has a normal ovarian reserve and lower numbers (<1 ng/mL) may indicate a woman with a low or diminished ovarian reserve (DOR)

Interpretation	AMH Blood Level
High (often an indicator of **PCOS**)	Over 3.0 ng/ml
Normal	Over 1.0 ng/ml
Low Normal Range	0.7 – 0.9 ng/ml
Low	0.3 – 0.6 ng/ml
Very Low	Less than 0.3 ng/ml

EXPLAINATION:

AMH or anti-mullerian hormone is a substance made by granulosa cells in ovarian follicles. It is first produced in primary follicles that move from the primary follicle stage. At these stages, follicles are microscopic and cannot be seen by ultrasound. AMH production is highest in preantral and small antral stages (less than 4 mm in diameter) of development. Almost no AMH was made in follicles of more than 8mm.

As a result, the levels are constant, and AMH testing can be performed on any day of the woman's cycle. AMH is an important fertility test to tell us about a woman's ovarian reserve as it stands today. It is a great tool to assess a woman's current ovarian reserve BUT it cannot predictor of whether a woman can get pregnant spontaneously in the future.

Women with higher AMH values will tend to have a better response to ovarian stimulation for **IVF (in vitro fertilization)**, with more eggs retrieved. Women with lower AMH have lower antral follicular counts and produce a lower number of oocytes (eggs).

INDICATIONS:

- Predict the start of **menopause**, a time in a woman's life when her menstrual periods have stopped and she can't become pregnant anymore. It usually starts when a woman is around 50 years old.
- Find out the reason for early menopause
- Help find out the reason for amenorrhea, the lack of menstruation.

- Help diagnose **polycystic ovary syndrome** (PCOS), a hormonal disorder that is a common cause of **female infertility**, the inability to get pregnant
- Check infants with genitals that are not clearly identified as male or female
- Monitor women who have certain types of ovarian cancer

NOTES

GASTROINTESTINAL AND HEPATOBILIARY SYSTEM

The gastrointestinal tract, (GI tract, GIT, digestive tract, digestion tract, alimentary canal) is the tract from the mouth to the anus which includes all the organs of the digestive system in humans and other animals. The human gastrointestinal tract consists of the esophagus, stomach, and intestines, and is divided into the upper and lower gastrointestinal tracts. The GI tract includes all structures between the mouth and the anus, forming a continuous passageway that includes the main organs of digestion, namely, the stomach, small intestine, and large intestine. However, the complete human digestive system is made up of the gastrointestinal tract plus the accessory organs of digestion (the tongue, salivary glands, pancreas, liver, and gallbladder)

NOTES

_____

_____

_____

_____

_____

_____

_____

_____

_____

_____

_____

_____

_____

AMMONIA (NH3):

SAMPLING:1ml of plasma is collected in a filled green-top (heparin) tube. Specimens should be transported tightly capped and in an ice slurry.

TECHNIQUE: Spectrophotometry

NORMAL VALUE:

Age	Conventional Units	SI Units (Conversion Factor 0.587)
Newborn	170–341 g/dL	100–200 mol/L
Adult	19–60 g/dL	11–35 mol/L

EXPLAINATION:

Blood ammonia (NH3) comes from two main sources: the deamination of amino acids during protein metabolism and the degradation of proteins by the colon bacteria. The liver converts the portal blood ammonia to urea, which is excreted by the kidneys. When liver function is severely impaired, especially in situations where the reduced hepatocellular function is combined with reduced portal blood flow, ammonia levels rise. Ammonia is possibly toxic to the central nervous system.

INDICATIONS:

- Predict possible advanced liver disease or other related disorders with altered serum ammonia levels.
- Identify potential hepatic encephalopathy with well-established liver disease.
- Monitor success of medication for hepatic encephalopathy reported decreased levels.
- Monitor patients receiving hyper-nutrition therapy.

RESULT

Increased in:
Gastrointestinal hemorrhage
Genitourinary tract infection along with distention and stasis
Inborn enzyme deficiency
Hepatic coma
Liver failure, late cirrhosis
Reye's syndrome
Total parenteral nutrition
Decreased in: **Not any specific condition**

IMPEDING FACTORS:

- Drugs that may increase the levels of ammonia include ammonium salts, asparaginase, barbiturates, diuretics, ethanol, fibrin hydrolysate, fluorides, furosemide, thiazides, and valproic acid.

- Drugs/organisms that may decrease the levels of ammonia include diphenhydramine, kanamycin, neomycin, tetracycline, and Lactobacillus acidophilus.
- Hemolysis falsely increases the level of ammonia.
- Prompt and proper processing, storage, and analysis of specimens are important for the achievement of accurate results. The specimen should be obtained on ice; the collection tube should be filled and kept tightly closed. Ammonia increases rapidly in the specimen collected, so the analysis should be carried out within 20 minutes of collection.

AMYLASE

SAMPLING:1ml of serum is collected in a red- or tiger-top tube. 1 ml plasma collected in a green-top (heparin) tube is also acceptable.

TECHNIQUE: Spectrophotometry

NORMAL VALUE:

Conventional Units	SI Units (Conversion Factor X0.017)
30–110 U/L	0.51–1.87 µKat/L

EXPLAINATION:

Amylase, a digestive enzyme, breaks starch into disaccharides. Even though many cells have amylase activity (e.g., liver, small intestine, ovaries, skeletal muscles), circulating amylase is produced from parotid and pancreatic glands. Amylase is a sensitive marker of pancreatic acinar cell damage and pancreatic obstruction. Newborns and infants up to 2 years of age have little detectable serum amylase. Salivary glands produce most of this enzyme in the early years of life.

INDICATIONS:

- Assist in the detection of acute pancreatitis; serum amylase begins to rise within 6 to 24 hours of onset and reverts to normal within 2 to 7 days.
- Assist in the diagnosis of macroamylasemia, alcohol disorder, malabsorption syndrome, and additional digestive problems.
- Help in the diagnosis of pancreatic duct obstruction, which tends to cause serum levels to remain elevated.
- Detect blunt trauma or accidental surgical trauma to the pancreas.

RESULT

Increased in:
• Diabetic ketoacidosis
• Duodenal obstruction
• Ectopic pregnancy
• Abdominal trauma
• Gastric resection

• Macroamylasemia
• Alcoholism
• Common bile duct obstruction
• Postoperative period
• Pancreatic cyst and pseudocyst
• Advanced Carcinoma involving the head of the pancreas
• Parotitis
• Peritonitis
• Mumps
• Pancreatitis
• Perforated peptic ulcer involving the pancreas
• Some tumors of the lung and ovaries
• Viral infections
Decreased in:
• Cystic fibrosis (advanced)
• Hepatic disease (severe)
• Pancreatic insufficiency
• Pancreatectomy

IMPEDING FACTORS:
- Drugs and substances that may raise amylase levels include asparaginase, captopril, cimetidine, clofibrate, corticosteroids, nitrofurantoin, oral contraceptives, estrogens, ethacrynic acid, furosemide, ibuprofen, methyldopa pentamidine, tetracycline, thiazide diuretics, sulfonamides, valproic acid, zalcitabine, and alcohol.
Drugs that may reduce amylase levels include anabolic steroids, citrates, and fluorides.

D-XYLOSE TOLERANCE TEST

SAMPLING: 1 mL of plasma is collected in a gray-top (fluoride/oxalate) tube and 10 mL of urine from a 5-hour collection from a timed collection in a clean amber plastic container.
TECHNIQUE: Spectrophotometry
NORMAL VALUE: Usually the test results are either positive or negative. A positive result means that D-xylose is found in the blood or urine and is therefore being absorbed by the intestines.

EXPLAINATION:
The test used to test for intestinal malabsorption of carbohydrates is D-xylose tolerance test. D-xylose is a pentose sugar that is not usually present in large amounts in the blood. It is partially absorbed as ingested and is usually unmetabolized in the urine.

INDICATIONS: Assist in the evaluation of malabsorption syndromes

RESULT:

Increased in: N/A
Decreased in:
• Nontropical sprue (celiac disease, gluten-induced enteropathy)
• Amyloidosis
• Bacterial overgrowth
• Eosinophilic gastroenteritis
• Lymphoma
• Parasitic infestations (*Giardia*, schistosomiasis, hookworm)
• Radiation enteritis
• Scleroderma
• Small bowel ischemia
• Tropical sprue
• Whipple's disease
• Zollinger-Ellison disease
• Postoperative period after huge resection of the intestine

IMPEDING FACTORS:
- Medications that may increase the levels of D-xylose in urine include phenazopyridine.
- Medications and compounds that may decrease the levels of D-xylose in the urine include acetylsalicylic acid, aminosalicylic acid, arsenic, colchicine, digitalis, ethionamide, gold indometacin, isocarboxazid, kanamycin, monoamine oxidase (MAO) inhibitors, neomycin, and phenelzine.
Poor renal function or vomiting can cause low levels of urine.

BILIRUBIN AND BILIRUBIN FRACTIONS

Conjugated/direct bilirubin, delta bilirubin, unconjugated/indirect bilirubin, TBil.

SAMPLING: 1 ml of serum is collected in a red- or tiger-top tube. 1mL of plasma collected in a green-top (heparin) tube, or a heparinized micro trainer is also acceptable.

TECHNIQUE: Spectrophotometry

NORMAL VALUE: Total bilirubin levels in babies should be lowered to adult levels by day ten as the function of the hepatic circulatory system matures. Values in breastfed infants can take longer to reach normal adult levels. Values in preterm infants may briefly be higher than in full-term infants and may also take longer to lower to normal levels.

Bilirubin	Conventional Units	SI Units (Conversion Factor X 17.1)
Total bilirubin		
Newborn–1 d	1.4–8.7 mg/dL	24–149 µmol/L
1–2 d	3.4–11.5 mg/dL	58–97 µmol/L
3–5 d	1.5–12.0 mg/dL	26–205 µmol/L
1 mo–adult	0.3–1.2 mg/dL	5–21 µmol/L
Unconjugated bilirubin	< 1.1 mg/dL	< 19 µmol/L
Conjugated bilirubin	< 0.3 mg/dL	< 5 µmol/L
Delta bilirubin	< 0.2 mg/dL	< 3 µmol/L

EXPLAINATION:

Bilirubin is a by-product of heme catabolism in old red blood cells. Bilirubin is mainly produced in the liver, spleen, and bone marrow. Total bilirubin is the sum of non-conjugated bilirubin, monoglucuronide and diglucuronide, conjugated bilirubin, and albumin-bound bilirubin delta. Unconjugated bilirubin is delivered to the liver by albumin, where it is conjugated. In the small intestine, conjugated bilirubin is converted to urobilinogen and then to urobilin. Urobilin is excreted in the feces. Increases in bilirubin levels may result from pre-hepatic and/or post-hepatic conditions, making fractionation useful in evaluating the cause of the increase in total bilirubin levels. Delta bilirubin has a longer half-life than other bilirubin fractions and thus remains elevated during recovery after the other fractions have reduced to normal levels. When the concentration of bilirubin rises, the yellowish pigment begins to deposit in the patient's skin and sclera. The increase in yellow pigmentation is called jaundice or icterus.

INDICATIONS:

- Support in the differential diagnosis of obstructive jaundice.

- Aid in the evaluation of liver and biliary disease.

- Examine the effects of drug reactions on liver function.

- Screen for jaundice in newborn patients.

- Scrutinize the effects of phototherapy on jaundiced newborns.

RESULT

Increased in:
Pre hepatic (hemolytic) jaundice
(1) The post–blood transfusion period, when several units are rapidly infused or in the case of a delayed transfusion reaction
(2) Erythroblastosis fetalis
(3) Hematoma
(4) Hemolytic anemias
(5) Pernicious anemia
(6) Red blood cell enzyme abnormalities (i.e., spherocytosis, G-6-PD, pyruvate kinase)
(7) Physiologic jaundice of the newborn
Hepatic jaundice—bilirubin conjugation failure
• Crigler-Najjar syndrome
Hepatic jaundice—a disturbance in bilirubin transport
• Dubin-Johnson syndrome (pre-conjugation transport failure)
• Gilbert's disease (post conjugation transport failure)
Hepatic jaundice—liver damage or necrosis
• Alcoholism
• Cholangitis
• Cholestatic drug reactions
• Cholecystitis
• Cirrhosis
• Hepatitis
• Hepatocellular damage
• Infectious mononucleosis
Posthepatic jaundice
• Advanced tumors of the liver
• Biliary obstruction
Other conditions
• Anorexia or starvation
• Breast milk jaundice
• Hypothyroidism
Decreased in:
Not any specific condition

CRITICAL VALUES:
Sustained hyperbilirubinemia can lead to brain damage. Kernicterus describes the deposition of bilirubin in the basal ganglia and the brainstem nuclei. There is no bilirubin level that places children at risk of developing kernicterus. Signs of kernicterus in babies involve lethargy, poor feeding, upward displacement of eyes, and fits. Amounts over 15 to 20 mg / dL are a cause for intervention. Interventions may include early repeated feeding to promote gastrointestinal motility, phototherapy, and exchange transfusion.

IMPEDING FACTORS:
- Drugs that may rise bilirubin levels by causing cholestasis include amitriptyline, anabolic steroids, androgens, estrogens, ethionamide, gold salts, chlorpropamide, dapsone, erythromycin, benzodiazepines, chlorothiazide, oral contraceptives, penicillins, imipramine, mercaptopurine, nitrofurans, sulfonamides, tamoxifen, phenothiazines, progesterone, propoxyphene, and tolbutamide.
- Medications that may raise bilirubin levels by causing hepatocellular damage include acetaminophen (toxic), acetylsalicylic acid, anabolic steroids, anticonvulsants, allopurinol, amiodarone, azithromycin, bromocriptine, asparaginase, captopril, cephalosporins, chloramphenicol, danazol, enflurane, ethambutol, clindamycin, clofibrate, fluoroquinolones, foscarnet, gentamicin, ethionamide, fenofibrate, fluconazole, interleukin-2, low-molecular-weight heparin, levamisole, levodopa, lincomycin, indomethacin, interferon, monoamine oxidase inhibitors, methyldopa, naproxen, nifedipine, nitrofurans, oral contraceptives, probenecid, procainamide, quinine, ranitidine, retinol, ritodrine, sulfonylureas, tetracyclines, tobramycin, and verapamil.
- Drugs that may raise bilirubin levels by causing hemolysis to include amphotericin B, cephaloridine, cephalothin, chlorpromazine, carbamazepine, carbutamide, chlorpropamide, dinitrophenol, ibuprofen, insulin, isoniazid, levodopa, mefenamic acid, melphalan, methotrexate, methyldopa, penicillin, quinine, rifampin, stibophen, sulfonamides, phenacetin, procainamide, quinidine, and tolbutamide.
- The bilirubin is sensitive to light. It is, therefore, necessary to cover the sample container to protect the sample from light between the time interval of collection and analysis.

HEPATITIS An ANTIBODY

HAV serology

SAMPLING: 1 mL of serum is collected in a red- or tiger-top tube.

TECHNIQUE: Enzyme immunoassay

NORMAL VALUE: Negative.

EXPLAINATION:

The type of hepatitis is also known as a picornavirus. The primary mode of spread is the fecal-oral route under conditions of poor personal hygiene or inadequate sanitation. The incubation period is roughly 28 days, varying from 15 days to 50 days. The onset is usually sudden, with acute illness occurring approximately one week. Therapy is positive, and there is no growth in chronic or carrier conditions. Full studies (immunoglobulin G [IgG] and IgM) of hepatitis A antibody and IgM-specific hepatitis A antibody help to distinguish new infections from prior exposure. If the findings of either IgM-specific or both tests are positive, a recent infection is presumed. If the IgM-specific test results are negative (-ve), and the total antibody test results are positive (+ve), prior contamination is suggested. The clinically relevant assay— IgM-specific antibody— is often the only test required. Jaundice appears in 70 to 80 percent of adult cases of HAV infection and 70 percent of pediatric cases.

INDICATIONS:

- Test individuals at high risk of exposure, such as those in hospitals or jails.
- Screen individuals suspected of having HAV infection.

RESULT:

Positive findings in:

- Individuals with recent hepatitis A infection
- Individuals with previous hepatitis A infection

HEPATITIS B, ANTIGEN AND ANTIBODY

HBeAg, HBeAb, HBcAb, HBsAb, HBsAg

SAMPLING: 1 mL of serum is collected in a red- or tiger-top tube.

TECHNIQUE: Enzyme immunoassay

NORMAL VALUE: Negative.

EXPLAINATION:

The hepatitis B virus (HBV) is known as a double-stranded retrovirus of the Hepadnaviridae family. Its main modes of transmission are parenteral, perinatal, and sexual contact. Serological profiles vary with different circumstances (i.e., asymptomatic infection, acute / resolved infection, coinfection, and chronic carrier status). The development and detectability of markers are also dose dependent. The following description applies to an HBV infection that is resolved. The incubation period is generally between 6 and 16 weeks.

A surface antigen of hepatitis B (HBsAg) is the first precursor to appear upon infection. It is visible 8 to 12 weeks after exposure and often pre-exists with symptoms. Approximately as liver enzymes return to normal levels, the HBsAg titer has fallen to non-detectable levels. When HBsAg is detectable after six months, the patient is likely to become a chronic carrier capable of transmitting the Virus. Hepatitis Antigen (HBeAg) occurs in the serum 10 to 12 weeks after exposure. HBeAg can be identified in the serum of patients with acute or persistent HBV infection and is a symptom of successful viral replication and infection. The rates of hepatitis A antibody (HBeAb) occur approximately 14 weeks after exposure, indicating that the virus is cured and that the patient's ability to spread the disease is gone. The quicker HBeAg fades, the shorter the acute phase of the illness. IgM-specific hepatitis B Core Antibody (HBcAb) emerges 6 to 14 weeks after exposure to HBsAg. It tends to be observable either until the infection is resolved or over a lifetime in patients as a chronic carrier state. In some instances, HBcAb may be the only detectable marker; thus, its sole presence has sometimes been referred to as the core opening.

HBcAb is not an indication of regeneration or immunity; however, it does suggest current or previous infections. Hepatitis B surface antibody (HBsAb) occurs 2 to 16 weeks after HBsAg is gone. The presence of HBsAb reflects the therapeutic recovery and immunity of the infection. The initiation of infection with HBV is usually insidious. Most children and half of the infected adults are asymptomatic. The signs range from mild too extreme during the acute phase of infection. Chronicity is increasing with age. The HBsAg and HBcAb examinations are used to screen donated blood before transfusion. HBsAg monitoring is often part of the routine prenatal screen.

INDICATIONS:
- Detecting exposure to HBV.
- Detecting possible carrier status.
- Screening of blood donated before transfusion.
- Check for persons at high risk of exposure, such as hemodialysis patients, people with multiple sex partners, people with a history of other sexually transmitted diseases, intravenous drug abusers, infants born to infected mothers, individuals residing in hospitals or correctional facilities, beneficiaries of blood or plasma-derived goods, associated health care workers and the public service.

RESULT:
Positive findings in:
- Patients recently infected with HBV
- Patients with a previous HBV infection

IMPEDING FACTORS:
Drugs that may reduce HBeAb and HBsAb include interferon.

HEPATITIS C ANTIBODY

HCV serology, hepatitis non-A/non-B.

SAMPLING: 1 mL of serum is collected in a red- or tiger-top tube.

NORMAL VALUE: Negative.

TECHNIQUE: polymerase chain reaction [PCR], Enzyme immunoassay, branch DNA [bDNA], recombinant immunoblot assay [RIBA]

EXPLAINATION:

Hepatitis C virus (HCV) causes the majority of non-A, non-B, bloodborne hepatitis. Its main modes of transmission are maternal, perinatal, and sexual contact. The virus is studied to be a flavivirus and contains a single-stranded RNA core. The period of incubation varies widely, from 2 to 52 weeks. Onset is progressive, and there is a high risk of chronic liver disease following infection. On average, hepatitis C antibodies are detected in approximately 45 percent of infected individuals within six weeks of infection. The remaining 55% will produce antibodies within the next 6 to 12 months. When infected with HCV, 50 % of patients will become chronic carriers. Infected individuals and carriers have a high incidence of chronic liver diseases, such as cirrhosis and chronic active hepatitis, and a higher risk of developing hepatocellular cancer. Hepatitis C transmission by blood transfusion has decreased dramatically since it became part of the routine blood donor screening panel. Pregnancy transmission is likely, especially in the presence of the human immunodeficiency virus (HIV) co-infection. This test is, therefore, often included in prenatal testing kits.

INDICATIONS:

- Assist in the evaluation of non-A, non-B viral hepatitis infection.
- Monitor patients suspected of being diagnosed with HCV but who have not yet developed an antibody.
- Monitoring of blood donated before transfusion.

RESULT:

Positive findings in:

- Patients presently infected with HCV
- Patients with a previous HCV infection

IMPEDING FACTORS:

Drugs that may reduce the levels of the hepatitis C antibody include interferon.

HEPATITIS D ANTIBODY
Delta hepatitis
SAMPLING:1 mL of serum is collected in a red- or tiger-top tube.
TECHNIQUE: Enzyme immunoassay, EIA
NORMAL VALUE: Negative.
EXPLAINATION:
Symptoms of hepatitis D virus (HDV) contamination are similar but often more severe than those of hepatitis B virus (HBV) infection. As with HBV, parenteral, perinatal, and sexual contact are the primary modes of HDV transmission. The virus has a single-stranded RNA core. To reproduce, it requires the presence of the outer coat of hepatitis B. Therefore, HDV infection can only appear with hepatitis B coinfection or superinfection. The start is abrupt, after an incubation period of between 3 and 13 weeks. Due to its dependence on HBV, prevention can be achieved by using the same pre-exposure and post-exposure protective measures used for HBV.
INDICATIONS: Establish the occurrence of coinfection or superinfection in patients with HBV (the clinical course of superinfection is more severe).
RESULT:
Positive findings in:
- Individuals currently infected with HDV
- Persons with a past HDV infection
IMPEDING FACTORS:
Medicines that may reduce the hepatitis D antibody levels include interferon.

HELICOBACTER PYLORI ANTIBODY (H. Pylori Antibody)
SAMPLING:1 mL of serum is collected in a plain red-top tube.
TECHNIQUE: Enzyme-linked immunosorbent assay [ELISA]
NORMAL VALUE: Negative.
EXPLAINATION:
There is a strong association between infection with Helicobacter pylori and gastric cancer, duodenal and gastric ulcer, and chronic gastritis. Immunoglobulin G (IgG) antibodies may be detected for up to 1 year after diagnosis. The H. Pylori can also be confirmed by a positive urea breath test, a positive stool sample, or a positive endoscopic biopsy. Patients with symptoms and H. Pylori infection is considered to have been infected with the organism; patients that show signs of H. Pylori, but without symptoms, is said to be colonized.
INDICATIONS:
- Attend the distinction between H. Pylori infection and nonsteroidal anti-inflammatory medication (NSAID) use as a source of gastritis or peptic or duodenal ulcer.
- Assist in the treatment of gastritis, gastric carcinoma or peptic or duodenal ulcer.

RESULT

Positive findings in:
• **H. Pylori infection**
• **H. Pylori colonization**
Negative findings in **N/A**

LIPASE

Triacylglycerol acylhydrolase

SAMPLING: 1 mL of serum is collected in a red- or tiger-top tube. 1 mL of plasma collected in a green-top (heparin) tube is also acceptable.

TECHNIQUE: Spectrophotometry

NORMAL VALUE: Plasma values may be 15 percent lower than serum values.

Conventional Units	SI Units (Conversion Factor X0.017)
40–375 U/L	0.68–6.38 µKat/L

EXPLAINATION:

Lipases are digestive enzymes that are secreted into the duodenum by the pancreas. Various lipolytic enzymes have specific substrates, but the aggregate function is collectively referred to as lipase. Lipase is active in fat digestion by breaking down triglycerides into fatty acids and glycerol. Lipase is released into the bloodstream when pancreatic acinar cells are damaged. The presence in the blood suggests a pancreatic disorder because it is the only organ that secretes the enzyme.

INDICATIONS:

- Assistance in the diagnosis of acute and chronic pancreatitis.

- Aid in the diagnosis of pancreatic carcinoma.

RESULT:

Increased in:
• **Acute cholecystitis**
• **Obstruction of the pancreatic duct**
• **Pancreatic cyst or pseudocyst**
• **Pancreatic carcinoma (early)**
• **Pancreatic inflammation**
• **Pancreatitis (acute and chronic)**
• **Renal failure (early)**
Decreased in: **N/A**

IMPEDING FACTORS:
- Drugs that may raise lipase levels include asparaginase, azathioprine, cholinergic, codeine, deoxycholate, didanosine, glycocholate, indometacin, methacholine, methylprednisolone, morphine, opioids, pancreozyme, pentazocine, and taurocholate.
- Products that may decrease lipase levels include protamine and saline (intravenous infusions).
- Endoscopic retrograde cholangiopancreatography can increase the levels of lipase.
- The amount of serum lipase increases with hemodialysis. Predialysis specimens should, therefore, be collected for analysis of lipase.

LACTOSE TOLERANCE TEST (LTT)

SAMPLING: 1 mL of plasma is collected in a gray-top (fluoride/oxalate) tube.
TECHNIQUE: Spectrophotometry
NORMAL VALUE:

Change in Glucose Value	Conventional Units	SI Units (Conversion Factor X0.0555)
Normal*	>30 mg/dL	>1.7 mmol/L
Inconclusive*	20–30 mg/dL	1.1–1.7 mmol/L
Abnormal*	< 20 mg/dL	< 1.1 mmol/L

EXPLAINATION:
Lactose is a disaccharide found in milk products. When ingested, lactose is broken down into glucose and galactose by the sugar-splitting enzyme lactase in the intestine. If sufficient lactase is not available, lactose is metabolized by intestinal bacteria, resulting in abdominal bloating, pain, flattening, and diarrhea. The lactose tolerance test tests for lactose intolerance by calculating glucose levels following the ingestion of the lactose dosage.

INDICATIONS: Assess patients for suspected lactose intolerance.
RESULT:

Glucose levels increased in N/A
Glucose levels decreased in Lactose intolerance

IMPEDING FACTORS:
- Various drugs that alter the level of glucose (see the monograph entitled "Glucose").
- Failure to limit diet and exercise can change the results of the tests.
- Delayed gastric emptying can reduce glucose levels.
- Smoking can falsely increase the level of glucose.

LACTATE DEHYDROGENASE AND ISOENZYMES

LDH and isos, LD, and isos

SAMPLING: 1 mL of serum is collected in a red- or tiger-top tube.

TECHNIQUE: Electrophoretic analysis for isoenzymes, Enzymatic analysis for lactate dehydrogenase

NORMAL VALUE: Normal ranges are method dependent and may vary from laboratory to laboratory.

Age	Conventional Units	SI Units (Conversion Factor X1)
1–3 y	500–920 U/L	500–920 U/L
4–6 y	470–900 U/L	470–900 U/L
7–9 y	420–750 U/L	420–750 U/L
10–13 y	432–750 U/L	432–750 U/L
14–15 y	360–730 U/L	360–730 U/L
16–19 y	340–670 U/L	340–670 U/L
Adult	313–618 U/L	313–618 U/L

EXPLAINATION:

Lactate dehydrogenase or LDH is an enzyme that catalyzes the reversible conversion of lactate to pyruvate in cells. Because many tissues produce LDH, elevated total LDH is considered a non-specific measure of cell damage unless other clinical data show the origin of the tissue. The determination of tissue origin is assisted by an electrophoretic study of the five isoenzymes unique to certain tissues. The heart and erythrocytes are abundant in LDH1, LDH2, and LDH3; the kidneys have large amounts of LDH3 and LDH4; and the liver and skeletal muscles are high in LDH4 and LDH5. Some glands (e.g., thyroid, adrenal, thymus), pancreas, spleen, lungs, lymph nodes, which white blood cells produce LDH3, while the ilium is an additional source of LDH5. Studies of the sixth isoenzyme of LDH have been published. This is seen in patients with severe liver disease and is a sign of an extremely poor prognosis. LDH is present in everybody's tissue. It is not used as a common diagnostic marker. Checking for the involvement of LDH and isoenzymes is increasingly used to validate acute myocardial infarction (MI), having been substituted by more sensitive and specific creatine kinase (CK-MB) and troponin assays.

INDICATIONS:

- Acute MI differentiation was shown by elevated LDH1 and LDH2, from pulmonary infarction and liver problems that increase LDH4 and LDH5.
- Evaluate the degree of muscle loss in muscular dystrophy (LDH levels rise early in this condition, and normal approach as muscle mass declines atrophy).
- Evaluate the efficacy of cancer chemotherapy (LDH levels should be decreased with successful treatment).

- Evaluate red cell hemolysis or renal infarction, particularly as suggested by the LDH1:LDH2 reversal ratio.
- Investigate acute MI or expansion, as shown by elevation (usually) of total LDH, the elevation of LDH1 and LDH2, and reversal of LDH1:LDH2 ratio within 48 hours of infarction.
- Investigate chronic liver, lung, and kidney disorders, as shown by LDH levels that remain persistently high.

RESULT:

Total LDH increased in:		
• Lukemias		
• MI or pulmonary infarction		
• Carcinoma of the liver		
• Chronic alcoholism		
• Cirrhosis		
• Congestive heart failure		
• Hemolytic anemias		
• Hypoxia		
• Megaloblastic and pernicious anemia		
• Musculoskeletal disease		
• Obstructive jaundice		
• Pancreatitis		
• Renal disease (severe)		
• Shock		
• Viral hepatitis		
Total LDH decreased in: **N/A**		
LDH Fraction	% of Total	Fraction of Total
LDH1	14–26	0.14–0.26
LDH2	29–39	0.29–0.39

LDH3	20–26	0.20–0.26
LDH4	8–16	0.08–0.16
LDH5	6–16	0.06–0.16

LDH Isoenzymes:

- LDH1 fraction elevated over LDH2 can be seen in acute MI, anemia (pernicious, hemolytic, acute sickle cell, megaloblastic, hemolytic), and acute renal cortical damage due to any cause. In specific, the LDH1 fraction is elevated in cases of germ cell tumors.
- Changes in the middle fractions are associated with conditions in which there has been massive destruction of platelets (e.g., pulmonary embolism, post-transfusion period) and lymphatic system disorders (e.g., viral mononucleosis, lymphomas, lymphocytic leukemia).

IMPEDING FACTORS:
- Drugs that may raise total LDH levels include amiodarone, etretinate, fluosol-DA, methotrexate, oxacillin, plicamycin, propoxyphene, and streptokinase.
- Medications that may decrease overall LDH levels include ascorbic acid, cefotaxime, enalapril, fluoride, naltrexone, and oxylate.
- Hemolysis can cause significant false elevations of total LDH and a false "flip" pattern of isoenzymes because the LDH1 fraction is of red blood cell origin.
- Certain isoenzymes are temperature sensitive; thus, prolonged storage at cooling temperatures can cause false decreases.

ALANINE AMINOTRANSFERASE
(ALT, Serum glutamic pyruvate transaminase (SGPT)).
SAMPLING: 1 ml serum is collected in a red- or tiger-top tube. 1 ml Plasma collected in a green-top (heparin) tube is also acceptable.
TECHNIQUE: Spectrophotometry
NORMAL value:

Age	Conventional Units	SI Units (Conversion Factor X0.017)
Newborn–1 y	13–45 U/L	0.22–0.77 µKat/L
2 y–adult		
Male	10–40 U/L	0.17–0.68 µKat/L
Female	7–35 U/L	0.12–0.60 µKat/L

EXPLAINATION:

Alanine aminotransferase (ALT), previously known as serum glutamic pyruvic transaminase (SGPT), is an enzyme produced by the liver. This acts as a catalyst for the reversible transition of the amino group between alanine and α-ketoglutarate. The highest concentration of ALT is present in liver cells, low levels are found in kidney cells, and smaller amounts are found in the heart and skeletal muscles. If liver damage occurs, serum ALT levels rise to 50 times average, making this an effective measure in the assessment of the liver injury. ALT is also used to assess and screen donated blood before transfusion, as the enzyme may be elevated in the absence of detectable serological markers for hepatitis.

INDICATIONS:

- Compare serially with aspartate aminotransferase (AST) rates to control the progression of liver disease.
- Control liver damage caused by hepatotoxic medications.
- Control response to liver disease therapy, with tissue repair indicating gradually declining levels.
- In blood banks, using hepatitis as a regular test in blood samples from donors.
Tests are excluded if they are more than 1.5 times the upper limits of standard.

RESULT
Increased in:
• **Acute pancreatitis**
• **Cirrhosis**
• **Fatty liver**
• **Hepatic Carcinoma**
• **Hepatitis**
• **Biliary tract obstruction**
• **Burns (severe)**
• **Chronic alcohol abuse**
• **Myocardial infarction**
• **Myositis**
• **Preeclampsia**
• **Shock (severe)**
• **Infectious mononucleosis**
• **After muscle injury from intramuscular injections, trauma, infection, and seizures (current)**
• **Muscular dystrophy**
Decreased in:
• **Pyridoxal phosphate deficiency**

IMPEDING FACTORS:

- Drugs that may increase ALT levels by producing cholestasis:
These include amitriptyline, anabolic steroids, androgens, benzodiazepines, chlorothiazide, chlorpropamide, dapsone, erythromycin, estrogens, ethionamide, progesterone, propoxyphene, sulfonamides, tamoxifen, gold salts, imipramine, mercaptopurine, nitrofurans, oral contraceptives, penicillins, phenothiazines, and tolbutamide.

Drugs that may raise ALT levels by causing hepatocellular damage:
These include acetaminophen (toxic), acetylsalicylic acid, allopurinol, amiodarone, anabolic steroids, anticonvulsants, asparaginase, clindamycin, clofibrate, danazol, enflurane, ethambutol, ethionamide, fenofibrate, fluconazole, azithromycin, bromocriptine, captopril, cephalosporins, chloramphenicol, fluoroquinolones, foscarnet, gentamicin, indomethacin, interferon, interleukin-2, levamisole, Levodopa, lincomycin, monoamine oxidase inhibitors, low-molecular-weight heparin, methyldopa, naproxen, nifedipine, nitrofurans, quinine, ranitidine, retinol, ritodrine, sulfonylureas, oral contraceptives, probenecid, procainamide, tetracyclines, tobramycin, and verapamil.

Drugs that may reduce ALT levels include cyclosporine and interferon.

ASPARTATE AMINOTRANSPEPTIDASE
(Serum glutamic-oxaloacetic transaminase, AST, SGOT)

SAMPLING: 1 mL of serum is collected in a red- or tiger-top tube.
TECHNIQUE: Spectrophotometry, enzymatic at 37ºC
NORMAL VALUE:

Age	Conventional Units	SI Units (Conversion Factor X0.17)
Newborn	47–150 U/L	0.80–2.55 Kat/L
10 d–23 m	9–80 U/L	0.15–1.36 Kat/L
2–59 y		
Male	15–40 U/L	0.26–0.68 Kat/L
Female	13–35 U/L	0.22–0.60 Kat/L
60–90 y		
Male	19–48 U/L	0.32–0.82 Kat/L
Female	9–36 U/L	0.15–0.61 Kat/L

EXPLAINATION:

Aspartate aminotransferase (AST) is an enzyme that catalyzes the reversible transfer of amino acids between aspartate and-ketoglutaric acid. Formerly known as serum glutamic-oxaloacetic transaminase (SGOT). AST occurs in large amounts in the liver and myocardial cells, and in smaller but significant concentrations in the skeletal muscles, the kidneys, the pancreas, and the brain. Serum AST increases when there is cell damage to the tissues where the enzyme is located. AST levels >500 U / L are typically associated with acute hepatitis and other hepatocellular diseases. AST levels are extremely high at birth and decrease with age. Note: AST calculation in the evaluation of myocardial infarction has been replaced by more sensitive tests, such as creatine kinase–MB fraction (CK-MB) and troponin.

INDICATIONS:

- Aid with the treatment of conditions or problems and wounds affecting organs, where AST is usually found.
- Assistance (formerly) in the diagnosis of Myocardial infarction (note: AST is rising). Within 6 to 8 hours, peaks at 24 to 48 hours, and it is dropping to normal inside 72 to 96 hours.
- Series comparison of alanine aminotransferase levels to monitor the course of action infection of the liver.
- Track reaction to therapy of potential hepatotoxic or nephrotoxic products.
- Track reaction to treatment of various conditions in which AST can be present and elevated, with tissue repair, suggested decreased rates.

RESULT

Meaningfully increased in (>five times normal levels):
• **Acute hepatitis**
• **Acute pancreatitis**
• **Liver tumors**
• **Acute hepatocellular disease**
Relatively increased in (three to five times normal levels):
• **Congestive heart failure**
• **Dermatomyositis• Biliary tract obstruction**
• **Cardiac arrhythmias**
• **Chronic hepatitis**
• **Shock**
• **Muscular dystrophy**
Slightly increased in (two to three times than normal):
• **Pericarditis**
• **Pulmonary infarction**

•	Cerebrovascular accident
•	Cirrhosis, fatty liver
•	Delirium tremens
•	Hemolytic anemia

IMPEDING FACTORS:
- Drugs that may rise AST levels by causing cholestasis include amitriptyline, anabolic steroids, androgens, benzodiazepines, estrogens, ethionamide, gold salts, nitrofurans, oral contraceptives, imipramine, mercaptopurine, penicillins, phenothiazines, chlorothiazide, chlorpropamide, dapsone, erythromycin, progesterone, propoxyphene, sulfonamides, tamoxifen, and tolbutamide.
- Drugs that may rise AST levels by causing hepatocellular damage consist of acetaminophen (toxic), acetylsalicylic acid, asparaginase, allopurinol, amiodarone, anabolic steroids, anticonvulsants, azithromycin, bromocriptine, captopril, cephalosporins, chloramphenicol, ethambutol, ethionamide, fenofibrate, clindamycin, clofibrate, danazol, enflurane, levodopa, lincomycin, low-molecular-weight heparin, methyldopa, monoamine, fluconazole, fluoroquinolones, probenecid, procainamide, quinine, ranitidine, retinol, ritodrine, sulfonylureas, foscarnet, gentamicin, indomethacin, interferon, interleukin-2, levamisole, oxidase inhibitors, naproxen, nifedipine, nitrofurans, oral contraceptives, tetracyclines, tobramycin, and verapamil.
- Hemolysis falsely rises the AST values.

ALBUMIN AND ALBUMIN/ GLOBULIN RATIO (Alb, A/G ratio)

SAMPLING:1ml serum is collected in a red- or tiger-top tube. 1ml plasma collected in a green-top (heparin) tube is also standard.

TECHNIQUE: Spectrophotometry

NORMAL value: Usually, the albumin/globulin (A/G) ratio is >1.

Age	Conventional Units	SI Units (Conversion Factor 10)
Newborn–4 d	2.8–4.4 g/dL	28–44 g/L
5 d–14 y	3.8–5.4 g/dL	38–54 g/L
15–18 y	3.2–4.5 g/dL	32–45 g/L
19–60 y	3.4–4.8 g/dL	34–48 g/L
61–90 y	3.2–4.6 g/dL	32–46 g/L
>90 y	2.9–4.5 g/dL	29–45 g/L

EXPLAINATION:

For most, the body's total protein is a combination of albumin and globulin. Albumin, the protein present at the highest concentrations, is the main transport protein in the body. Albumin also retains oncotic plasma pressure. Serum albumin values are affected by the synthesis, distribution, and degradation process. Low levels may be the consequence of either inadequate production or excessive losses. Albumin levels are more useful as a sign of chronic deficiency than short-term deficiency.

The amount of albumin is affected by posture. The findings of specimens collected in an upright position are higher than the results of samples collected in a supine posture. The A/G ratio is helpful in the assessment of liver and kidney disease. The ratio is analyzed using the following formula:

albumin/(total protein-albumin),

where globulin is the variation between the total protein value and the albumin value. For instance, with a total protein of 7 g / dL and albumin of 4 g / dL, the ratio of A/G is measured as 4/(7–4) or 4/3= 1.33. The reverse of the ratio where globulin equals albumin (i.e., the ratio of < 1.0) is clinically significant.

INDICATIONS:
- Evaluate the nutritional status of hospitalized patients, especially geriatric patients
- Evaluate chronic illness
-Any condition that results in a decrease in plasma water (e.g., dehydration)
- Hyperinflation of albumin

Results:

Decreased in:
• **Insufficient intake**
• **Malabsorption malnutrition**
• **Decreased synthesis by the liver**
• **Neoplasm**
• **Inflammation and chronic ailments**
• **Amyloidosis Bacterial Monoclonal gammopathies (e.g., multiple myeloma, Waldenström's macroglobulinemia)**
• **Parasitic infestations**
• **Peptic ulcer**
• **Sustaine infections**
• **Immobilization**

• Rheumatic diseases
• Severe skin disease
• Acute and chronic liver ailments (e.g., alcoholism, cirrhosis, and hepatitis)
Increased loss over body surface:
• Rapid hydration or overhydration Burns
• Enteropathies due to vulnerability to swallowed substances (e.g., gluten allergy, Crohn's disease, ulcerative Colitis)
• Fistula (gastrointestinal or lymphatic)
• Decreased catabolism in Cushing's disease and Preeclampsia
• Hemorrhage
• Kidney diseaes
• Renal protein dificiency
• Recurrent thoracentesis or paracentesis
• Damage and crushing accidents
Increased in:
• Thyroid dysfunction
• Increased blood volume (hypervolemia)
• Congestive heart failure
• Pregnancy
• Monoclonal gammopathies (Waldenström's disease, myeloma)

IMPEDING FACTORS:

- Medications that may increase the level of albumin include enalapril.
- Drugs that may decrease albumin levels consist of acetaminophen (poisoning), dapsone, dextran, estrogens, prednisone (high doses), trazodone, ibuprofen, nitrofurantoin, oral contraceptives, phenytoin, and valproic acid.
- The effectiveness of drugs administered is affected by variations in albumin levels

.

OVA AND PARASITES, STOOL
SAMPLING: Stool is collected in clean plastic, tightly capped container.
TECHNIQUE: Macroscopic and microscopic examination
NORMAL VALUE: No presence of parasites, ova, or larvae.

EXPLAINATION:
This test evaluates stools for the involvement of intestinal parasites and their larvae. Some parasites are non-pathogenic; others, such as protozoa and worms, can cause serious illness.

INDICATIONS: Aid in the diagnosis of parasitic infestation.

RESULT:

Positive findings in:
• Amebiasis—*Entamoeba histolytica* infection
• Ascariasis—*Ascaris lumbricoides* infection
• Schistosomiasis—*Schistosoma haematobium, Schistosoma japonicum, Schistosoma mansoni* infection
• Strongyloidiasis—*Strongyloides stercoralis* infection
• Blastocystis—*Blastocystis hominis* infection
• Giardiasis—*Giardia lamblia* infection
• Hookworm disease—*Ancylostoma duodenale, Necator americanus* infection
• Isospora—*Isospora Belli* infection
• Cryptosporidiosis—*Cryptosporidium parvum* infection
• Enterobiasis—*Enterobius vermicularis* (pinworm) infection
• Tapeworm disease—*Diphyllobothrium, Hymenolepiasis, Taenia solium* infection, *Taenia saginata*
• Trematode disease—*Clonorchis Sinensis, Fasciolopsis buski* infection, *Fasciola hepatica*
• Trichuriasis—*Trichuris trichiura* infection

IMPEDING FACTORS:
- Failure to test a fresh specimen can result in a false-negative result.
- Antimicrobial or anti-amebic therapy can yield false-negative results within ten days of the study.
- Failure to wait one week after a gastrointestinal analysis using barium or after laxative use may influence test results.
- Medications such as antacids, bismuth, antibiotics, castor oil, antidiarrheal compounds, iron, magnesia, or psyllium (Metamucil) can interfere with the analysis.

PERITONEAL FLUID ANALYSIS (Ascites fluid analysis)

SAMPLING: 5 mL of peritoneal fluid is obtained in a red-or green-top (heparin) tube for amylase, glucose, and alkaline phosphatase; lavender-top (ethylenediaminetetraacetic acid[EDTA]) cell count tube; sterile tubes for microbiological specimens; 200 to 500 mL of liquid in a transparent cytological anticoagulant jar.

TECHNIQUE: Glucose, amylase, and alkaline phosphatase spectrophotometry; automatic or manual cell count, a macroscopic inspection of cultured organisms, and microscopic examination of specimens for microbiology, cytology, and study of cultured microorganisms

NORMAL VALUE:

Peritoneal Fluid	NORMAL Value
Appearance	Clear
Color	Pale yellow
Amylase	Parallel serum values
Alkaline phosphatase	Parallel serum values
Glucose	Parallel serum values
Red blood cell count	< 100,000/mm^3
White blood cell count	< 300/mm^3
Culture	No growth
Acid-fast stain	No organisms are seen
Gram stain	No organisms are seen
Cytology	No abnormal cells are seen

EXPLAINATION: The peritoneal cavity and the organs inside it are covered with a protective membrane. The fluid between the membranes is called fluid. Usually, only a small amount of fluid is present because the rate of fluid production and absorption is roughly the same. Some pathological conditions can lead to fluid build-up in the peritoneal cavity. Specific tests are usually performed in addition to a standard set of tests used to differentiate a transudate from an exudate. Transudates are just like effusions that form because of systemic dysfunction that disrupts fluid balance regulation such as alleged perforation. Exudates are caused by conditions involving the membrane tissue itself, such as infection or malignancy. The fluid is removed by needle aspiration from the peritoneal cavity.

Characteristic	Transudate	Exudate
Appearance	Clear	Cloudy or turbid
Specific gravity	< 1.015	>1.015

Total protein	< 2.5 g/dL	>3.0 g/dL
Fluid-to-serum protein ratio	< 0.5	>0.5
LDH	Parallels serum value	< 200 U/L
Fluid-to-serum LDH ratio	< 0.6	>0.6
Fluid cholesterol	< 55 mg/dL	>55 mg/dL
White blood cell count	< 100/mm³	>1000/mm³

INDICATIONS:

- Ascites of unknown cause.
- Evaluate alleged peritoneal rupture, perforation, malignancy, or infection.

RESULT:

Increased in (condition/test showing increased result):
Abdominal malignancy (red blood cell count [RBC], carcinoembryonic antigen, anomalous cytology)
Abdominal trauma (RBC count >100,000 / mm3)
Cirrhosis-related ascites (white blood cell count [WBC], neutrophils >25% but < 50%, total granulocyte count >250 / mm3)
Bacterial peritonitis (WBC count, neutrophils >50%, total granulocyte count >250 / mm3)
Peritoneal effusion due to perforation, gastric strangulation, or necrosis (amylase, ammonia, alkaline phosphatase)
Peritoneal effusion due to pancreatic trauma, pancreatitis, or pancreatic pseudocyst (amylase)
Rupture or perforation of the urinary bladder (ammonia, creatinine, urea)
Tuberculosis (high lymphocyte count, positive acid-fast bacillus, and culture [25 to 50 percent of cases])
Decreased in (condition/test showing decreased result):
Abdominal malignancy (glucose)
Tuberculous effusion (glucose)

IMPEDING FACTORS:

A traumatic tap may obtain

- Bloody fluids.
- Unexplained hyperglycemia or hypoglycemia may be confusing when measuring fluid and blood glucose levels. It is therefore recommended to obtain comparative serum samples a few hours before paracentesis is done.

PSEUDOCHOLINESTERASE AND DIBUCAINE NUMBER (CHS, PCHE, AcCHS)

SAMPLING: 1 mL of plasma is collected in a lavender-top (ethylenediaminetetraacetic acid [EDTA]) tube. 1 mL of serum collected in a red-top tube is also acceptable.

TECHNIQUE: Spectrophotometry, kinetic

NORMAL VALUE:

Test	Conventional Units	SI Units (Conversion Factor 1)
Pseudocholinesterase	2–11 U/mL	2–11 kU/L
Dibucaine Number	**Fraction (%) of Activity Inhibited**	**SI Units (Conversion Factor 0.01)**
Normal homozygote	79–84%	0.79–0.84 kU/L
Heterozygote	55–70%	0.55–0.70 kU/L
Abnormal homozygote	16–28%	0.16–0.28 kU/L

INDICATIONS:

- Assist in the assessment of liver function.

- Screening of pathological pseudocholinesterase genotypes in people with a family history of succinylcholine exposure who are about to undergo succinylcholine anesthesia.

RESULT:

Increased in:
• **Diabetes**
• **Hyperthyroidism**
• **Nephrotic syndrome**
• **Obesity**
Decreased in:
• **Congenital deficiency**
• **Acute infection**
• **Anemia (severe)**
• **Carcinomatosis**
• **Cirrhosis**
• **Hepatic carcinoma**
• **Hepatocellular disease**
• **Infectious hepatitis**
• **Malnutrition**
• **Muscular dystrophy**

•	Myocardial infarction
•	Plasmapheresis
•	Succinylcholine hypersensitivity
•	Insecticide exposure (organic phosphate)
•	Tuberculosis
•	Uremia

CRITICAL VALUES:

If the test result is positive and surgery is set, inform the anesthesiologist. A positive result indicates that the patient is at risk of chronic or unrecoverable apnea due to the inability to metabolize succinylcholine.

IMPEDING FACTORS:

- Medications and compounds that may decrease the level of pseudocholinesterase include ambenonium, barbiturates, cyclophosphamide, echothiophate, edrophonium, fluorides, ibuprofen, iodipamide, iopanoic acid, isofluorphate, neostigmine, parathion, procainamide, physostigmine, pyridostigmine, estrogens, and oral contraceptives.

- Medications that may increase the level of pseudocholinesterase include carbamazepine, phenytoin, and valproic acid.

- Pregnancy lowers the value of pseudocholinesterase by about 30%.

- Improper anticoagulant: fluoride interferes with the calculation and induces a misleading decrease in value

CERULOPLASMIN (Copper oxidase, Cp.)

SAMPLING: 1 mL of serum is collected in a red- or tiger-top tube.

TECHNIQUE: Nephelometry

NORMAL VALUE:

Age	Conventional Units	SI Units (Conversion Factor 10)
Newborn–3 mo	5–18 mg/dL	50–180 mg/L
6–2 mo	33–43 mg/dL	330–430 mg/L
1–3 y	26–55 mg/dL	260–550 mg/Lg
4–5 y	27–56 mg/dL	270–560 mg/L
6–7 y	24–48 mg/dL	240–480 mg/L
>7 y	20–54 mg/dL	200–540 mg/L

EXPLAINATION:

Ceruloplasmin is an α2-globulin generated by the liver that binds copper into the blood after it is absorbed from the gastrointestinal system. Decreased production of this globulin allows copper to be stored in body tissues such as the brain, kidneys, liver, and cornea.

INDICATIONS:

- Help in the diagnosis of Menkes (Kinky Hair) Syndrome aid in the diagnosis of Wilson's disease.
- Determine genetic predisposition to Wilson's disease.
- Regularly monitor response to total parenteral nutrition (hyperalimentation).

RESULT:

Increased in:
Acute infections
Biliary cirrhosis
Copper intoxication
Hodgkin's disease
Leukemia
Pregnancy (last trimester)
Cancer of the bone, lung, stomach
Rheumatoid arthritis
Tissue necrosis
Decreased in:
Menkes syndrome
Nutritional deficiency of copper
Wilson's disease

IMPEDING FACTORS:

- Drugs that may enhance the level of ceruloplasmin include anticonvulsants, norethindrone, oral contraceptives, and tamoxifen.
- Medications that may decrease the levels of ceruloplasmin include asparaginase and levonorgestrel (Norplant).
- Excessive therapeutic consumption of zinc can interfere with copper intestinal absorption.

RESPIRATORY SYSTEM

The respiratory system (also respiratory apparatus, ventilatory system) is a biological system consisting of specific organs and structures used for gas exchange in animals

In humans and other mammals, the anatomy of a typical respiratory system is the respiratory tract. The tract is divided into an upper and a lower respiratory tract. The upper tract includes the nose, nasal cavities, sinuses, pharynx, and the part of the larynx above the vocal folds. The lower tract includes the lower part of the larynx, the trachea, bronchi, bronchioles, and the alveoli.

The branching airways of the lower tract are often described as the respiratory tree or tracheobronchial tree. The alveoli are the dead-end terminals of the "tree"where final gaseous exchange takes place.

NOTES

_____

_____

_____

_____

_____

_____

_____

_____

_____

_____

_____

_____

_____

_____

_____

_____

BLOOD GASES

Arterial blood gases (ABGs), capillary blood gases, venous blood gases, cord blood gases.

SAMPLING: Whole blood. Specimen volume and collection containers may vary with the collection method. See the interest section for specific collection instructions. Specimens should be tightly capped and transported in an ice slurry.
TECHNIQUE: Selective electrodes for pH, pO2, and pCO2
NORMAL VALUE:

Blood Gas Value (pH)	Birth, Cord, Full Term	Adult/Child
Arterial	7.11–7.36	7.35–7.45
Venous	7.25–7.45	7.32–7.43
Capillary	7.32–7.49	7.35–7.45
Scalp	7.25–7.40	N/A

pCO2	Arterial	SI Units (Conversion Factor X 0.133)	Venous	SI Units (Conversion Factor X 0.133)	Capillary	SI Units (Conversion Factor X 0.133)
Birth, cord, full-term	32–66 mm Hg	4.3–8.8 kPa	27–49 mm Hg	3.6–6.5 kPa	—	—
Adult/child	35–45 mm Hg	4.66–5.98 kPa	41–51 mm Hg	5.4–6.8 kPa	26–41 mm Hg	3.5–5.4 kPa

pO2	Arterial	SI Units (Conversion Factor 0.133)	Venous	SI Units (Conversion Factor 0.133)	Capillary	SI Units (Conversion Factor 0.133)
Birth, cord, full-term	8–24 mm Hg	1.1–3.2 kPa	17–41 mm Hg	2.3–5.4 kPa	—	—
Adult/child	80–95 mm Hg	10.6–12.6 kPa	20–49 mm Hg	2.6–6.5 kPa	80–95 mm Hg	10.6–12.6 kPa

HCO₃	The Arterial SI Units mmol/L (Conversion Factor X1)	The Venous SI Units mmol/L (Conversion Factor X1)	Capillary SI Units mmol/L (Conversion Factor X 1)
Birth, cord, full term	17–24 mEq/L	17–24 mEq/L	N/A
Adult/child	18–23 mEq/L	24–28 mEq/L	18–23 mEq/L
O² Sat	**Arterial**	**Venous**	**Capillary**
Birth, cord, full-term	40–90%	40–70%	—
Adult/child	95–99%	70–75%	95–98%
SI Units (conversion factor x .01)			
tCO₂	**Arterial** SI Units mmol/L (Conversion FactorX 1)	**Venous** SI Units mmol/L (Conversion Factor 1)	
Birth, cord, full-term	13–22 mEq/L	14–22 mEq/L	
Adult/child	22–29 mEq/L	25–30 mEq/L	
BE Arterial	**SI Units mmol/L (Conversion Factor X1)**		
Birth, cord, full-term	(10)–(2) mEq/L		
Adult/child	(2)–(3) mEq/L		

EXPLAINATION:

Blood gas analysis is used to evaluate the respiratory function and to provide an acid-base balance scale. Respiratory and cardiovascular system activities are combined with maintaining a normal acid-base balance. Respiratory or metabolic disorders may, therefore, cause abnormal blood gas findings. Blood gas quantities commonly reported are pH, partial blood carbon dioxide pressure (pCO2), partial blood oxygen pressure (pO2), bicarbonate (HCO3), O2 saturation, and base excess (BE) or base deficiency (BD). pH is a representation of the number of free hydrogen ions (H) in the body. A pH of < 7.35 suggests acidosis.

The pH value >7.45 suggests alkalosis. Improvements in the ratio of free hydrogen ions to bicarbonate can result in a counterbalancing response from the lungs or kidneys to maintain proper acid-base balance. PCO2 is an important indicator of ventilation. The pCO2 level is controlled mainly by the lungs and is referred to as the respiratory portion of the acid-base balance. The body's main buffer system is the bicarbonate–carbonic acid system.

Bicarbonate (HCO3) is an essential alkaline ion that participates in acid neutralization along with other anions such as hemoglobin, proteins, and phosphates. To maintain proper electrolyte balance, the body must have a ratio of 20 parts of bicarbonate to one part of carbonic acid (20:1).

Carbonic acid levels are partially calculated by pCO2. The amount of bicarbonate is partially measured by the total carbon dioxide content (tCO2).

Carbonic acid levels are not evaluated directly but can be calculated at 3% of pCO2. Bicarbonate can also be determined from these figures once the carbonic acid content has been obtained, leading to the 20:1 ratio. For, e.g., if pCO2 is 40, the carbonic acid would be 1.2 (3 percent 40), and the HCO3 would be 24 (20 1.2). The key acid in the acid-based system is carbonic acid. It is a metabolic or non-respiratory portion of the acid-based mechanism and is regulated by the kidney. The levels of bicarbonate can either be measured directly or inferred from tCO2 in the blood. BE/BD reflects the number of anions present in the blood to help buffer pH changes. BD (negative BE) indicates metabolic acidosis, while positive BE indicates metabolic alkalosis.

In general, the spikes in acidosis are more life-threatening than alkalosis.

Acidosis can progress either very rapidly (e.g., cardiac arrest) or over a prolonged period (e.g., renal failure).

Children can develop acidosis very easily if they are not kept warm and given enough calories. Kids with diabetes tend to get more easily into acidosis than people who have been living with the condition for a longer period. In many cases, a venous or capillary test is sufficient to obtain the necessary details on the acid-base balance without subjecting the patient to an arterial puncture with its associated risks. As shown in the comparison range table, pO2 is smaller in babies than in children and adults due to the respective level of lung maturation at birth. After 30 years of age, pO2 tends to fall by about 3 to 5 mm Hg per decade as organs mature and begin to lose elasticity. There is a method that can be used to approximate the age-to-po2 relationship: pO2 104 (age 0.27). Like carbon dioxide, Oxygen is transported to the body in a dissolved and combined form (oxyhemoglobin).

Total Oxygen is the sum of Oxygen dissolved and combined. The oxygen-carrying potential of the blood shows how much Oxygen could be transported if all hemoglobin become filled with Oxygen. Maximum oxygen saturation is oxygen content separated by 100 times of oxygen content. Specimens other than arterial specimens are often provided where oxygen measurements are not needed or when information on Oxygen can be collected by non-invasive techniques such as pulse oximetry.

Capillary blood is satisfactory for most pH and pCO2 purposes; the use of capillary pO2 is limited to the exclusion of hypoxia. Measurements containing Oxygen are typically not helpful when conducted on venous samples; arterial blood is required for accurate calculation of pO2 and oxygen saturation.

There is considerable evidence that prolonged acquaintance to high levels of Oxygen may result in injuries, such as prematurity retinopathy in infants or airway drying in any patient. In such cases, the measurement of pO2 from blood gases is particularly appropriate.

INDICATIONS:
- Classification of assessments is used to evaluate symptoms such as asthma, chronic obstructive pulmonary disease (COPD), embolism (e.g., fatty, or other embolisms) after coronary artery bypass surgery, and hypoxia. It is also used to help diagnose respiratory failure identified as pO2 < 50 mm Hg and pCO2 >50 mm Hg.
- Blood gasses may be useful in the management of patients on ventilators or in the weaning off from ventilation. Blood gas values are used to assess the acid-base state, the degree of disparity, and the level of compensation, as outlined in the following section. The return of pH to near-normal levels is referred to as a fully balanced equilibrium.
- When pH Values move in the same direction (i.e., increasing or decreasing) aspCO2 or HCO3⁻, the difference is metabolic. If pH values shift in the opposite direction from pCO2 or HCO3, the deficiency is triggered by respiratory disruptions. The following mnemonic can be helpful: MeTRO = Metabolic Together, Respiratory Opposite

Acid-Base Disturbance	pH	pCO$_2$	pO$_2$	BE
Respiratory Acidosis				
Uncompensated	Decreased	Increased	Normal	Normal
Compensated	Normal	Increased	Increased	Increased
Respiratory Alkalosis				
Uncompensated	Increased	Decreased	Normal	Normal
Compensated	Normal	Decreased	Decreased	Decreased
Metabolic (Nonrespiratory) Acidosis				
Uncompensated	Decreased	Normal	Decreased	Decreased
Metabolic (Nonrespiratory) Alkalosis				
Uncompensated	Increased	Normal	Increased	Increased
Compensated	Normal	Increased	Increased	Increased

RESULT:

The acid-base ratio is calculated by the measurement of pH, pCO2, and HCO3 levels. pH < 7.35 indicates an acidic state, while a pH higher than 7.45 reflects alkalosis. PCO2 and HCO3 decide whether the imbalance is respiratory or non-respiratory. Since a patient might have more than one imbalance and may also be in the course of being compensated, the definition of blood gas levels may not always appear clear.

Respiratory disorders that interfere with normal breathing can allow CO2 to stay in the blood. It increases endogenous carbonic acid and a corresponding reduction in pH (respiratory acidosis). Acute respiratory acidosis can happen in acute pulmonary edema, severe respiratory infections, bronchial obstruction, pneumothorax, hemothorax, open chest wounds, opiate overdose, respiratory depression treatment, and high CO2 air inhalation.

Chronic respiratory acidosis can be seen in asthma pulmonary fibrosis, emphysema, bronchiectasis, and respiratory depressive therapy. In turn, respiratory conditions that increase the breathing rate can cause CO2 to be released from the alveoli more rapidly than is generated. This will result in alkaline pH. Acute respiratory alkalosis can be seen in agitation, hysteria, hyperventilation, pulmonary embolus, and decreased artificial ventilation.

Chronic respiratory alkalosis may be seen in case of high fever, administration of medications (e.g., salicylate and sulfate) that activate the respiratory system, hepatic coma, high-altitude hypoxia, and central nervous system (CNS) lesions, or injury resulting in activation of the respiratory center.

Metabolic (non-respiratory) conditions that cause inappropriate accumulation or reduced excretion of organic or inorganic acids result in metabolic acidosis.

Some of these disorders include consumption of salicylates, ethylene glycol, and methanol, as well as uncontrolled diabetes, malnutrition, pain, kidney disease, vomiting, and biliary or pancreatic fistula. Metabolic alkalosis arises from conditions that increase pHs, such as excessive intake of antacids to cure gastritis or peptic ulcers, excessive intake of HCO3, lack of stomach acid due to prolonged diarrhea, cystic fibrosis, or potassium and chloride deficits.

pH INCREASE:

Alkali ingestion (excessive)

> Gastric suctioning

- Potassium depletion: Cushing's disease, excessive ingestion of licorice, inadequate potassium intake, potassium losing nephropathy, diarrhea, diuresis, excessive vomiting, steroid administration

pH (respiratory alkalosis):

- Fever
- Hyperventilation
- Hysteria
- Salicylate intoxication
- CNS lesions or injuries that stimulate the respiratory center
- Excessive artificial ventilation

pH DECREASE:

pH (metabolic acidosis):

- Decreased formation of acids: diabetic ketoacidosis, high fat/low-carbohydrate diets
- Decreased excretion of H+ ion:
- acquired (e.g., drugs, hypercalcemia), Fanconi's syndrome, Addison's disease
- inherited (e.g., cystinosis, Wilson's disease), renal tubular acidosis, renal failure
- Increased acid intake
- Increased loss of alkaline body fluids: excess potassium loss through fistula and diarrhea

pH (respiratory acidosis):

- Drugs depressing the respiratory system
- Emphysema
- Pneumonia
- Pulmonary edema
- Asthma

INCREASED pO2:

- Hyperbaric oxygenation
- Hyperventilation

DECREASED pO2:

- Decreased alveolar gas exchange:
- cancer, compression or resection of the lung, respiratory distress syndrome (newborns), sarcoidosis
- Reduced ventilation or perfusion:
- asthma, bronchitis, cystic fibrosis (mucoviscidosis), emphysema, bronchiectasis, cancer, croup, granulomata, pulmonary infarction, shock
- Hypoxemia: pneumonia, anesthesia, cardiac disorders, high altitudes, near drowning, carbon monoxide exposure, presence of abnormal hemoglobins
- Hypoventilation:
- The cerebrovascular incident, drugs depressing the respiratory system, head injury
- Right to left shunt: congenital heart disease, intrapulmonary venoarterial shunting

INCREASED pCO2 (respiratory acidosis):

- Acute intermittent porphyria
- Asthma
- Bronchitis
- Cardiac disorders
- Congestive heart failure
- Cystic fibrosis
- Depression of the respiratory center

- Electrolyte disturbances (severe)
- Emphysema
- Hypothyroidism (severe)
- Near drowning
- Pneumonia
- Pneumothorax
- Poliomyelitis
- Pulmonary edema
- Pulmonary tuberculosis
- Respiratory failure
- Respiratory disorders
- Tumor

tCO2 (metabolic alkalosis):
- Alkali ingestion (excessive)
- Hypochloremic states
- Hypokalemic states
- Salicylate intoxication
- Shock
- Vomiting

DECREASED pCO2 (respiratory alkalosis):
- Anxiety
- Fever
- Head injury
- Hyperthermia
- Hyperventilation
- Salicylate intoxication
- **tCO2 (metabolic acidosis):**
- Diabetic ketoacidosis
- Renal disease

INCREASED HCO3⁻:
- Anoxia
- Metabolic alkalosis
- Respiratory acidosis

DECREASED HCO3⁻:
- Hypocapnia
- Metabolic acidosis
- Respiratory alkalosis

INCREASED O2 saturation:
- Hyperbaric oxygenation
- Hypocapnia
- Hypothermia
- Oxygen therapy
- Respiratory alkalosis

DECREASED O2 saturation:
- Anemia (severe)
- Anorexia
- Anoxia
- Atelectasis
- Carbon monoxide poisoning
- Cardiac disorders
- Congenital heart defects
- COPD
- Fever
- Head injury
- Hypercapnia
- Near drowning
- Pleural effusion
- Poisoning
- Pneumonia
- Pneumothorax
- Pulmonary embolism
- Respiratory distress syndrome (adult and neonatal)
- Sarcoidosis

INCREASED:
• Base excess: Metabolic alkalosis
DECREASED:
• Base excess: Metabolic acidosis
CRITICAL VALUES:

Arterial Blood Gas Parameter	Less than	Greater Than
pH	7.20	7.60
HCO_3	10 mmol/L	40 mmol/L
pCO_2	20 mm Hg	55 mm Hg
pO_2	45 mm Hg	

IMPEDING FACTORS:
- Medications that may induce an increase in pH include antacids, acetylsalicylic acid (primarily), carbenicillin, carbenoxolone, laxatives, mafenide, ethacrynic acid, glycyrrhiza (licorice), and sodium bicarbonate.
- Medications that may induce a pH fall include acetazolamide, acetylsalicylic acid (long-term or heavy doses), citrate, trimethadione, creatine, ethylene glycol, fluoride, mercury compounds (laxatives), methylenedioxyamphetamine, paraldehyde, and xylitol.

- Drugs that may cause pCO2 to raise include acetylsalicylic acid, aldosterone bicarbonate, carbenicillin, carbenoxolone, ethacrynic acid, laxatives (chronic abuse), corticosteroids, dexamethasone, and x-ray contrast agents.
- Medications that may cause a reduction in pCO2 include acetazolamide, acetylsalicylic acid ethamivan, NSD 3004 (arterial long-acting carbonic anhydrase inhibitor), neuromuscular relaxants (secondary to postoperative hyperventilation), theophylline, tromethamine, and xylitol.
- Drugs that can cause an increase in pO2 include theophylline and urokinase.
- Medications that may cause a reduction in pO2 include althesin, barbiturates, GM-CSF, isoproterenol, and meperidine.
- Blood gas samples are obtained by arterial puncture, which carries a risk of bleeding, especially in patients who have bleeding diathesis or who are taking medication for bleeding disorders.
- Recent blood transfusions can yield misleading values.
- Specimens with exceptionally high white blood cell counts will experience false pH declines due to cell metabolism if delivery to the laboratory is postponed.
- Specimens acquired soon after a shift of inspired Oxygen has occurred will not accurately reflect the state of oxygenation of the individual.
- Specimens obtained within 20 to 30 minutes of suction of respiratory passage or other respiratory therapy will not be correct.
- Excessive variations in actual body temperature compared to normal body temperature are not reflected in the results. Temperature affects the quantity of gas in the solution. Blood gas analyzers measure samples at 37°C (98.6°F); thus, if the patient is hyperthermic or hypothermic, it is important to inform the laboratory of the exact body temperature of the patient at the time the specimen was taken. Fever raises the true pO2 and pCO2 values; thus, the uncorrected values measured at 37°C will be wrongly reduced.
- Hypothermia reduces the actual pO2 and pCO2 values; thus, the erroneous values measured at 37°C will be incorrectly raised.
- Falsely increased O2 saturation can occur due to elevated levels of carbon monoxide in the blood.
- O2 saturation is a measured parameter based on the 100 percent hemoglobin A assumption. Values may be inaccurate when types of hemoglobin with different oxygen dissociation curves are present. Hemoglobin S induces a shift to the right, suggesting a reduced oxygen binding. Methemoglobin and Fetal hemoglobin will cause a shift to the left, suggesting an increase in oxygen binding.
- Unnecessary amounts of heparin in the sample may falsely reduce pH, pCO2, and pO2.
- The Citrates should never be used as an anticoagulant in evacuated blood gas collection tubes because citrates can induce a pronounced analytic decrease in pH.

- Air bubbles or blood clots in the test are the reason for rejection. Air bubbles in the specimen can falsely increase or decrease the results depending on the status of the patient's blood gas. If the evacuated tubing is used for the processing of venous blood gas tests, the tube must be separated from the needle before the needle is withdrawn from the arm or the sample becomes polluted with room air.
- Specimens should be put in ice slurry shortly following sampling, as the blood cells continue to perform metabolic processes in the specimen after withdrawal from the individual. These natural life processes can influence pH, pO2, pCO2, and other calculated values over a short period. The cold temperature of the ice slurry slows down but does not completely stop the molecular changes occurring in the sample over time.
- Iced specimens not tested within 60 minutes of collection should be refused for examination.

ANION GAP

(AG, A-gap)
SAMPLING:
1 ml of serum for electrolytes is collected in a red- or tiger-top tube. 1 mL of plasma collected in a green-top (heparin) tube is also acceptable.
TECHNIQUE:
The anion gap is mathematically derived from direct measurements of sodium, chloride, and gross carbon dioxide. For some electrolytes, there are variations in serum and plasma values.
NORMAL VALUE:

Age	Conventional Units	SI Units (Conversion Factor X1)
Child	8–16 mEq/L	8–16 mmol/L
Adult	8–16 mEq/L	8–16 mmol/L

EXPLANATION:
The anion gap is most widely used as a clinical indicator of metabolic acidosis. It does not include the calculation of essential cations, such as calcium, potassium (usually) and magnesium, or anions, such as proteins, phosphorus derivatives, sulfur, and organic acids.
The anion gap is calculated as follows:
(sodium - [chloride + HCO3-])
Since HCO3 - is not directly measured by most multichannel chemistry analyzers, HCO3 - is determined by substituting the total carbon dioxide content in the equation. Many laboratories may include potassium in anion gap measurement. Calculations like potassium may be invalidated since small amounts of hemolysis can lead to massive levels of potassium leaked to the serum due to cell breakup.

The anion gap is also commonly used as a laboratory quality control measure since small gaps usually indicate a reagent, sensor, or instrument defect.

INDICATIONS:

- Calculate metabolic acidosis.

- Signify the presence of a disturbance in electrolyte balance.

- Signify the need for laboratory instrument recalibration or evaluation of electrolyte reagent preparation and stability.

RESULT:

Increased in:
Dehydration (severe)
Excessive exercise
Poisoning (salicylate, methanol, ethylene glycol, or paraldehyde)
Renal failure
Uremia
Ketoacidosis triggered by starvation, high-protein/low-carbohydrate diet, diabetes, and alcoholism
Lactic acidosis
Decreased in:
Hypergammaglobulinemia (multiple myeloma) • Hyperchloremia
Hypoalbuminemia
Hyponatremia (hyperviscosity syndromes)

TCO_2 is widely used to supplement HCO_3- in anion gap measurements. It is important to note the clinical significance of excessive HCO_3- in the case of renal alkalosis, gastrointestinal alkalosis, and excessive intake of exogenous alkali sources, the results of which may not be accurately reflected in the measured anion gap.

IMPEDING FACTORS:

- Products that may raise or lower the anion gap include those specified in the individual electrolytes (i.e., sodium, calcium, magnesium, chloride, and total carbon dioxide), total protein, lactic acid, and phosphorus monographs. Samples should never be obtained over the intravenous line due to the risk for dilution as the specimen and the intravenous solution is mixed in the sample tube, wrongly reducing the outcome. There is also the ability to contaminate the sample with the agent of interest present in the intravenous solution, wrongly raising the outcome.

ARTERIAL/ALVEOLAR OXYGEN RATIO OR ALVEOLAR/ARTERIAL GRADIENT

(a/A ratio, Alveolar-arterial difference, A/a gradient)

SAMPLING: 1 ml of Arterial blood is collected in a heparinized syringe. Samples should be transferred tightly capped and in an ice slurry.

TECHNIQUE: Selective electrodes that calculate pO2 and pCO2

NORMAL VALUE:

Alveolar/arterial gradient	< 10 mm Hg at rest
	(room air)
	20–30 mm Hg at maximum
	exercise activity (room air)
Arterial/alveolar oxygen ratio	>0.75 (75%)

EXPLAINATION:

The capacity of oxygen to move from the alveoli to the lungs is used when determining the extent of oxygenation of the patient. This examination may help to identify the cause of hypoxemia (low oxygen levels in the blood) and intrapulmonary shunting that may occur from one of the following three conditions: ventilated alveoli without perfusion, unventilated alveoli with adequate perfusion, or collapse of alveoli and adjoining blood vessels. Data on the alveolar/arterial gradient (A/a) can be measured indirectly using partial oxygen pressure (pO2) (derived from a blood gas analysis) in a basic mathematical formula:

A/a gradient = pO2 in alveolar air (expected) - pO2 in arterial blood (measured)

The measurement of alveolar pO2 is accomplished by subtracting the water vapor pressure from the barometric pressure, multiplying the resultant pressure by the fraction of inhaled oxygen (FIO2; the percentage of oxygen the patient breathes), and subtracting it from $1^{1/4}$ times the partial arterial pressure of carbon dioxide (pCO2). The gradient is obtained by subtracting from the determined alveolar pO2, the arterial pO2 of the patient.

Alveolar pO2 = [(barometric or atmospheric pressure - water vapor pressure) X FIO2] - [$1^{1/4}$ X pCO2]

A/a gradient = arterial pO2 (measured) - alveolar pO2 (estimated)

The ratio of arterial to alveolar (a/A) reflects the percentage of alveolar pO2 found in arterial pO2. It is calculated by dividing the pO2 arterial by the pO2 alveolar:

a/A = paO2/pAO2

The level of A/a decreases as the concentration of oxygen the patient induces increases. If the gradient is unusually high, either there is an issue with the capacity of oxygen to flow through the alveolar membrane, or oxygenated blood is combined with non-oxygenated blood. The ratio of a/A does not depend on FIO2; it does not increase with the corresponding increase in inhaled oxygen. In patients on a mechanical FIO2 ventilator, the ratio of a/A can be used to determine whether the diffusion of oxygen is increasing.

INDICATIONS:
- Assist in identifying the cause of hypoxemia.
- Assess intrapulmonary or coronary artery shunting.

RESULT
Increased in:
• **Acute respiratory distress syndrome**
• **Atelectasis**
• **Atrial venous shunts**
• **Bronchospasm**
• **Pneumothorax**
• **Pulmonary edema**
• **Chronic obstructive pulmonary disease**
• **Congenital cardiac septal defects**
• **Underventilated alveoli (mucus plugs)**
• **Pulmonary embolus**
• **Pulmonary fibrosis**

IMPEDING FACTORS:
- Specimens should be gathered before the administration of oxygen therapy.
- The patient's temperature should be observed and submitted to the laboratory if it is significantly elevated or lowered so that the measured values can be calibrated to the actual body temperature.
- The sensitivity of the sample to room air impacts the results of the test.
- Values usually increase with increasing age (see the monograph entitled "Blood Gasses").
- Samples for A/a gradient testing are collected by arterial puncture, which carries a risk of bleeding, particularly in patients with bleeding disorders or who are taking medication for bleeding disorders.
- Fast and proper processing, storage, and analysis of specimens are essential for the achievement of accurate results. Samples should always be transported to the laboratory as soon as possible after collection. Delay in shipping the sample or transporting it without ice may affect the test results.

HYPERSENSITIVITY PNEUMONITIS SEROLOGY

Farmer's lung disease serology, extrinsic allergic alveolitis
SAMPLING: 2 mL of serum is collected in a red-top tube.
TECHNIQUE: Immunodiffusion
NORMAL VALUE: Negative.

EXPLAINATION:

Hypersensitivity pneumonia is a respiratory disease caused by the inhalation of bacteria from an organic source. Compromised and symptomatic individuals will display acute bronchospastic reactions 4 to 6 hours after contact with the offending antigen. Inhalation of the antigen promotes the production of antibodies to immunoglobulin G (IgG).

The application of immune complexing and cell-mediated immunopathogenesis contributes to chronic granulomatous pneumonia in the interstitial lung. Hypersensitivity Pneumonia Serology includes the detection of antibodies to Aspergillus fumigatus, Micropolyspora faeni, Thermoactinomyces Vulgaris, and T. Candidus. A negative test result will not rule out hypersensitivity pneumonia as a possible diagnosis, nor does a positive test result verify the diagnosis. However, people with a positive test result may not have typical symptoms, and patients with severe symptoms may not have detectable levels of antibodies while their infection is latent.

It is necessary to get a sputum culture and chest x-rays to confirm the diagnosis.
INDICATIONS: Assist in the detection of hypersensitivity pneumonia in patients with fever, chills, and dyspnea after repeated exposure to moist organic sources.
RESULT:
Increased in: Hypersensitivity pneumonitis

LECITHIN/SPHINGOMYELIN RATIO (L/S ratio)

SAMPLING: 10 ml of amniotic fluid is collected in sterile, brown glass or plastic tube or bottle protected from light.
TECHNIQUE: Thin-layer chromatography
NORMAL VALUE:
- Mature (nondiabetic): >2:1 in the presence of phosphatidylglycerol
- Borderline: 1.5 to 1.9:1
- Immature: < 1.5:1

EXPLAINATION:

RDS or Respiratory distress syndrome is the most frequent problem faced in the treatment of premature infants. RDS, also known as hyaline membrane syndrome, is the result of a lack of phospholipid lung surfactants. Surfactant phospholipids are formed by specialized alveolar cells and deposited in granular lamella cells in the lung. In the naturally formed lungs, the surfactant coats the alveoli sheet. When breathing, the surfactant reduces the surface tension of the alveolar wall.

When the amount of surfactant is inadequate, the alveoli cannot normally extend, and the flow of gas is hindered. Amniocentesis is a procedure that takes out fluid from the amniotic sac to determine fetal lung maturity. Lecithin is the main surfactant phospholipids and is a stabilizing agent for alveoli. It is produced at a slow but constant rate until the 35th week of gestation, after which its production increases dramatically. Sphingomyelin, another surfactant phospholipids component, is also produced at a constant rate after the 26th week of gestation.

Before the 35th week, the ratio of lecithin/sphingomyelin (L/S) is normally < 1.6:1. The ratio increases to 2.0 or higher when the lecithin production rate increases after the 35th week of gestation. Many phospholipids, such as phosphatidylglycerol (PG) and phosphatidylinositol (PI), also rise in amniotic fluid over time. The presence of PG suggests that the fetus is within 2 to 6 weeks of pulmonary maturity (i.e., full-term). The simultaneous measurement of the L/S ratio of PG increases diagnostic accuracy. In diabetic mothers, the production of phospholipid surfactants is delayed. Caution must, therefore, be used when assessing the results obtained from a diabetic patient, and a higher ratio is supposed to indicate maturity.

INDICATIONS:

- Help in the determination of fetal lung development.
- Determine the optimal period for obstetric interventions in situations of risk of fetal survival due to trauma related to maternal diabetes, toxemia, hemolytic diseases of the newborn or post-maturity.
- Identify fetuses at risk of acquiring respiratory distress syndrome (RDS).

RESULT:

Increased in:
• Malnutrition
• Premature rupture of the membranes
• Maternal diabetes
• Placenta previa
• Placental infarction
• Hypertension
• Intrauterine growth retardation
Decreased in:
• Polyhydramnios

• Immature fetal lungs	
• Advanced maternal age	
• Multiple gestations	

CRITICAL VALUES:

The L/S ratio of < 1.5:1 is indicative of RDS at the time of delivery. Infants considered to be at risk for RDS may be treated with a surfactant by intratracheal administration at birth.

IMPEDING FACTORS:

- Fetal blood mistakenly raises the L/S ratio.
- Exposing the specimen to light can give abnormal reduced values.
- There is a possibility that an amniocentesis will be performed, and this should be weighed against the need to acquire the necessary diagnostic information. A small percentage (0.5%) of patients experienced complications, including premature membrane rupture, premature labor, spontaneous abortion, and stillbirth.

PLEURAL FLUID ANALYSIS (Thoracentesis fluid analysis)

SAMPLING:

5 ml of pleural fluid is collected in a green-top (heparin) tube for amylase, cholesterol, glucose, lactate dehydrogenase (LDH), protein, pH, and triglycerides; lavender-top (ethylenediaminetetra-acetic acid [EDTA]) tube for cell count; sterile containers for microbiology specimens; equal amounts of fixative and fluid in plastic containers for cytology.

TECHNIQUE:

 Spectrophotometry for amylase, automated or manual cell count; cholesterol, glucose, LDH, protein, and triglycerides; ion-selective electrode for pH; macroscopic and microscopic examination of cultured microorganisms; microscopic examination of specimen for microbiology and cytology

NORMAL VALUE:

Pleural Fluid	NORMAL Value
Appearance	Clear
Color	Pale yellow
Amylase	Comparable to serum values
Cholesterol	Comparable to serum values
Glucose	Comparable to serum values
LDH	< 200 U/L
Fluid LDH–to–serum LDH ratio	0.6 >
Protein	3.0 g/dL

Fluid protein–to–serum protein ratio	0.5 >
Triglycerides	Comparable to serum values
pH	7.37–7.43
RBC count	< 1000/mm^3
WBC count	< 1000/mm^3
Culture	No growth
Gram stain	No organisms are detected
Cytology	No abnormal cells are seen

EXPLAINATION:

The pleural cavity and the organs within it (lungs) are covered with a protective membrane. The fluid between the membranes is called pleural fluid. Typically, only a small amount of fluid is present because the rate of fluid production and absorption is roughly the same. Many pathological conditions can lead to fluid build-up in the pleural cavity. Relevant tests are usually performed in addition to the normal set of tests used to make a distinction transudate from exudate. Transudates are effusions that build up as an outcome of a condition that disrupts the control of the fluid balance, such as the alleged perforation. Exudates are triggered by conditions that affect the membrane tissue itself, like cancer or malignancy. The fluid is pumped out of the pleural cavity by needle aspiration and tested, as shown in the tables above.

INDICATIONS:

- Distinction transudates from exudates.
- Evaluate effusion of unknown disease.
- Investigate suspected rupture immune disorder, malignancy, or infection.

RESULT:

Bacterial or tuberculous empyema:
• Red blood cell (RBC) count 5000/mm3
• White blood cell (WBC) count 25,000 to 100,000/mm3 with a predominance of neutrophils, increased protein-to serum ratio
• Increased LDH-to-serum ratio
• Decreased glucose
• pH < 7.3
Chylous pleural effusion:
• A marked rise in both triglycerides (two to three times serum level) and chylomicrons
Effusion caused by pneumonia:
• Raised protein-to-serum ratio
• Raised LDH-to-serum ratio
• RBC count 5000/mm3
• pH < 7.4

• Decreased glucose if bacterial pneumonia is suspected
• WBC count 5000 to 25,000/mm3 with a high proportion of neutrophils and some eosinophils
Esophageal rupture:
• Significantly reduced pH (6.0) and elevated amylase
Hemothorax:
• Bloody appearance
• Increased RBC count
• Elevated hematocrit
Malignancy:
• Abnormal cytology
• Raised protein-to-serum ratio
• Raised LDH-to-serum ratio
• Reduced glucose
• pH < 7.3
• WBC count 5000 to 10,000/mm3 with a predominance of lymphocytes
• RBC count 1000 to 100,000/mm3
Pancreatitis:
• RBC count 1000 to 10,000/mm3
• WBC count 5000 to 20,000/mm3 with a predominance of neutrophils
• Enhanced protein-to-serum ratio
• Increased LDH-to-serum ratio
• Increased amylase
• pH >7.3
Pulmonary infarction:
• Regular/normal glucose
• Increased fluid protein–to–serum protein ratio
• Increased fluid LDH–to–serum LDH ratio
• WBC count 5000 to 15,000/mm3 with a predominance of neutrophils
• RBC count 10,000 to 100,000/mm3
• pH >7.3
Pulmonary tuberculosis:
• RBC count 10,000/mm3
• Decreased glucose
• pH < 7.3
• WBC count 5000 to 10,000/mm3 with a predominance of lymphocytes, positive acid-fast bacillus stain and culture, increased protein
Rheumatoid disease:

• Normal RBC count
• WBC count 1000 to 20,000/mm3 with a predominance of either lymphocytes or neutrophils
• pH < 7.3
• Decreased glucose
• Increased protein-to-serum ratio
• Increased LDH-to-serum ratio
• Increased immunoglobulins
Systemic lupus erythematosus:
Similar findings of rheumatoid arthritis, except that glucose is not normally reduced.

IMPEDING FACTORS:

- Blood fluids may be the consequence of a traumatic tap.
- Unknown hyperglycemia or hypoglycemia may be misleading when comparing fluid and serum glucose levels. It is best to obtain similar serum samples a few hours before thoracentesis.

α1-ANTITRYPSIN AND α 1-ANTITRYPSIN PHENOTYPING

α 1-antitrypsin: A1AT, α 1-AT, AAT; α 1-AT phenotype, AAT phenotype, α 1-antitrypsin phenotyping: A1AT phenotype, Pi phenotype.

SAMPLING: 1 mL serum is collected for α 1-AT phenotype, AAT phenotype, α 1-antitrypsin, and 2 mL of serum for α 1-AT phenotyping collected in a red- or tiger-top tube.

TECHNIQUE: isoelectric focusing/high-resolution electrophoresis for α 1-AT phenotyping, Rate nephelometry for α 1-AT

NORMAL VALUE:

Age	Conventional Units	SI Units (Conversion Factor 0.01)
0–1 mo	124–348 mg/dL	1.24–3.48 g/L
2–6 mo	111–297 mg/dL	1.11–2.97 g/L
7 mo–2 y	95–251 mg/dL	0.95–2.51 g/L
3 y–19 y	110–279 mg/dL	1.10–2.79 g/L
Adult	126–226 mg/dL	1.26–2.26 g/L

α1-Antitrypsin Phenotyping

There are three key protease inhibitor phenotypes:

MM—Normal

SS—Intermediate; heterozygous

ZZ—Markedly abnormal; homozygous

The overall level of quantifiable α1-AT varies with the genotype. Symptoms of an α1-AT deficiency depends on the patient's conduct but are most severe in patients who smoke tobacco.

INDICATIONS:
- Assist in forming a diagnosis of COPD.
- Assist in forming a diagnosis of liver disease.
- Spot hereditary absence or deficiency of α1-AT.

RESULT

Increased in:
• **Estrogen therapy**
• **Postoperative recovery**
• **Acute and chronic inflammatory conditions**
• **Carcinomas**
• **Pregnancy**
• **Steroid therapy**
• **Stress (extreme physical)**
Decreased in:
• **COPD**
• **Liver disease (severe)**
• **Homozygous α1-AT–deficient patients**
• **Liver cirrhosis (child)**
• **Malnutrition**
• **Nephrotic syndrome**

IMPEDING FACTORS:

- α1-AT is an acute phase-reacting protein, and every inflammatory reaction increases rates. If the serum C-reactive protein is obtained simultaneously and is stable, the patient will be retested for α1-AT within 10 to 14 days.
- The rheumatoid factor causes false-positive elevations.
- Medications that may raise serum α1-AT levels include aminocaproic acid, estrogen therapy, oral contraceptives (high dose preparations), oxymetholone, streptokinase, tamoxifen, and typhoid vaccine.

CENTRAL NERVOUS SYSTEM

The central nervous system (CNS) is the part of the nervous system consisting primarily of the brain and spinal cord. The CNS is so named because it integrates the received information and coordinates and influences the activity of all parts of the bodies of bilaterally symmetric animals.

The CNS is contained within the dorsal body cavity, with the brain housed in the cranial cavity and the spinal cord in the spinal canal. In vertebrates, the brain is protected by the skull, while the spinal cord is protected by the vertebrae. The brain and spinal cord are both enclosed in the meninges while CSF runs as shock absorbing fluids between mengies

NOTES

_____
_____
_____
_____
_____
_____
_____
_____
_____
_____
_____
_____
_____
_____
_____

CEREBROSPINAL FLUID ANALYSIS (CSF analysis)

SAMPLING: 1 to 3 ml of CSF is stored in three or four distinct conical plastic tubes. Tube 1 is used for serological and chemical analysis, tube 2 is used for microbiological assessment, tube 3 is used for cell count, and tube 4 is used for other tests.

TECHNIQUE: Macroscopic appearance assessment; myelin basic protein radioimmunoassay; IgG nephelometry; electrophoresis for oligoclonal banding; examination of fluid for cell count; glucose, lactic acid, and protein spectrophotometry; Gram stain, India ink preparation, and culture for microbiology, microscopic, flocculation for Venereal Disease Research Laboratory [VDRL].

NORMAL VALUE:

Lumbar Puncture	Conventional Units	SI Units
Color and appearance	Crystal clear	
		(Conversion FactorX 10)
Protein	15–45 mg/dL	150–450 mg/L
		(Conversion Factor X0.0555)
Glucose		
Infant or child	60–80 mg/dL	3.3–4.4 mmol/L
Adult	40–70 mg/dL	2.2–3.9 mmol/L

Lactic acid		*(Conversion Factor X0.111)*
Neonate	10–60 mg/dL	1.1–6.7 mmol/L
3–10 days of lofe	10–40 mg/dL	1.1–4.4 mmol/L
Adult	<25.2 mg/dL	< 2.8 mmol/L
		(Conversion Factor X1)
Myelin basic protein	<2.5 ng/mL	< 2.5 g/L
Oligoclonal bands	Absent	
	(Conversion Factor X 10)	
IgG	<3.4 mg/dL	< 34 mg/L
Gram stain	Negative	
India ink	Negative	
Culture	No growth	

RBC count	0		0	
WBC count			(Conversion Factor X 1)	
< 1 y	0–30/mL		0–30 10^6/L	
1–4 y	0–20/mL		0–20 10^6/L	
5–12 y	0–10/mL		0–10 10^6/L	
Adult	0–5/mL		0–5 10^6/L	
WBC Differential	Adult	Children	Adult	Children
Lymphocytes	40–80%	5–13%	0.4–0.8	0.55–0.35
Monocytes	15–45%	50–90%	0.15–0.45	0.50–0.90
Neutrophils	0–6%	0–8%	0–0.6	0–0.8
VDRL	Nonreactive			
Cytology	No abnormal cells are seen			

WBC Differential	Adult	Children
Lymphocytes	40%–80%	5%–13%
Monocytes	15%–45%	50%–90%
Neutrophils	0%–6%	0%–8%

EXPLAINATION:

Cerebrospinal fluid (CSF) circulates in subarachnoid space and has a dual function: to shield the brain and spinal cord from damage and to carry cell metabolism and neurosecretion materials.

CSF analysis helps establish the presence and cause of bleeding and helps diagnose cancer, infections, and autoimmune and degenerative disorders of the brain and spinal cord. Specimens for study are most frequently obtained by lumbar puncture and sometimes by ventricular or cistern puncture. A lumbar puncture may also have therapeutic uses, including injections of medications and anesthesia.

INDICATIONS:

- Aid in the diagnosis and differential of subarachnoid or intracranial hemorrhage.
-Assist in the diagnosis and distinction of viral or bacterial meningitis or encephalitis.
- Aid in the evaluation of diseases such as multiple sclerosis, autoimmune, or degenerative brain disorders.
- Help in making the diagnosis of neurosyphilis and chronic central nervous system (CNS) infections.
- Detection of disruption of CSF circulation due to hemorrhage, tumor, or edema.
- Determination of any disease that hampers the delivery of oxygen to the brain.

- Monitoring of cancer metastases to the CNS.
- Monitoring of severe brain injury.

RESULT:

Increases in:

- Color and appearance:
- bloody hemorrhage
- xanthochromic—old hemorrhage, methemoglobin, red blood cell (RBC) breakdown, bilirubin (>6 mg/dL), increased protein (>150 mg/dL), melanin (meningeal melanosarcoma), carotene (systemic carotenemia).
- hazy meningitis
- pink to dark yellow aspiration of epidural fat.
- turbid—cells, microorganisms, protein, fat, or contrast medium.
- Protein: encephalitis, meningitis.
- Lactic acid: bacterial, tubercular, fungal meningitis.
- Myelin basic protein: trauma, stroke, multiple sclerosis, tumor, subacute sclerosing panencephalitis.
- IgG and oligoclonal banding: CNS syphilis, multiple sclerosis, and subacute sclerosing panencephalitis.
- Gram stain: establishing the causative organism of meningitis:
- *Streptococcus pneumoniae,*
- *Neisseria meningitidis,*
- *Cryptococcus neoformans*
- *Haemophilus influenzae,*
- India ink preparation: diagnosing meningitis due to *C. neoformans.*
- Culture: encephalitis or meningitis caused by herpes simplex virus, *H. influenzae, S. pneumoniae, N. meningitidis, C. neoformans.*
- RBC count: hemorrhage.
- White blood cell (WBC) count:
- **General increase—**

injection of contrast media or anticancer medications in subarachnoid space; CSF infarct; a metastatic tumor in link with CSF; reaction to repeated lumbar puncture

- **Raised WBC count with a majority of neutrophils**

indicative of bacterial meningitis

- **Raised WBC count with a majority of lymphocytes**

indicative of tubercular, viral, parasitic, or fungal meningitis; multiple sclerosis

- **Raised WBC count with a majority of monocytes**

indicative of chronic bacterial meningitis, multiple sclerosis, amebic meningitis, toxoplasmosis

- **Raised plasma cells**

indicative of multiple sclerosis, sarcoidosis, acute viral infections, syphilitic meningoencephalitis, subacute sclerosing parasitic infections, Guillain-Barré syndrome panencephalitis, tubercular meningitis.

The appearance of eosinophils in the sample is suggestive of parasites and fungal infections, acute polyneuritis, idiopathic hypereosinophilic disease, drug reactions or shunt in CSF.

- VDRL: syphilis

Positive findings in:

- Cytology: malignant cells

Decreases in:

- Glucose: bacterial and tubercular meningitis

CRITICAL VALUES:

- Presence of malignant cells - Any of the above-listed results should be communicated to the requesting health care practitioner immediately.
- India ink preparation, Positive Gram stain, or culture.

IMPEDING FACTORS:

- Medications that may decrease CSF protein levels include cefotaxime and dexamethasone.
- Interferon-β can increase the basic protein levels of myelin.
- Drugs that may increase the level of CSF glucose include cefotaxime and dexamethasone.
- The RBC count may be inappropriately raised with a traumatic spinal tap.
- This procedure is contraindicated if the infection is present at the site of needle insertion.
- Recent radioactive scans or radiation exposure within one week of the test may conflict with the test results, while radioimmunoassay is the test method.
- Note any recent practices that may conflict with the results of the test.
- It may also be contraindicated in patients along with degenerative joint disease or coagulation deficiency and in patients who are non-cooperative during the procedure.
- Use with great caution in patients with increased intracranial pressure as overly rapid removal of CSF can result in herniation.

NOTES

MUSCULOSKELETAL SYSTEM

The human musculoskeletal system (also known as the locomotor system, and previously the activity system is an organ system that gives humans the ability to move using their muscular and skeletal systems. The musculoskeletal system provides form, support, stability, and movement to the body.
It is made up of the bones of the skeleton, muscles, cartilage, tendons, ligaments, joints, and other connective tissue that supports and binds tissues and organs together. The musculoskeletal system's primary functions include supporting the body, allowing motion, and protecting vital organs. The skeletal portion of the system serves as the main storage system for calcium and phosphorus and contains critical components of the hematopoietic system.

NOTES

URIC ACID, BLOOD (Urate)

SAMPLING: 1 mL of serum is collected in a red- or tiger-top tube. 1 mL of plasma collected in a green-top (heparin) tube is also acceptable.

TECHNIQUE: Spectrophotometry

NORMAL VALUE:

Age	Conventional Units	SI Units (Conversion Factor X0.059)
Child < 12 y	2.0–5.5 mg/dL	0.12–0.32 mmol/L
Adult younger than 60 y		
Male	4.4–7.6 mg/dL	0.26–0.45 mmol/L
Female	2.3–6.6 mg/dL	0.14–0.39 mmol/L
Adult older than 60 y		
Male	4.2–8.0 mg/dL	0.25–0.48 mmol/L
Female	3.5–7.3 mg/dL	0.21–0.43 mmol/L

EXPLAINATION:

Purins are important components of nucleic acids; the purine turnover constantly occurs in the body, producing substantial amounts of uric acid even in the absence of purine intake from dietary sources such as organ meat (e.g., liver, thymus gland and pancreas, kidney), legumes and yeast. Uric acid is filtered, absorbed, and excreted by the kidneys and is a common urinary constituent.

INDICATIONS:

- Assist in the diagnosis of gout when elevated uric acid levels indicate a family history (autosomal-dominant genetic disorder) or signs and symptoms of gout.
- Determine the cause of known or suspected kidney stones.
- Assess the extent of tissue destruction in infection, starvation, over-exercise, malignancies, chemotherapy, or radiation therapy.
- Assess possible damage to the liver due to increased levels of uric acid.
- Scrutinize the effects of drugs known to alter uric acid levels, either as side effects or therapeutic effects.

RESULT:

Increased in:
• Glucose-6-phosphate dehydrogenase deficiency
• Acute tissue damage because of starvation or excessive exercise
• Alcoholism
• Chemotherapy and radiation therapy
• Chronic lead toxicity
• Congestive heart failure

•	Diabetes
•	Down's syndrome
•	Eclampsia
•	Excessive dietary purines
•	Gout
•	Hyperparathyroidism
•	Hypertension
•	Hypoparathyroidism
•	Lactic acidosis
•	Lead poisoning
•	Sickle cell anemia
•	Type III hyperlipidemia
•	Lesch-Nyhan syndrome
•	Multiple myeloma
•	Pernicious anemia
•	Polycystic kidney disease
•	Polycythemia
•	Psoriasis
Decreased in:	
•	Wilson's disease
•	Fanconi's syndrome
•	Low-purine diet
•	Severe liver disease

IMPEDING FACTORS:

- Medications and substances that may increase uric acid levels consist of acetylsalicylic acid (low doses), aldatense, hydroflumethiazide, hydroxyurea, ibufenac, ibuprofen, levarterenol, levodopa, mefruside, mercaptopurine, cisplatin, corn oil, cyclosporine, ethacrynic acid, ethambutol, ethoxzolamide, etoposide, flumethiazide, cyclothiazide, cytarabine, diapamide, aminothiadiazole, anabolic steroids, antineoplastic agents, ascorbic acid, chlorambucil, chlorthalidone, diazoxide, diuretics, ergothioneine, methicillin, methotrexate, methoxyflurane, methyclothiazide, mitomycin, morinamide, polythiazide, prednisone, pyrazinamide, salicylate, spironolactone, triamterene, trichlormethiazide, vincristine, theophylline, thiazide diuretics, thioguanine, thiotepa, thiouric acid, warfarin, and xylitol.

- Medicines that may reduce uric acid levels include allopurinol, aspirin (high doses), chlorpromazine, chlorprothixene, azathioprine, acetohexamide, benzbromaron, benziodarone, canola oil, chlorothiazide (given intravenously), cinchophen, corticotropin, lisinopril, mefenamic acid, mersalyl, methotrexate, oxyphenbutazone, phenindione, phenolsulfonphthalein, probenecid, seclazone, sulfinpyrazone, corticosteroids, clofibrate, coumarin, diatrizoic acid, dicumarol, dipyrone, enalapril, fenofibrate, flufenamic acid, guaifenesin, hydralazine, iodipamide, iodopyracet, iopanoic acid, ipodate, and verapamil.

COLLAGEN CROSSLINKED N-TELOPEPTIDE (NTx)

SAMPLING:2 mL of urine from a random specimen collected in a clean plastic container.

TECHNIQUE: Immunoassay

NORMAL VALUE:

Male	0–85 nmol bone collagen equivalents/mmol creatinine
Female (premenopausal)	14–76 nmol bone collagen equivalents/mmol creatinine

EXPLAINATION:

Osteoporosis is more frequently seen in women than in men. Other risk factors include thin, small-frame body structure; family history of osteoporosis; low-calcium diet; Caucasian or Asian race; excessive alcohol use; cigarette smoking; sedentary lifestyle; long-term use of corticosteroids, thyroid replacement drugs, or antiepileptic drugs; the history of bulimia, anorexia nervosa, chronic liver disease, or malabsorption disorders; and postmenopausal disorder osteoporosis is a major consequence of menopause in women due to a decline in estrogen production.

The most prevalent bone disease in the western world is Osteoporosis. It is often termed as a "silent disease" because bone loss occurs without symptoms. The formation and maintenance of bone mass depend on a combination of factors, including genetics, nutrition, exercise, and hormonal activity. Normally, the rate of bone development is like that of bone resorption. After midlife, the bone loss rate begins to increase.

Osteoporosis is rarely seen in premenopausal women. Estrogen replacement therapy (after menopause) is a strategy that has been commonly used to prevent osteoporosis, although its exact protective mechanism is unknown. Results of some recently published studies suggest that there may be major adverse effects of estrogen replacement therapy; further research is needed to understand the long-term (positive and negative) effects of estrogen replacement therapy. Other treatment options include raloxifene (selectively modulates estrogen receptors), calcitonin (directly interacting with osteoclasts), and bisphosphates (inhibit osteoclast-mediated bone resorption).

A non-invasive test to detect the presence of collagen cross-linked N-telopeptide (NTx) is used to monitor the improvement of patients who have started treatment for osteoporosis. When collagenase acts on the bone, NTx is formed. Small fragments of NTx are excreted in the urine after bone resorption. An appropriate response, 2 to 3 months after initiation of therapy, is a 30 percent reduction in NTx and a 50 percent reduction below baseline by 12 months.

INDICATIONS:
- Assist in the determination of osteoporosis.
- Help in the management and treatment of osteoporosis.
- Monitor the effects of osteoporosis replacement therapy.

RESULT:
Increased in:

• **Hyperparathyroidism**
• **Osteomalacia**
• **Osteoporosis**
• **Paget's disease**
Decreased in:
Effective therapy for osteoporosis

IMPEDING FACTORS:
NTx levels are influenced by urinary excretion and may be affected by renal impairment or illness.

CREATINE KINASE AND ISOENZYMES (CK and isos)

SAMPLING: 1 mL of serum is collected in a red- or tiger-top tube. Serial samples are highly recommended. Care must be taken to utilize the same type of collection container if serial measurements are to be taken.

TECHNIQUE: Enzymatic for CK, enzyme immunoassay techniques electrophoresis for isoenzymes are in common use for CK-MB

NORMAL VALUE:

	Conventional Units	SI Units (Conversion Factor X 0.017)
Total CK		
Newborn	3 adult values	3 adult values
Children and men	38–174 U/L	0.65–2.96 µKat/L
Children and women	26–140 U/L	0.46–2.38 µKat/L

	Conventional Units
CK isoenzymes by electrophoresis	
CK-BB	Absent
CK-MB	< 4–6%
CK-MM	94–96%
CK-MB by immunoassay	< 10 ng/mL

EXPLAINATION:

CK or Creatine kinase is an enzyme that occurs almost entirely in the skeletal muscle, the heart muscle, and, to a lesser extent, the brain. This enzyme is vital for the storage and release of energy within the cell. Three isoenzymes have been identified by electrophoresis. These are classified according to the organ in which they are present: CK-BB brain, CK-MB cardiac, and CK-MM skeletal muscle. When these tissues are damaged, the enzymes are released into the bloodstream. Enzyme Levels increase and decrease within a predictable timeframe. Quantity of serum levels can help to calculate the extent and timing of damage. Noting the presence of a particular isoenzyme helps to conclude the location of tissue damage. Acute myocardial infarction (MI) discharges CK to the blood within the first 48 hours; the values become normal within 3 days. The isoenzyme CK-MB appears within the first 6 to 24 hours and is usually gone within 72 hours.

Recurrent elevation of CK indicates re-infarction or extension of ischemic damage. Significant increases in CK are expected in the early stages of muscular dystrophy, even before clinical signs and symptoms appear. CK increases decrease as the disease progresses, and muscle mass decreases. The differences in total CK with age and gender relate to the fact that the predominant isoenzyme is the origin of the muscle. Bodybuilders have higher values, while older individuals have lower values due to muscle mass deterioration. In the MI assessment, the use of the mass assay for CK-MB with cardiac troponin, I have largely replaced the use of CK isoenzymes with electrophoresis. CK-MB mass assays are more sensitive and faster than electrophoresis. It is highly recommended that serial samples for CK-MB be evaluated.

INDICATIONS:
- Help in the diagnosis of acute MI and assess cardiac ischemia (CK-MB).
- Detect musculoskeletal disorders, such as dermatomyositis or Duchenne muscular dystrophy (CK-MM).
- Establish the success of coronary artery reperfusion after streptokinase infusion or percutaneous transluminal angioplasty, as demonstrated by a decrease in CK-MB.

RESULT:

Increased in:
• **Alcoholism**
• **Brain infarction (extensive)**
• **Congestive heart failure**
• **Delirium tremens**
• **Dermatomyositis**
• **Head injury**
• **Hypothyroidism**
• **Hypoxic shock**
• **Infectious diseases**
• **Gastrointestinal (GI) tract infarction**
• **Loss of blood supply to any muscle**
• **Malignant hyperpyrexia**
• **Muscular dystrophies**
• **MI**
• **Myocarditis**
• **Polymyositis**
• **Pregnancy**
• **Prolonged hypothermia**

•	Pulmonary edema
•	Pulmonary embolism
•	Reye's syndrome
•	Rhabdomyolysis
•	Surgery
•	Tachycardia
•	Tetanus
•	Trauma
•	Neoplasms of the bladder, prostate, and GI tract
	Decreased in:
•	Small stature
•	Sedentary lifestyle

IMPEDING FACTORS:
- Medications that may increase total CK levels include any intramuscularly administered formulations related to tissue trauma caused by the injection.
- Drugs that may reduce total CK levels include dantrolene and dobesilate.

ALDOLASE (ALD)

SAMPLING: 1 ml serum is collected in a red- or tiger-top tube.
TECHNIQUE: Spectrophotometry
NORMAL value:

Age	Conventional Units	SI Units (Conversion Factor X 0.017)
Newborn–2 y	3.4–11.8 U/L	0.06–0.20 µKat/L
25 m–16 y	1.2–8.8 U/L	0.02–0.15 µKat/L
Adult	< 7.4 U/L	< 0.13 µKat/L

EXPLAINATION:
Aldolase (ALD), an enzyme found all over the body, catalyzes the breakdown of glucose into lactate. The highest level of this enzyme is found in the skeletal and cardiac muscles, the liver, and the pancreas. If damage or injury causes the cellular breakdown of these muscles or tissues, large amounts of ALDs are released into the blood. Measuring serum levels helps to establish the presence and, in some cases, the progression of the disease. This test is not commonly demanded because the testing of other liver enzymes and creatine kinase is generally sufficient to provide the necessary information.

INDICATIONS:
- Assist in the evaluation of Duchenne muscular dystrophy.
- Distinguish neuromuscular conditions from neurological disorders such as multiple sclerosis or myasthenia gravis.

RESULT

Increased in:
• Carcinoma (lung, breast, genitourinary tract, and metastasis to the liver)
• Central nervous system tumors
• Delirium tremens
• Hepatitis (acute viral or toxic)
• Infectious mononucleosis
• Leukemia (granulocytic and megaloblastic)
• Limb-girdle muscular dystrophy
• Myocardial infarction
• Dermatomyositis
• Duchenne's muscular dystrophy
• Gangrene
• Hemolytic anemias
• Pancreatitis (acute)
• Polymyositis
• Psychoses and schizophrenia (acute)
Decreased in:
• Hereditary fructose intolerance

IMPEDING FACTORS:
- Drugs that may increase the levels of aldolase include aminocaproic acid, carbenoxolone, clofibrate, chlorinated and organophosphorus insecticides, labetalol, and thiabendazole.
- Drugs that may reduce aldolase levels include phenothiazines (in schizophrenic patients with high initial values) and probucol.
- Intramuscular injections may increase the level of aldolase due to muscle trauma.
- Red blood cells contain aldolases; hemolysis may cause a false elevation of values.

SYNOVIAL FLUID ANALYSIS

(Arthrocentesis, joint fluid analysis, knee fluid analysis)
SPECIMEN:
Synovial fluid obtained in a red-top tube for antinuclear antibodies (ANAs), supplement, crystal analysis, calcium, rheumatoid factor (RF) and uric acid; lavender-top (ethylenediaminetetraacetic acid [EDTA]) tube for complete blood count (CBC); sterile (red-top) tube for microbiological testing and differential; gray-top (sodium fluoride [NaFl]) tube for glucose; a green-top (heparin) tube for whole blood count (CBC) and differential; green-top(heparin) tube for lactic acidosis and pH.

TECHNIQUE:
Macroscopic assessment of appearance; spectrophotometry for glucose, lactic acid, protein, and uric acid; ion-selective electrode for pH; Gram stain, acid-fast stain, and culture for microbiology; microscopic examination of fluid for cell count and evaluation of crystals; nephelometry for RF and C3; indirect fluorescence for ANAs.

NORMAL VALUE:

Color	Colorless to pale yellow
Clarity	Clear
Viscosity	High
ANA	Parallels serum level
C3	Parallels serum level
Glucose	< 10 mg/dL of the blood level
Lactic acid	5–20 mg/dL
pH	7.2–7.4
Protein	< 3 g/dL
RF	Parallels serum level
Uric acid	Parallels serum level
Crystals	None present
RBC count	None
WBC count	< 200/mm3
Neutrophils	< 25%
WBC morphology	No abnormal cells or inclusions
Gram stain and culture	No organisms present
AFB smear and culture	No AFB present

ANA = antinuclear antibodies; C3 = complement; RF = rheumatoid factor; RBC = red blood cell; WBC = white blood cell; AFB = acid-fast bacilli.

EXPLAINATION:

Synovial fluid analysis is performed through arthrocentesis, an invasive procedure requiring the introduction of a needle into the joint space. Synovial effusions are correlated with joint disorders or injuries. The most often aspirated joint is the knee, while samples may also be obtained from the shoulder, elbow, wrist, hip, and ankle if clinically indicated. Joint disorders can be divided into the following categories: non-inflammatory, inflammatory septic, crystal-induced, and hemorrhagic.

INDICATIONS:

- Support in the evaluation of joint effusions.
- Distinguish gout from pseudogout.

RESULT:

Fluid values increased in:

- *Acute bacterial arthritis*:

White blood cell counts 10,000 to 200,000 / mm3, reported neutrophil predominance (90 percent of cases), positive Gram stain (50 percent of cases), positive cultures (30 to 80 percent of cases), probable involvement of Rice bodies, elevated lactic acid, and serum complement levels (may be increased or decreased).

- *Gout*: WBC counts 500 to 200,000/mm3 with a predominance of neutrophils (approximately 70%), presence of monosodium urate crystals, raised uric acid, and complement levels parallel to serum (may be elevated or decreased).
- *Osteoarthritis, degenerative joint disease*:

WBC numbers < 5,000/mm3 for regular differential and cartilage cells

- *Pseudogout*: Presence of calcium pyrophosphate crystals.
- *Rheumatoid arthritis*: WBC counts 2,000 to 100,000/mm3 with the predominance of neutrophils (30 to 50 percent), presence of phagocyte cells and possibly Rice bodies, presence of cholesterol crystals when the effusion is chronic, increased lactic acid, increased protein, and presence of rheumatoid factor (60 percent of cases).
- *Systemic lupus erythematosus (SLE)*:

WBC counts 2,000 to 100,000/mm3 with a predominance of neutrophils (30 to 40 percent), presence of SLE cells and occurrence of antinuclear antibodies (20 percent of cases).

- *Trauma, joint tumors, or hemophilic arthritis*:

Elevated RBC count, elevated protein levels and appearance of fat droplets (if trauma is involved).

- *Tuberculous arthritis*:

WBC counts 2,000 to 100,000/mm3 with the predominance of neutrophils (30 to 60 percent), the possible presence of Rice bodies, presence of cholesterol crystals when the effusion is chronic, in some cases positive culture and acid-fast bacilli (frequently negative results), and lactic acid.

Fluid values reduced in (analytes in parentheses are decreased):
- Gout (glucose)
- Acute bacterial arthritis (glucose and pH)
- SLE (glucose, pH, and complement)
- Tuberculous arthritis (glucose and pH)
- Rheumatoid arthritis (glucose, pH, and complement)

IMPEDING FACTORS:
- Blood in the traumatic arthrocentesis sample may falsely increase the RBC count.
- Undetected hypoglycemia or hyperglycemia can produce misleading glucose levels.
- Sample refrigeration can result in an increase in monosodium urate crystals due to a decrease in uric acid solubility, exposure of the sample to room air resulting in a loss of carbon dioxide, and an increase in pH promotes the formation of calcium pyrophosphate crystals.

ACETYLCHOLINE RECEPTOR ANTI-BODY (AchR antibody)

SAMPLING: 1 mL of serum is received in a red-top tube.
Technique: Radioimmunoassay
NORMAL value: < 0.03 nmol/L.
EXPLAINATION:
When present, acetylcholine receptor Antibody (AChR) blocks the binding of acetylcholine at the muscle binding sites on the Cell Membrane. AChR destroys acetylcholine, interferes with neuromuscular Transmission, and triggers muscle fatigue. Antibodies of the Acetylcholine receptor sites present in 90 % of patients with Myasthenia gravis (MG), and 75 to 80 percent of patients with one of these, face types of MG remission.

INDICATIONS:
- Confirm the presence, but not the seriousness, of myasthenia gravis (MG)
- Make a distinction between generalized and ocular forms of MG because patients with the ocular form have lower titers
- Monitor the efficacy of immunosuppressive therapy for MG
- Monitor the remission stage of MG

RESULTS:

Raised in:
• Lateral amyotrophic syndrome
• MG (4.8 nmol / L) suggests generalized MG, 1.2 nmol / L suggests MG of the eye, 0.9 nmol / L suggests the remission)
• Thymoma like MG
Decreased in:
not any cause

IMPEDING FACTORS:
- Products that can develop false-positive effects contain muscle relaxants, including metocurin and succinylcholine.
- Products that can raise the levels of AChR contains penicillamine.
- Past treatment of immunosuppressive medications may result in adverse test outcomes.
- Past radioactive or nuclear scans as these tests could intervene with results if done within the past week.

NOTES

SERUM ELECTROLYTES

Electrolytes are minerals that carry an electric charge when they are dissolved in a liquid such as blood. The blood electrolytes—sodium, potassium, chloride, and bicarbonate—help regulate nerve and muscle function and maintain **acid-base balance** and **water balance**.

If the balance of electrolytes is disturbed, disorders can develop. For example, an electrolyte imbalance can result from the following:

- Becoming **dehydrated** or **overhydrated**
- Taking certain drugs
- Having certain heart, kidney, or liver disorders
- Being given intravenous fluids or feedings in inappropriate amounts

NOTES

_____

_____

_____

_____

_____

_____

_____

_____

_____

_____

_____

_____

_____

_____

_____

_____

CALCIUM, SERUM (total calcium, Ca)

SAMPLING:1 mL of serum is collected in a red- or tiger-top tube. 1 mL of plasma collected in a green-top (heparin) tube is also acceptable.

TECHNIQUE: Spectrophotometry

NORMAL VALUE:

Age	Conventional Units	SI Units (Conversion Factor X0.25)
Cord	8.2–11.2 mg/dL	2.05–2.80 mmol/L
0–10 d	7.6–10.4 mg/dL	1.90–2.60 mmol/L
11 d–2 y	9.0–11.0 mg/dL	2.25–2.75 mmol/L
3–12 y	8.8–10.8 mg/dL	2.20–2.70 mmol/L
13–18 y	8.4–10.2 mg/dL	2.10–2.55 mmol/L
Adult	8.2–10.2 mg/dL	2.05–2.55 mmol/L
Adult older than 90 y	8.2–9.6 mg/dL	2.05–2.40 mmol/L

EXPLAINATION:

Calcium, the most common cation in the body, is active in almost all vital processes. The parathyroid glands largely regulate the production of calcium and the activity of vitamin D. 98 to 99 percent of the body's calcium stores are concentrated in the teeth and skeleton. Calcium levels are higher in children due to growth and healthy bone formation. Approximately 45 percent of the total quantity of blood calcium circulates as free ions that participate in coagulation, intracellular modulation, glandular secretion, neuromuscular conduction, and skeletal and cardiac muscle contractility function.

The rest is attached to circulating proteins (40 percent bound mostly to albumin) and anions (15 percent bound to anions such as phosphate, bicarbonate, citrate, and lactate) and does not play a physiological role. Calcium levels may be revised up or down by 0.8 mg / dL for every 1 g / dL. The albumin is higher than or < 4 g / dL. Calcium and phosphorus are inversely related.

Fluid and electrolyte imbalances are frequently seen in people with serious illness or injury; the natural homeostatic equilibrium of the body is disrupted in these clinical situations.

During surgery or in the case of critical illness, bicarbonate, phosphate, and lactate concentrations can change dramatically. Therapeutic therapies may also cause or contribute to electrolyte imbalances. Therefore, total body calcium levels can sometimes be misleading. Abnormal levels of calcium are used to imply general malfunctions in various body systems. Measurement of Ionized calcium is used under more specific conditions.

Calcium values should be viewed following other test results. Normal calcium with a high phosphorus value indicates decreased calcium absorption (possibly due to altered parathyroid hormone levels or activity). Normal calcium with an elevated value of urea nitrogen indicates possible hyperparathyroidism (primary or secondary). Standard calcium with decreased albumin content is an indicator of hypercalcemia. Hypoalbuminemia is the most frequent cause of hypocalcemia (low calcium levels). Hyperparathyroidism and cancer are the most common causes of hypercalcemia (high calcium levels).

INDICATIONS:

- Identify the failure of the parathyroid gland following thyroid or other neck surgery, as demonstrated by decreased levels.
- Assess cardiac arrhythmias and coagulation disorders to determine whether the altered serum calcium level contributes to the problem.
- Evaluate the effects of various diseases on calcium metabolism bone disorders.
- Monitor the effects of renal failure and various drugs on calcium levels.
- Monitor the efficacy of treatment to correct elevated calcium levels, in particular calcium deficiencies.

RESULT:

Increased in:
Acidosis
Acromegaly
Cancers (bone, Burkitt lymphoma, Hodgkin lymphoma, leukemia, myeloma, and other organ metastases)
Dehydration
Excessive intake (milk, antacids)
Hyperparathyroidism
Idiopathic hypercalcemia of infancy
Malignant tumor without bone involvement (pulmonary squamous cell carcinoma, kidney cancer)
Milk alkali syndrome (Burnett's syndrome)
Paget's disease
Pheochromocytoma
Polycythemia vera
Renal transplant
Sarcoidosis
Thyrotoxicosis
Vitamin D toxicity
Decreased in:
Acute pancreatitis
Alcoholism
Alkalosis
Chronic renal failure

Cystinosis
Hepatic cirrhosis
Hyperphosphatemia
Hypoalbuminemia
Inadequate nutrition
Leprosy
Long-term anticonvulsant therapy
Magnesium deficiency
Malabsorption (celiac disease, tropical sprue, pancreatic insufficiency)
Massive blood transfusion
Neonatal prematurity
Osteomalacia (advanced)
Renal tubular disease
Vitamin D deficiency (rickets)
Hypoparathyroidism (congenital, idiopathic, surgical)

CRITICAL VALUES:
< 7 mg/dL
>12 mg/dL (some patients can bear higher concentrations)
Monitor signs with substantially reduced or elevated levels of calcium in the patient. Clinically convulsions, facial spasms (positive Chvostek sign), numbness in the extremities, tetany, muscle cramps, tingling, and muscle twitching (positive Trousseau sign) marks hypocalcemia. Arrhythmias indicate hypocalcemia along with electrocardiogram (ECG) changes in the form of prolonged ST-segment and Q-T interval.

Possible interventions include seizure protection, improved ECG monitoring, and administration of calcium or magnesium.

Extreme hypercalcemia is characterized by polyuria, lethargy, constipation, ECG changes (shortened ST segment), muscle fatigue, apathy, anorexia, vomiting, and nausea, which can eventually lead to coma. Possible treatments include the administration of regular saline and diuretics to enhance the excretion or administration of calcitonin or hormones that allow calcium to accumulate in the cells.

IMPEDING FACTORS:
- Medications that may raise calcium levels include anabolic steroids, certain antacids, calcitriol, calcium salts, danazol, diuretics (long-term), ergocalciferol, isotretinoin, lithium, oral contraceptives, parathyroid extract, parathyroid hormone, prednisone, progesterone, tamoxifen, vitamin A, and vitamin D.

- Medications that may reduce calcium levels include albuterol, alprostadil, aminoglycosides, anticonvulsants, calcitonin, diuretics (initially), glucagon, glucocorticoids, leptin, laxatives (excessive use), magnesium salts, methicillin, phosphates, plicamycin, sodium sulfate (intravenous), tetracycline (in pregnancy), trazodone, and viomycin.
- Calcium demonstrates diurnal variation; repeated samples should be collected for analysis at the same time of day.
- Venous hemostasis caused by persistent use of a tourniquet during venipuncture can artificially increase calcium levels.
- Patients with ethylenediaminetetraacetic acid (EDTA) treatment (chelation) may have mistakenly reduced calcium levels.
- Specimens should never be obtained above the intravenous (IV) line due to the potential for dilution when the specimen and the IV solution are mixed in the collection container, inappropriately reducing the outcome.

CALCIUM, URINE

SAMPLING: 5 mL of urine from a fresh random sample or timely marked specimen is collected in a clean plastic container.

TECHNIQUE: Spectrophotometry

NORMAL VALUE:

Age	Conventional Units*	SI Units (Conversion Factor X0.025) *
Infant and children	Around 6 mg/kg/day	Around 0.15 mmol/kg/day
Adult on the standard diet	100–300 mg/day	2.5–7.5 mmol/day

* Values vary according to dietary intake. Normal daily consumption of calcium: 600–800 mg/day.

EXPLAINATION:

The control of electrolyte balance is a major function of the kidneys. Of normal functioning kidneys, urinary levels rise when serum levels are high and decline when serum levels are low to conserve homeostasis. Evaluating the levels of urinary electrolytes can provide important cues to the activity of the kidneys and other major organs. Calcium checks of urine usually involve timed collecting of urine over a 12-or 24-hour period. Measurements of random samples may also be required. Urinary calcium excretion might also be expressed as a calcium-to-creatinine ratio: the ratio is < 0.14 for a healthy individual with steady muscle mass.

INDICATIONS:
- Assess bone disease.
- Evaluate food consumption and absorption.
- Evaluate renal impairment.
- Monitor calcium replacement therapy in patients.
- Assist in establishing the presence of kidney stones.

RESULT:

Increased in:
Acromegaly
Diabetes
Some instances of leukemia and lymphoma
Fanconi's syndrome
Glucocorticoid excess
Hepatolenticular degeneration
Hyperparathyroidism
Hyperthyroidism
Idiopathic hypercalciuria
Immobilization
Kidney stones
Myeloma
Neoplasm of the breast or bladder
Osteitis deformans
Osteoporosis
Paget's disease
Renal tubular acidosis
Sarcoidosis
Schistosomiasis
Thyrotoxicosis
Vitamin D intoxication
Osteolytic bone metastases (carcinoma, sarcoma)
Decreased in:
Hypocalcemia (other than a renal disease)
Malabsorption (celiac disease, tropical sprue)
Hypocalciuric hypercalcemia (familial, nonfamilial)
Hypoparathyroidism
Hypothyroidism
Malignant bone neoplasm
Nephrosis and acute nephritis
Osteoblastic metastases
Osteomalacia
Preeclampsia
Pseudohypoparathyroidism
Renal osteodystrophy
Rickets
Vitamin D deficiency

IMPEDING FACTORS:
- Drugs that may increase urinary calcium levels include acetazolamide, ammonium chloride, corticotropin, dexamethasone, asparaginase, calcitonin, calcitriol, corticosteroids, diuretics (initially), ergocalciferol, ethacrynic acid, mannitol (initially), meralluride, mersalyl, nandrolone, mercaptopurine, sodium sulfate, sulfate, triamterene, parathyroid extract, parathyroid hormone, plicamycin, viomycin, and Vit D.
- Medications that may decrease calcium levels in the urine include angiotensin, bicarbonate, calcitonin, citrate, diuretics (chronic), lithium neomycin, oral contraceptives, and spironolactone.
- Failed to collect all the urine and safely store the specimen during the 24-hour test period invalidates the findings.

SODIUM, SERUM (Serum Na⁺)

SAMPLING: 1 mL of serum is collected in a red- or tiger-top tube. 1mL of plasma collected in a green-top (heparin) tube is also acceptable.
TECHNIQUE: Ion-selective electrode
NORMAL VALUE:
EXPLAINATION:
Sodium (Na+) is the most abundant cation present in extracellular fluid, and together with corresponding chloride and bicarbonate anions, it accounts for 92% of serum osmolality. Sodium plays a key role in maintaining homeostasis in a variety of ways, including maintaining the osmotic pressure of the extracellular fluid, controlling renal retention and excretion in water, retaining acid-base balance, managing potassium and chloride levels, triggering neuromuscular reactions, and maintaining systemic blood pressure.
Hypernatremia (high sodium level) occurs when there is excessive water loss or excessive sodium retention. Hyponatremia (low sodium level) occurs when sodium retention or absorption becomes insufficient.
INDICATIONS:
- Evaluate sodium in the whole body because the ion is primarily extracellular.
- Monitor the effectiveness of drug therapy, especially diuretics, on serum sodium levels.
RESULT:

	Increased in:
•	**Azotemia**
•	**Burns**
•	**Cushing's disease**
•	**Dehydration**
•	**Diabetes**
•	**Excessive intake**

•	Excessive saline therapy
•	Excessive sweating
•	Fever
•	Hyperaldosteronism
•	Lactic acidosis
•	Nasogastric feeding with inadequate fluid
•	Diarrhea (water loss over the salt loss)
•	Vomiting
	Decreased in:
•	Central nervous system disease
•	Congestive heart failure
•	Cystic fibrosis
•	Excessive use of diuretics
•	Hepatic failure
•	Hypoproteinemia
•	Insufficient intake
•	Intravenous (IV) glucose infusion
•	Metabolic acidosis
•	Mineralocorticoid deficiency (Addison's disease)
•	Excessive antidiuretic hormone production
•	Nephrotic syndrome

CRITICAL VALUES:
Hyponatremia: <120 mmol/L
Hypernatremia: >160 mmol/L

Age	Conventional Units	SI Units (Conversion Factor X1)
Newborn	133–146 mEq/L	133–146 mmol/L
Infant	133–144 mEq/L	133–144 mmol/L
Child	135–145 mEq/L	135–145 mmol/L
Adult	135–145 mEq/L	135–145 mmol/L

Note and record increased or decreased values and signs of fluid imbalance to the patient health care practitioner. Signs and symptoms of hyponatremia include agitation, irritability, seizure, tachycardia, nausea, vomiting, and loss of consciousness. Possible interventions include airway maintenance, convulsion management, fluid restraint, and regular neurological checks. The application of saline for replacement requires close attention to plasma and urinary osmolality. Signs and symptoms of hypernatremia include restlessness, intense thirst, exhaustion, swollen tongue, fits, and coma. Possible interventions include management of the root cause of water loss or sodium toxicity, which involves sodium restriction and application of diuretics in conjunction with IV solutions of 5% dextrose in water (D5W).

IMPEDING FACTORS:
- Drugs that can increase serum sodium levels include anabolic steroids, angiotensin, bicarbonate, carbenoxolone, cisplatin, corticotropin, cortisone, gamma globulin, and mannitol.
- Substances that may reduce serum sodium levels include amphotericin B, bicarbonate, cathartic (excessive use), chlorpropamide, chlorthalidone, diuretics, ethacrynic acid, fluoxetine, furosemide, laxative (excessive use), methyclothiazide, metolazone, nicardipine, quinethazone, theophylline (IV infusion), thiazides, and triamterene.
- Specimens should never be obtained above the IV line due to the potential for dilution when the specimen and the IV solution are mixed in the collection container, incorrectly reducing the outcome. The probability of contaminating the sample with the substance of interest contained in the IV solution is also falsely increasing.

SODIUM, URINE (Urine Na+)

SAMPLING: 5 mL of urine from an unpreserved random or timed specimen is collected in a clean, plastic collection container.

NORMAL VALUE:

Age	Conventional Units	SI Units (Conversion Factor X1)
6–10 y		
Male	41–115 mEq/24 h	41–115 mmol/24 h
Female	20–69 mEq/24 h	20–69 mmol/24 h
10–14 y		
Male	63–177 mEq/24 h	63–177 mmol/24 h
Female	48–168 mEq/24 h	48–168 mmol/24 h
Adult	27–287 mEq/24 h	27–287 mmol/24 h

Values vary depending on dietary intake and hydration state.

EXPLAINATION:
The regulation of electrolyte balance is a major function of the kidneys. In normally functioning kidneys, sodium levels of urine increase when serum levels are high and reduce when serum levels are low to preserve homeostasis. Analyzing these urinary levels can present important insights into the functioning of the kidneys and other major organs. Diurnal variation in sodium excretion is observed, with values lower at night. Urine sodium tests usually involve a timed collection of urine over a 12- or 24-hour period. Measurements of arbitrary specimens may also be required.

INDICATIONS:
- Determine the potential cause of kidney stones.
- Evaluate known or suspected endocrine disorder.
- Assess known or suspected renal disease.
- Evaluate malabsorption disorders.

RESULT:

Increased in:
• Adrenal failure
• Alkalosis
• Diabetes
• Diuretic therapy
• Excessive intake
• Renal tubular acidosis
• Salt-losing nephritis
Decreased in:
• Excessive sweating hydration
• Extrarenal sodium loss with adequate
• Adrenal hyperfunction
• Congestive heart failure
• Diarrhea
• Insufficient intake
• Prerenal azotemia
• Sodium retention (premenstrual)
• Postoperative period (first 24 to 48 hours)

IMPEDING FACTORS:

- Medicines that may increase urine sodium levels include acetazolamide, diapamide, dopamine, ethacrynic acid, furosemide, hydrocortisone, hydroflumethiazide, bumetanide, calcitonin, chlorothiazide, clopamide, cyclothiazide, isosorbide, levodopa, mercurial diuretics, methyclothiazide, amiloride, ammonium chloride, acetylsalicylic acid, azosemide, benzthiazide, metolazone, polythiazide, quinethazone, trichlormethiazide, triflocin, verapamil, spironolactone, sulfates, tetracycline, thiazides, torasemide, triamterene, and vincristine.

- Medications that may decrease sodium levels in the urine include aldosterone, anesthetics, angiotensin, corticosteroids, cortisone, etodolac, indomethacin, levarterenol, lithium, and propranolol.

- Sodium levels are subject to diurnal variation (the level being the lowest at night), which is why 24-hour collections are recommended.

POTASSIUM, SERUM (Serum K+)

SAMPLING: 1 mL of serum is collected in a red- or tiger-top tube. 1 mL of plasma collected in a green-top (heparin) tube is also acceptable.

TECHNIQUE: Ion-selective electrode

NORMAL VALUE:

Serum	SI Units (Conversion Factor X1)
Newborn	3.7–5.9 mmol/L or mEq/L
Infant	4.1–5.3 mmol/L or mEq/L
Child	3.4–4.7 mmol/L or mEq/L
Adult	3.5–5.0 mmol/L or mEq/L

EXPLAINATION:

Electrolytes dissolve into electrically charged ions. Cations, like potassium, are positively charged. Body fluids contain approximately equal amounts of anions and cations, although the existence and mobility of the ions differ between intracellular and extracellular compartments. The electrical and osmolar processes of the body are affected by both types of ions. Electrolyte concentrations and the equilibrium between them are regulated by the exchange of oxygen and carbon dioxide in the lungs, the absorption secretion and excretion of many compounds by the kidneys, and the secretion of hormonal hormones by the endocrine glands. Potassium is the most plentiful intracellular cation in the blood. It is important for the propagation of electrical impulses in the cardiac and skeletal muscles.

It also acts in enzymatic reactions that transform glucose into energy as well as amino acids into proteins. Potassium helps to maintain the acid-base balance and also has a significant and inverse relation to pH: apH decrease of 0.1 increases the potassium level by 0.6 mEq / L. Potassium deficiency can be caused by several underlying factors and can be described as follows: impaired renal excretion: typically 80 to 90% of the body's potassium passes into the kidneys every day (the remainder is excreted in sweat and feces); kidney failure can lead to unusually high potassium rates. Altered dietary intake: severe potassium deficit can be caused by low oral potassium intake. Changes in cell metabolism: damaged red blood cells (RBCs) leak potassium into the circulating plasma, resulting in elevated serum potassium.

INDICATIONS:

- Evaluate documented or suspected conditions associated with renal dysfunction, glucose metabolism, trauma, or burns.
- Aid in the assessment of electrolyte imbalances; this examination is particularly indicated in elderly patients, patients taking supplementation, patients on hemodialysis, and patients with hypertension.
- Assess cardiac arrhythmia to decide whether the altered potassium levels contribute to the problem, particularly during digitalis therapy, which contributes to ventricular irritability.
- Estimate the effects of drug therapy, especially diuretics.

- Evaluate the response to treatment for elevated potassium levels.
- Monitor known or presumed acidosis, as potassium moves from RBCs to extracellular fluids in acidic states.
- Routine electrolyte screening in acute and chronic conditions.

RESULT:

Increased in:
• Diet (too much intake of salt substitutes or potassium salts of medications)
• Acidosis
• Acute renal failure
• Addison's disease
• Asthma
• Burns
• Chronic interstitial nephritis
• Dehydration
• Dialysis
• Excessive theophylline administration
• Exercise
• Hemolysis (massive)
• Hyperventilation
• Hypoaldosteronism
• Insulin deficiency
• Uremia
• Ketoacidosis
• Leukocytosis
• Muscle necrosis
• Near-drowning
• Pregnancy
• Prolonged periods of standing
• Tissue trauma
• Transfusion of old banked blood
• Tubular unresponsiveness to aldosterone
Decreased in:
• Gastrointestinal loss caused by vomiting, diarrhea, nasogastric suction, or intestinal fistula
• Alcoholism
• Alkalosis
• Anorexia nervosa
• Bradycardia
• Congestive heart failure
• Crohn's disease

•	Cushing's syndrome
•	Diet deficient in meat and vegetables
•	Excess insulin
•	Familial periodic paralysis
•	Hyperaldosteronism
•	Hypertension
•	Hypomagnesemia
•	Chronic, excessive licorice ingestion (from licorice root)
•	Laxative abuse
•	Malabsorption
•	Pica (clay eating)
•	Renal tubular acidosis
•	Stress
•	Sweating
•	Thyrotoxicosis
•	Toxic shock syndrome
•	Intravenous (IV) therapy with inadequate potassium supplementation

CRITICAL VALUES:
Newborns:
< 2.5 mmol/L
>7.0 mmol/L
Adults:
< 2.5 mmol/L
More than 6.5 mmol/L
Report and record elevated or reduced levels and signs of fluid imbalance to the patient health care professional. Hyperkalemia symptoms include irritability, diarrhea, cramps, oliguria, speech impairment, and cardiac arrhythmias (peak T waves and ventricular fibrillation). Continuous cardiac monitoring is suggested. The use of sodium bicarbonate or calcium chloride can be required. When the patient requires an IV replacement, verify if the patient is voiding.
Symptoms of hypokalemia involve malaise, anorexia, thirst, polyuria, weak pulse, low blood pressure, vomiting, diminished reflexes, and electrocardiographic changes (depressed T-wave and ventricular ectopy). Replacement therapy has been suggested.
IMPEDING FACTORS:
- Medicines that can cause a rise in potassium levels include dexamethasone, some drugs with potassium salts, propranolol, enalapril, mannitol, methicillin, metoprolol, nonsteroidal anti-inflammatory drugs, spironolactone, and succinylcholine.

- Medications that may cause a decrease in potassium levels include acetazolamide, dexamethasone, alanine, albuterol, aldosterone, ammonium chloride, amphotericin B, acetylsalicylic acid, bicarbonate, digoxin, diuretics, enalapril, bisacodyl, captopril, carbenicillin, cathartics, cisplatin, chlorexolone, desoxycorticosterone, furosemide, hydrocortisone, hydroflumethiazide, laxatives, moxalactam (common w). Many of these medications increase serum potassium levels. However, they also have a diuretic effect that promotes the loss of potassium in the urine, except in cases of renal insufficiency.
- Leukocytosis, as seen in leukemia, causes elevated potassium levels.
- False elevations can occur with intense hand pumping during venipuncture. Sample hemolysis and high platelet count may increase potassium levels as follows: (1) Since potassium is an intracellular ion and the concentrations are approximately 150 times extracellular, even a small amount of hemolysis may cause a significant increase in levels. (2) Platelets discharge potassium during the clotting process, and therefore serum samples collected from patients with elevated platelet counts can yield spuriously high levels of potassium. Plasma would be the ideal medium in patients known to have elevated platelet counts.
- Collection of unprocessed blood allows potassium levels to increase as a significant amount of potassium spills out of the cells in just a few hours. Plasma or serum should be separated from the cells within four hours of collection.
- Specimens should never be collected above the IV line due to the potential for dilution when the sample and the IV solution are mixed in the collection container, falsely reducing the result. The ability to contaminate the sample with the substance of interest present in the IV solution is also unfairly increasing

POTASSIUM, URINE (Urine K+)

SAMPLING: 5 mL of urine from an unpreserved random or timed specimen is collected in a clean, plastic collection container.
TECHNIQUE: Ion-selective electrode
NORMAL VALUE:

Age	Conventional Units	SI Units (Conversion Factor X1)
6–10 y		
Male	17–54 mEq/24 h	17–54 mmol/24 h
Female	8–37 mEq/24 h	8–37 mmol/24 h
10–14 y		
Male	22–57 mEq/24 h	22–57 mmol/24 h
Female	18–58 mEq/24 h	18–58 mmol/24 h
Adult	26–123 mEq/24 h	26–123 mmol/24 h

EXPLAINATION:

Electrolytes dissolve into electrically charged ions. Cations, including potassium, are positively charged. Body fluids contain approximately equal amounts of anions and cations, although the existence and mobility of the ions differ between intracellular and extracellular compartments. The electrical and osmolar processes of the body are affected by both types of ions. Electrolyte concentrations and the equilibrium between them are regulated by the exchange of oxygen and carbon dioxide in the lungs, the absorption secretion and excretion of many substances by the kidneys, and the secretion of hormonal hormones by the endocrine glands.

Potassium is the most readily available intracellular cation in the body. It is important for the propagation of electrical impulses in the cardiac and skeletal muscles. It also acts in enzyme reactions that turn glucose into energy and amino acids into proteins. Potassium helps maintain acid-base balance and has a major and opposite relation to pH: a pH decreases of 0.1 raises the potassium level by 0.6 mEq / L.

Abnormal potassium can be caused by several contributing factors, which can be categorized as follows: impaired renal excretion: usually 80 to 90 percent of the body's potassium is absorbed through the kidneys each day (the rest is excreted in sweat and stool); kidney disease can lead to abnormally high potassium levels.

Impaired dietary intake: extreme potassium deficit may be caused by inadequate dietary potassium intake.

Altered cell metabolism: injured red blood cells (RBCs) leak potassium into the circulating fluid, resulting in increased potassium levels. The regulation of electrolyte balance is one of the main functions of the kidneys. For normal functioning kidneys, urinary potassium levels increase when serum levels are high and decline when serum levels are low to maintain homeostasis. The kidneys react to alkalosis by excreting potassium to retain hydrogen ions and increase acidity. In the case of acidosis, the body excretes hydrogen ions and retains potassium. Analyzing these urinary levels can provide important insights into the functioning of the kidneys and other major organs. Urinary potassium tests usually involve timed processing of urine over a 12-or 24-hour period. Measurement of arbitrary measurements may also be required.

INDICATIONS:

- Determine the potential cause of kidney stones.
- Evaluate known or suspected endocrine disorder.
- Evaluate known or suspected renal disease.
- Evaluate malabsorption disorders.

RESULT:

Increased in:
• **Hyperaldosteronism**
• **Cushing's syndrome**
• **Diabetic ketoacidosis**
• **Diuretic therapy**

• Starvation (onset)	
• Vomiting	
• Albright-type renal disease	
Decreased in:	
• Addison's disease	
• Potassium deficiency (chronic)	
• Renal failure with decreased urine flow	

IMPEDING FACTORS:

- Medications and compounds that may induce a rise in urinary potassium levels include acetazolamide, acetylsalicylic acid, ammonium chloride, bendroflumethiazide, carbenoxolone, chlorthalidone, citrate, clopamide, corticosteroids, cortisone, desoxycorticosterone, dexamethasone, diuretics, dopamine, ethacrynic acid, glycyrrhiza, mefruside, niacinamide, certain oral contraceptives.

- Products that may decrease the levels of potassium in the urine include alanine, amiloride, anesthetic agents, cyclosporine, felodipine, levarterenol, and ramipril.

- Dietary deficiency or excess potassium can lead to false outcomes.

- Diuretic therapy with excessive electrolyte loss in the urine can wrongly increase results.

- All urine that has been voided for the scheduled collection period must be included in the sample, or incorrectly reduced values may be obtained. Compare output records with the amount obtained to ensure that all voids have been included in the sample.

- Potassium levels are subject to diurnal variation (the production being the highest at night), which is why 24-hour collections are recommended.

PHOSPHORUS, SERUM (Inorganic phosphorus, phosphate, PO4)

SAMPLING: 1 mL of serum is collected in a red- or tiger-top tube. 1 mL of plasma collected in a green-top (heparin) tube is also acceptable

TECHNIQUE: Spectrophotometry

NORMAL VALUE:

Age	Conventional Units	SI Units (Conversion Factor 0.323)
0–5 days	4.6–8.0 mg/dL	1.5–2.6 mmol/L
1–3 years	3.9–6.5 mg/dL	1.3–2.1 mmol/L
4–6 years	4.0–5.4 mg/dL	1.3–1.7 mmol/L
7–11 years	3.7–5.6 mg/dL	1.2–1.8 mmol/L
12–13 years	3.3–5.4 mg/dL	1.1–1.7 mmol/L
14–15 years	2.9–5.4 mg/dL	0.9–1.7 mmol/L
16–19 years	2.8–4.6 mg/dL	0.9–1.5 mmol/L

>19 years	2.5–4.5 mg/dL	0.8–1.4 mmol/L

EXPLAINATION:

Phosphorus, as phosphate ion, is spread across the human body. About 85 percent of body phosphorus is contained in bones; the rest is found in cells and body fluids. It is a major intracellular anion and plays a key role in cell metabolism, cell membrane maintenance, and bone and teeth formation. Phosphorus also indirectly affects the release of hemoglobin associated oxygen by affecting the production of 2,3-bisphosphoglycerate.

Phosphorus levels depend on dietary intake.

The kidneys regulate the excretion of phosphorous. Calcium and phosphorus are related to absorption and metabolic function.

They have an opposite concentration relationship: serum phosphorus is decreased as serum calcium is increasing. Hyperphosphatemia may be caused by the baby being fed cow's milk only during the first few weeks of life, due to the combination of high phosphorus content in cow's milk and the inability of an infant's kidneys to remove excess phosphorus.

INDICATIONS:

- Aid in the diagnosis of hyperparathyroidism.
- Help in the determination of renal failure.

RESULT:

Increased in:
• Acromegaly
• Bone metastases
• Diabetic ketoacidosis
• Hyperthermia
• Hypocalcemia
• Hypoparathyroidism
• Lactic acidosis
• Milk alkali syndrome
• Pulmonary embolism
• Excessive levels of vitamin D
• Pseudohypoparathyroidism
• Renal failure
• Respiratory acidosis
Decreased in:
• Acute gout
• Alcohol withdrawal
• Gram-negative bacterial septicemia
• Growth hormone deficiency
• Hyperalimentation therapy
• Hypercalcemia

• Hyperinsulinism
• Hyperparathyroidism
• Hypokalemia
• Impaired renal absorption
• Malabsorption syndromes
• Malnutrition
• Osteomalacia
• Parathyroid hormone-producing tumors
• Primary hyperparathyroidism
• Renal tubular acidosis
• Renal tubular defects
• Respiratory alkalosis
• Respiratory infections
• Rickets
• Salicylate poisoning
• Severe burns
• Severe vomiting and diarrhea
• Vitamin D deficiency

CRITICAL VALUES: Values of < 1.0 mg / dL may have significant effects on the neuromuscular, gastrointestinal, cardiopulmonary, and skeletal systems. Interventions include intravenous (IV) sodium or potassium phosphate replacement therapy may be needed. Close monitoring of both phosphorus and calcium during replacement therapy is necessary.

IMPEDING FACTORS:

- Products that may raise phosphorus levels include anabolic steroids, -adrenergic antagonists, ergocalciferol, furosemide, hydrochlorothiazide, methicillin (a nephrotoxicity event), oral contraceptives, parathyroid extract, phosphates, sodium etidronate, tetracycline (a nephrotoxicity event), and vitamin D.

- Medications that may reduce phosphorus levels include acetazolamide, albuterol, fibrin hydrolysate, fructose, glucocorticoids, glucose, insulin, mannitol, oral contraceptives, pamidronate, phenothiazine, phytate, aluminum salts, amino acids (via IV), anesthetic agents, anticonvulsants, calcitonin, epinephrine, and plicamycin.

- Serum phosphorus levels are subjected to diurnal variation: the highest in the late morning and the lowest in the evening; thus, serial samples should be collected at the same time of day for continuity of perception.

- Hemolysis will mistakenly increase the value of phosphorus.

- Samples should never be collected above the IV because of the possibility for dilution when the specimen and the IV solution are mixed in the collection container, thus wrongly lowering the test result.

PHOSPHORUS, URINE (Urine phosphate)

SAMPLING: 5 mL of urine from an unpreserved random or timed specimen is collected in a clean, plastic collection container.

TECHNIQUE: Spectrophotometry

NORMAL VALUE: NORMAL values are dependent on the intake of phosphorus and calcium. Phosphate excretion has diurnal variation and is significantly greater at night.

Conventional Units	SI Units (Conversion Factor X32.3)
0.4–1.3 g/24 h	12.9–42.0 g/24 h

EXPLAINATION:

Phosphorus, in the way of phosphate, is distributed across the body. Approximately 85 percent of body phosphorus is contained in bones; the rest is found in cells and body fluids. It is a major intracellular anion and plays a key role in cell metabolism, cell membrane repair, and bone and teeth formation. Phosphorus also indirectly affects the release of hemoglobin oxygen by causing the development of 2,3-bisphosphoglycerate. Phosphorus levels are dependent on dietary intake. Analyzing the levels of urinary phosphorus can provide important clues to the activity of the kidneys and other major organs. Urine phosphorus measurements usually involve the timed accumulation of urine over a 12-or 24-hour period. Measurements of arbitrary specimens may also be required. Children with thalassemia may have an average absorption of phosphorus with increased excretion, which may lead to a phosphorous deficiency.

INDICATIONS:

- Assist in the detection of hyperparathyroidism.
- AID in the evaluation of calcium and phosphorus hemostasis.
- Assist in the assessment of nephrolithiasis.
- Assist in the assessment of renal tubular disorder.

RESULT:

Increased in:	
•	Abuse of diuretics
•	Renal tubular acidosis
•	Vitamin D deficiency
•	Primary hyperparathyroidism
Decreased in:	
•	Hypoparathyroidism
•	Vitamin D intoxication
•	Pseudohypoparathyroidism

IMPEDING FACTORS:

- Medications and vitamins that can cause an increase in urine phosphorus levels include acetazolamide, corticosteroids, dihydrotachysterol, glycine, hydrochlorothiazide, metolazone, parathyroid extract, parathyroid hormone, phosphates, tryptophan, acetylsalicylic acid, alanine, bismuth salts, calcitonin, valine, and vitamin D.
- Products that may cause a decline in the total of urinary phosphorus include antacids containing aluminum.
- Urinary phosphorus levels are subject to diurnal variation: the output is highest in the afternoon, which is why a 24-hour collection of urine is required.
- All urine that has been voided for the scheduled collection period must be included in the sample, or wrongly reduced values may be obtained. Match output records with the amount collected to ensure that all voids have been included in the sample.

MAGNESIUM, SERUM (Serum Mg++)

SAMPLING: 1 mL of serum is collected in a red- or tiger-top tube.
TECHNIQUE: Spectrophotometry
NORMAL VALUE:

Age	Conventional Units	Alternative Units (Conversion Factor X0.8229)	SI Units (Conversion Factor X0.4114)
Newborn	1.5–2.2 mg/dL	1.23–1.81 mEq/L	0.62–0.91 mmol/L
Child	1.7–2.1 mg/dL	1.40–1.73 mEq/L	0.70–0.86 mmol/L
Adult	1.6–2.6 mg/dL	1.32–2.14 mEq/L	0.66–1.07 mmol/L

DESCRIPTION

Magnesium is necessary as a cofactor in several key enzymatic processes, like nucleic acid synthesis, protein synthesis, and muscle contraction. Magnesium is also needed for the use of adenosine diphosphate as an energy source. Magnesium is needed for nerve impulse propagation and muscle relaxation. Controls the absorption of sodium, potassium, calcium, and phosphorus; the use of carbohydrates, lipids, and proteins; and the activation of enzyme systems that allow B vitamins to function. Magnesium is also vital for oxidative phosphorylation, nucleic acid synthesis, and blood coagulation. Urine magnesium levels indicate magnesium deficiency before serum levels. Magnesium deficiency can be severe enough to cause hypocalcemia and cardiac arrhythmias despite normal serum magnesium levels.

INDICATIONS:

- Establish electrolyte balance in renal failure and chronic alcoholism.
- Assess cardiac arrhythmias (lower magnesium levels can lead to excessive ventricular irritability).

- Evaluate known or suspected conditions correlated with altered magnesium levels.
- Monitor the effects of various medications on magnesium levels.

RESULT:

Increased in:
• Addison's disease
• Adrenocortical insufficiency
• Dehydration
• Diabetic acidosis (severe)
• Hypothyroidism
• Systemic lupus erythematosus (SLE)
• Multiple myeloma
• Overuse of antacids
• Renal insufficiency
• Tissue trauma
Decreased in:
• Glomerulonephritis (chronic)
• Hemodialysis
• Alcoholism
• Diabetic acidosis
• Hyperaldosteronism
• Hypercalcemia
• Hypoparathyroidism
• Inadequate intake
• Long-term hyperalimentation
• Malabsorption
• Pancreatitis
• Pregnancy
• Inappropriate secretion of antidiuretic hormone
• Severe loss of body fluids (diarrhea, laxative abuse, lactation, sweating)

CRITICAL VALUES:

< 1.2 mg/dL

>6.1 mg/dL

• Symptoms such as tetany, weakness, dizziness, tremor, hyperactivity, nausea, vomiting, and seizures occur at reduced (< 1.2 mg / dL) levels.

- Electrocardiographic (ECG) changes (prolonged P-R and Q-T periods, wide flat T waves, and ventricular tachycardia) may also occur. Therapy may include administration of magnesium salts, monitoring of respiratory depression and areflexia (intravenous [IV] administration of magnesium salts), and management of diarrhea and metabolic alkalosis (oral administration to substitute magnesium).
- Respiratory paralysis, reduced reflexes, and cardiac arrest arise at extremely elevated levels (more than 15 mg / dL). Changes in ECGs, such as lengthy P-R and Q-T intervals and bradycardia, may be seen. Toxic levels of magnesium may be corrected with the administering of calcium, dialysis, and elimination of the source of excessive intake.

IMPEDING FACTORS:
- Drugs that can increase the levels of magnesium include acetylsalicylic acid and progesterone.
- Medications that may decrease magnesium levels include albuterol, aminoglycosides, amphotericin B, bendroflumethiazide, chlorthalidone, citrate, cyclosporine, cisplatin, digoxin, gentamicin, glucagon, and oral contraceptives.
- Hemolysis results in a misleading elevation of values; these specimens should be refused for review.
- Specimens should never be obtained above the IV line due to the potential for dilution when the specimen and the IV solution are mixed in the collection container, wrongly reducing the outcome. The risk to contaminate the sample with the substance of interest present in the IV solution is also mistakenly raising.

MAGNESIUM, URINE (Urine Mg++)

SAMPLING: 5 mL of urine from a random or timed sample collected in a clean plastic collection container along with 6N hydrochloride as a preservative.
TECHNIQUE: Spectrophotometry
NORMAL VALUE:

Conventional Units	Alternative Units (Conversion Factor X0.8229)	SI Units (Conversion Factor X0.4114)
7.3–12.2 mg/24 h	6.0–10.0 mEq/24 h	3.0–5.0 mmol/24 h

EXPLAINATION:
Magnesium is needed as a cofactor in many key enzymatic processes, like protein synthesis, nucleic acid synthesis, and muscle contraction.
Magnesium is also essential for the use of adenosine diphosphate as an energy source. Magnesium is needed for nerve impulse transmission and muscle relaxation. It controls the absorption of sodium, potassium, calcium, and phosphorus; the use of carbohydrates, lipids, and proteins; and the activation of enzyme systems that allow B vitamins to function.

Magnesium is also vital for oxidative phosphorylation, nucleic acid synthesis, and blood coagulation. Urine magnesium levels indicate magnesium deficiency before serum levels.

Magnesium deficiency can be severe enough to cause hypocalcemia and cardiac arrhythmias despite normal serum magnesium levels. The regulation of electrolyte balance is one of the main functions of the kidneys. In normal functioning kidneys, urine levels increase when serum levels are high, and decline when serum levels are low, to maintain homeostasis. Analyzing these urinary levels can provide important insights into the workings of the kidneys and other major organs. Electrolyte tests, such as magnesium, usually involve the accumulation of measured urine over a 12-or 24-hour period. Measurements of random specimens may also be required.

INDICATIONS:
- Determine the potential source of kidney stones.
- Evaluate known or suspected endocrine condition.
- Evaluate established or suspected renal dysfunction.
- Evaluate magnesium deficiency.
- Evaluate malabsorption issues.

RESULT:

Increased in:
• Alcoholism
• Bartter's syndrome
• Use of diuretics
• Use of corticosteroids
• Transplant recipients on cyclosporine and prednisone
Decreased in:
• Abnormal renal function
• Crohn's disease
• Salt-losing conditions
• Inappropriate secretion of antidiuretic hormone

IMPEDING FACTORS:
- Medications that may increase the levels of urinary magnesium include cisplatin, cyclosporine, ethacrynic acid, furosemide, mercaptomerine, mercurial diuretics, and thiazides.
- Pharmaceutical products that may decrease the levels of urinary magnesium include amiloride, angiotensin, oral contraceptives, parathyroid extract, and phosphates.
- The magnesium levels match the circadian rhythm, and therefore 24-hour collections are recommended.

- Any urine that has been voided for the scheduled collection period must be included in the sample, or incorrectly lowered values may be collected. Compare output records with the amount obtained to ensure that all voids have been included in the sample.

CARBON DIOXIDE: (CO2 combining power, CO2, tCO2)

SAMPLING: 1 mL of serum is collected in a red- or tiger-top tube, 1 mL of plasma is collected in a green-top (lithium or sodium heparin) tube; or 1 mL of whole blood collected in a green-top (lithium or sodium heparin) tube or heparinized syringe.

TECHNIQUE: Colorimetry, enzyme assay, or pCO2 electrode

NORMAL VALUE:

Carbon Dioxide	Conventional Units	SI Units (Conversion Factor X1)
Plasma or serum (venous)		
Infant–2 y	13–29 mmol/L	13–29 mmol/L
2 y and older	23–29 mmol/L	23–29 mmol/L
Whole blood (venous)		
Infant–2 y	18–28 mmol/L	18–28 mmol/L
2 y and older	22–26 mmol/L	22–26 mmol/L

EXPLAINATION:

Serum or plasma carbon dioxide (CO2) measurements are usually performed as part of an electrolyte screen. Total CO2 (tCO2) is an important factor of the body's buffering capacity, and tests are used specifically in the evaluation of the acid-base balance. It is important to understand the differences between tCO2 (CO2 content) and CO2 (pCO2 content). Total CO2 forms the concentration of CO2 in the body, mainly in the form of bicarbonate (HCO_3-), which is present as a base and is regulated by the kidneys. CO2 gas adds little to the level of tCO2, is acidic, and is regulated by the lungs.

CO2 provides the basis for the primary buffering system of the extracellular fluid system, the bicarbonate-carbonic acid buffer system. CO2 circulates in the body, either tied to protein or dissolved physically. Blood components that contribute to tCO2 levels include bicarbonate, carbamino compounds, and carbonic acid (carbonic acid contains uncoupled carbonic acid and dissolved CO2). Bicarbonate (HCO_3-) is the second-largest group of anions in extracellular fluids (chloride being the largest group of extracellular anions). tCO2 levels closely reflect bicarbonate (HCO_3) levels in the blood, as 90 to 95 percent of CO2 circulates as HCO_3.

INDICATIONS:
- Evaluate reduced venous CO_2 in the case of compensated metabolic acidosis.
- Evaluate reduced venous CO_2 in the case of compensated metabolic alkalosis.
- Monitor reduced venous CO_2 because of compensated respiratory alkalosis.
- Monitor raised venous CO_2 as a result of compensation for respiratory acidosis due to central respiratory system failure or cancer, drop-in respiratory rate.

RESULT:

Increased in:
• Acute intermittent porphyria
• Airway obstruction
• Asthmatic shock
• Brain tumor
• Bronchitis (chronic)
• Cardiac disorders
• Electrolyte disturbance (severe)
• Emphysema
• Hypothyroidism
• Hypoventilation
• Metabolic alkalosis
• Myopathy
• Poliomyelitis
• Pneumonia
• Respiratory acidosis
• Tuberculosis (pulmonary)
• Depression of the respiratory center
Decreased in:
• Acute renal failure
• Anxiety
• Dehydration
• Diabetic ketoacidosis
• Salicylate intoxication
• Diarrhea (severe)
• High fever
• Metabolic acidosis
• Respiratory alkalosis

CRITICAL VALUES:

< 15 mmol/L

>50 mmol/L

Strictly Monitor the individual for signs and symptoms of elevated or low levels of CO2 and report these results to the health care practitioner. If the individual has been vomiting for several days and breathes shallowly, or if the patient has had gastric suction and breathes shallowly, this may suggest an elevated level of CO2. Decreased levels of CO2 are evidenced by deep rapid breathing and flushed skin.

IMPEDING FACTORS:

- Medicines that may lead to an increase in tCO2 levels include acetylsalicylic acid, aldosterone, corticosteroids, dexamethasone, bicarbonate, carbenicillin, carbenoxolone, ethacrynic acid, laxatives (chronic abuse), and x-ray contrast agents.

- Medications that may cause a reduction in tCO2 levels to include acetazolamide, acetylsalicylic acid (initially), amiloride, ammonium chloride, fluoride, metformin, methicillin, nitrofurantoin, NSD 3004 (a long-acting carbonic anhydrase inhibitor), paraldehyde, tetracycline, triamterene, and xylitol.

- Fast and proper processing, storage, and analysis of samples are important for the achievement of accurate results. The specimen should be processed under anaerobic conditions following selection to prevent the release of CO2 gas from the specimen.

Falsely diminished values are the product of exposed specimens. It is estimated that CO2 is emitted from the sample at a rate of 6 mmol / h.

NOTES

_____

_____

_____

_____

_____

_____

_____

_____

_____

VITAMINS AND TRACE ELEMENTS

Vitamins and minerals are regarded as essential nutrients—because acting in harmony, they play different roles in the body. They help make bones strong, heal wounds, and support the immune system. They also turn food into energy and fix cellular damage.

NOTES

VITAMIN B12 (Cyanocobalamin)

SAMPLING:1 mL of serum collected in a red- or tiger-top tube.
TECHNIQUE: Radioimmunoassay
NORMAL VALUE:

Age	Conventional Units	SI Units (Conversion Factor X0.738)
Newborn	160–1300 pg/mL	118–959 pmol/L
Adult	200–900 pg/mL	148–664 pmol/L

EXPLAINATION:
Vitamin B12 has a ringed crystalline structure that surrounds the cobalt atom. It is important for DNA synthesis, hematopoiesis, and integrity of the central nervous system. It is derived solely from dietary intake. Animal products are an abundant source of B12 vitamins. The absorption depends on the availability of an intrinsic factor. Circumstances that may result in a deficiency of this vitamin include the presence of stomach or intestinal disorder, as well as inadequate dietary intake of vitamin B12 products. A significant increase in RBCs means that body volume may be an important indicator of vitamin B12 deficiency.

INDICATIONS:
- Aid in the assessment of central nervous system disorders.
- Help in the evaluation of megaloblastic anemia.
- Assess alcoholism.
- Analyze malabsorption syndromes.

RESULT:

Increased in:
Chronic obstructive pulmonary disease (COPD)
Chronic granulocytic leukemia
Chronic renal failure
Diabetes
Leukocytosis
Obesity
Polycythemia vera
Protein malnutrition
Severe congestive heart failure
Liver cell damage (hepatitis, cirrhosis)
Some carcinomas
Decreased in:
Defects of cobalamin transport or metabolism
Bacterial overgrowth
Crohn's disease
Hypochlorhydria
Inflammatory bowel disease
Late pregnancy

Pernicious anemia
Intestinal malabsorption
Dietary deficiency (e.g., in vegetarians)
Diphyllobothrium (fish tapeworm) infestation
Gastric or small intestine surgery
Intrinsic factor deficiency

IMPEDING FACTORS:

- Drugs that may raise the level of vitamin B12 include chloral hydrate.

- Drugs that may significantly reduce vitamin B12 include alcohol, aminosalicylic acid, anticonvulsants, ascorbic acid, cholestyramine, cimetidine, colchicine, metformin, neomycin, oral contraceptives, ranitidine, and triamterene.

- Hemolysis or exposure of the specimen to light invalidates the result.

- Recent radioactive scans or exposure to radiation within one week of the test can interfere with the test results when radioimmunoassay is the test method.

- The collection of specimens shortly after a blood transfusion may falsely increase vitamin B12 levels.

VITAMIN D

Cholecalciferol, vitamin D,25-dihydroxy

SAMPLING: 1 mL of serum is collected in a red-top tube. 1 mL of plasma collected in a green-top (heparin) tube is also acceptable.

TECHNIQUE: Radioreceptor assay for vitamin D 1,25-dihydroxy, Radiobinding assay for vitamin D 25-dihydroxy

NORMAL VALUE:

Form	Conventional Units	SI Units (Conversion Factor X2.496)
Vitamin D 25-dihydroxy	9–52 ng/mL	22.5–129.8 nmol/L
Vitamin D 1,25-dihydroxy	15–60 pg/mL	37.4–149.8 pmol/L

EXPLAINATION:

There are two metabolic forms of vitamin D. Ergocalciferol (vitamin D2) is produced when ergosterol is exposed to sunlight in plants. Ergocalciferol is absorbed by the stomach and intestine as ingested orally. Cholecalciferol (vitamin D3) is formed when the skin is exposed to sunlight or ultraviolet light.

Upon absorption, vitamins D2 and D3 enter the bloodstream. Vitamin D3 is converted to 25-hydroxy vitamin D by the liver and is the major circulating source of the vitamin.

Vitamin D2 is converted by the kidneys to vitamin D 1,25-dihydroxy and is a more biologically active type.

Vitamin D acts with parathyroid hormone and calcitonin to control calcium metabolism and osteoblast activity.

INDICATIONS:

- Differential diagnosis of calcium and phosphorus metabolism disorders.

- Determination of deficiency or potential poisoning.

- Evaluation of bone disease.

- Analysis of malabsorption.

RESULT:

Increased in:
Vitamin D intoxication
Decreased in:
Bowel resection
Celiac disease
Malabsorption
Osteitis fibrosa cystica
Osteomalacia
Pancreatic insufficiency
Rickets
Inflammatory bowel disease
Thyrotoxicosis

CRITICAL VALUES:

Vitamin toxicity can be as significant as the problems caused by vitamin deficiencies. The possibility of toxicity is especially important concerning fat-soluble vitamins, which are not removed from the body as easily as water-soluble vitamins and may accumulate in the body.

Most cases of toxicity are caused by over-supplement and can be avoided by consulting a qualified nutritionist for recommended daily dietary and supplemental allowances.

Signs and symptoms of vitamin D toxicity consist of nausea, loss of appetite, vomiting, polyuria, weakness of the body, and constipation.

IMPEDING FACTORS:

Medications that may raise the levels of vitamin D include etidronate disodium and pravastatin.

Drugs and compounds that may reduce vitamin D levels include aluminum hydroxide, anticonvulsants, cholestyramine, colestipol, glucocorticoids, isoniazid, mineral oil, and rifampin.

Recent radioactive scans or exposure to radiation within one week of the test can conflict with the test results when radioimmunoassay is the test method.

VITAMIN E (α-Tocopherol)

SAMPLING: 1 mL of serum is collected in a red- or tiger-top tube.

TECHNIQUE: High-performance liquid chromatography

NORMAL VALUE:

Age	Conventional Units	SI Units (Conversion Factor X23.22)
1–12 y	0.3–0.9 mg/dL	7–21 µmol/L
13–19 y	0.6–1.0 mg/dL	14–23 µmol/L
Adult	0.5–1.8 mg/dL	12–42 µmol/L

INDICATIONS:

- Evaluate neuromuscular disorders in preterm infants and adults.

- Examine individuals with malabsorption disorders.

- Evaluate possible hemolytic anemia in preterm infants and adults.

- Monitor long-term parenteral feeding.

RESULT:

Increased in:
Obstructive liver disease
Vitamin E intoxication
Decreased in:
A-β-lipoproteinemia
Hemolytic anemia
Malabsorption disorders, such as biliary atresia, cirrhosis, pancreatic carcinoma, cystic fibrosis, chronic pancreatitis, and chronic cholestasis

EXPLAINATION:

Vitamin E is a strong fat-soluble antioxidant that inhibits the degradation of unsaturated fatty acids, which can be mixed with polysaccharides to build tissue deposits. For this cause, vitamin E is thought to reduce the risk of coronary artery disease. Vitamin E deposits in lung tissue provide a buffer against air pollution and protect the integrity of the red blood cell membrane from oxidation.

Degradation of fatty acids in red blood cell membranes can lead to irreversible membrane damage and hemolysis. Studies are underway to support the hypothesis that oxidation also leads to the development of cataracts and macular retinal degeneration. Since vitamin E is present in a wide range of foods, a deficiency due to inadequate dietary intake is uncommon.

CRITICAL VALUES:

Vitamin toxicity can be as important as the issues caused by vitamin deficiency. The potential for toxicity is especially important concerning fat-soluble vitamins, which are not removed from the body as easily as water-soluble vitamins and may accumulate in the body. Most cases of toxicity are caused by over-supplement and can be prevented by contacting a professional nutritionist for recommended daily dietary and supplementary allowances.

Note: Excessive dosage (more than 60 times the recommended dietary amount for one year or longer) may result in excessive bleeding, delayed wound healing, and depression.

IMPEDING FACTORS:

- Medications that can increase vitamin E levels include anticonvulsants (in women).
- Drugs that may reduce vitamin E levels include anticonvulsants (male).
- The exposure of the specimen to light reduces the level of vitamin E, resulting in a falsely low result.

VITAMIN K (Phylloquinone, phytonadione)

SAMPLING: 1 mL of serum is collected in a red-top tube.

TECHNIQUE: High-performance liquid chromatography

NORMAL VALUE:

Conventional Units	SI Units (Conversion Factor X2.22)
0.13–1.19 ng/mL	0.29–2.64 nmol/L

EXPLAINATION:

Vitamin K is also one of the major fat-soluble vitamins in the body. It is essential for the formation of prothrombin, factors VII, IX, and X, and proteins C and S. Vitamin K also works with vitamin D to synthesize bone protein and regulate calcium levels. Vitamin K levels are not often requested, but vitamin K is often prescribed as a medicine. Intestinal bacteria provide about one-half of the body's vitamin K; the other half is obtained from dietary sources.

There are three varieties of vitamin K: vitamin K1 or phylloquinone found in foods; vitamin K2 or menaquinone, which is synthesized by intestinal bacteria; and vitamin K3 or menadione, which is a synthetic, water-soluble, prescription form of vitamin K. Vitamin K3 is two or three times more potent than naturally occurring forms.

INDICATIONS:
- Evaluation of bleeding of unknown cause (e.g., frequent nosebleeds, bruising).
RESULT:

Increased in:
Excessive administration of vitamin K
Decreased in:
Chronic fat malabsorption
Cystic fibrosis
Diarrhea (in infants)
Gastrointestinal disease
Antibiotic therapy (by decreasing intestinal flora)
Hypoprothrombinemia
Liver disease
Obstructive jaundice
Pancreatic disease
Hemorrhagic disease of the newborn

CRITICAL VALUES:
Vitamin toxicity can be as critical as the problems caused by vitamin deficits. The potential for toxicity is particularly important concerning fat-soluble vitamins, which are not removed from the body as quickly as water-soluble vitamins and may accumulate in the body.
 Natural forms, vitamins K1 and K2, do not cause toxicity. Signs and symptoms of the intoxication of vitamin K3 include bleeding and jaundice. Possible interventions include removing/stopping the source.
IMPEDING FACTORS:
Drugs and substances that may reduce vitamin K levels include antibiotics, cholestyramine, coumarin, mineral oil, and warfarin.

VITAMINS A, B1, B6, & C

Vitamin A: retinol, carotene; vitamin B6: niacin, pyroxidine, P-5'-P, pyridoxyl-5-phosphate; vitamin B1: thiamine; vitamin C: ascorbic acid.

SAMPLING: 1 mL of serum is collected in a red-top tube each for vitamins A and C; 1 mL of plasma is collected in a lavender-top (ethylenediaminetetraacetic acid [EDTA]) tube for vitamins B1 and B6.

TECHNIQUE: Capillary electrophoresis for vitamin C, Chromatography for vitamins A, B1, and B6

NORMAL VALUE:

Vitamin	Age	Conventional Units	SI Units (Conversion Factor 0.0349)
Vitamin A	1–6 y	20–43 µg/dL	0.70–1.50 µmol/L
	7–12 y	26–49 µg/dL	0.91–1.71 µmol/L
	13–19 y	26–72 µg/dL	0.91–2.51 µmol/L
	Adult	30–80 µg/dL	1.05–2.80 µmol/L (Conversion Factor 29.6)
Vitamin B$_1$		0.21–0.43 µg/dL	6.2–12.8 µmol/L (Conversion Factor 4.046)
Vitamin B$_6$		5–30 ng/mL	20–121 nmol/L (Conversion Factor 56.78)
Vitamin C		0.2–1.9 mg/dL	11.4–107.9 µmol/L

EXPLAINATION:

Vitamin assays are used to assess nutritional status. Low levels suggest inadequate oral intake, poor nutritional status, or malabsorption problems. High levels indicate excessive intake, deficiency of vitamins, or difficulties with absorption. Vitamin A is a fat-soluble nutrient that stimulates normal vision and prevents night-time blindness; contributes to the bone, teeth, and soft tissue growth; promotes the formation of thyroxine; maintains epithelial cell membranes, skin, and all mucous membranes; and acts as an anti-infection agent.

The vitamins B1, B6, and C are water-soluble. Vitamin B1 functions as an antioxidant and plays a key role in the Krebs cycle.

Vitamin B6 is essential in heme synthesis and acts as a coenzyme in the metabolism and glycogenolysis of amino acids. It includes pyridoxine, pyridoxal, and pyridoxamine. Vitamin C stimulates collagen synthesis, retains capillary energy, encourages iron release from ferritin to form hemoglobin, and functions in response to stress.

INDICATIONS:
Vitamin A:
- Evaluate skin disorders.
- Aid in the diagnosis of night blindness.
- Investigate alleged vitamin A deficiency.

Vitamin B1:
- Explore suspected cases of beriberi.
- Supervise the effects of chronic alcoholism.

Vitamin B6:
- Investigate suspected vitamin B6 deficiency.
- Investigate suspected malabsorption or malnutrition.

Vitamin C:
- Investigate suspected metabolic or malabsorptive disorders.
- Investigate suspected scurvy.

RESULT:
Increases in:
Vitamin A:
- Chronic kidney disease
- Idiopathic hypercalcemia in infants
- Vitamin A toxicity

Decreases in:
Vitamin A:
- A-β-lipoproteinemia
- Carcinoid syndrome
- Chronic infections
- Cystic fibrosis
- Disseminated tuberculosis
- Hypothyroidism
- Infantile blindness
- Liver, gastrointestinal, or pancreatic disease
- Night blindness
- Protein malnutrition
- Sterility and teratogenesis
- Zinc deficiency

Vitamin B1:
- Alcoholism
- Carcinoid syndrome
- Hartnup's disease
- Pellagra

Vitamin B6:
- Alcoholism
- Asthma

- Carpal tunnel syndrome
- Gestational diabetes
- Lactation
- Malabsorption
- Malnutrition
- Neonatal seizures
- Normal pregnancies
- Occupational exposure to hydrazine compounds
- Pellagra
- Preeclamptic edema
- Renal dialysis
- Uremia

Vitamin C:
- Alcoholism
- Anemia
- Cancer
- Hemodialysis
- Hyperthyroidism
- Malabsorption
- Pregnancy
- Rheumatoid disease
- Scurvy

CRITICAL VALUES:

Vitamin toxicity can be as significant as the problems caused by vitamin deficiencies. The potential for toxicity is especially important concerning fat-soluble vitamins, which are not removed from the body as easily as water-soluble vitamins and may accumulate in the body. Most cases of toxicity are caused by over-supplement and can be avoided by discussing with a qualified nutritionist for a recommended daily dietary and supplemental allowances. The following signs and symptoms represent vitamin A toxicity. These include headaches, blurred vision, joint pain, bone pain, dry skin, and appetite loss.

IMPEDING FACTORS:

- Medications and substances that may increase vitamin A levels include probucol, alcohol (moderate consumption), and oral contraceptives. Drugs and compounds that may decrease vitamin A levels include alcohol (chronic intake, alcoholism), allopurinol, cholestyramine, colestipol, and mineral oil.
- Drugs that may reduce vitamin B1 levels include glibenclamide, isoniazid, and valproic acid.
- Drugs that may decrease vitamin B6 include amiodarone, anticonvulsants, cycloserine, disulfiram, ethanol, hydralazine, isoniazid, levodopa, oral contraceptives, penicillamine, pyrazinoic acid, and theophylline.

- Drugs and substances that may reduce vitamin C levels include aminopyrine, acetylsalicylic acid, barbiturates, estrogens, heavy metals, oral contraceptives, nitrosamines, and paraldehyde. Vitamin levels may be affected by various diseases (see Results section).
- Diets high in freshwater fish and tea, which are thiamine antagonists, may cause a decrease in vitamin B1 levels.
- Long-term hyperailment may result in lower levels of vitamins.
- The sensitivity of the specimen to light decreases the vitamin levels, resulting in falsely low results.
- Chronic tobacco smoking lowers vitamin C levels.

COPPER (Cu)

SAMPLING: 1 mL of serum is collected in a royal blue–top, trace element–free tube.

TECHNIQUE: Atomic absorption spectrophotometry

NORMAL VALUE:

Age	Conventional Units	SI Units (Conversion Factor _0.157)
Newborn–5 d	9–46 µg/dL	1.4–7.2 µmol/L
1–5 y	80–150 µg/dL	12.6–23.6 µmol/L
6–9 y	84–136 µg/dL	13.2–21.4 µmol/L
10–14 y	80–121 µg/dL	12.6–19.0 µmol/L
15–19 y	80–171 µg/dL	10.1–18.4 µmol/L
Adult		
Men	70–140 µg/dL	11.0–22.0 µmol/L
Women	80–155 µg/dL	12.6–24.3 µmol/L
Pregnant women	118–302 µg/dL	18.5–47.4 µmol/L

Values for the African American population are 8% to 12% higher.

EXPLAINATION:

Copper is an important cofactor for enzymes involved in the formation of hemoglobin and collagen. Copper is also a component of the coagulation factor V, helps in the oxidation of glucose, is used for the production of melanin pigment, is used for the synthesis of ceruloplasmin, and is necessary for the conservation of healthy myelin sheaths. The amount of copper varies with the intake. This element is absorbed in the stomach and duodenum, deposited in the intestine, and excreted in urine and feces with bile salts. Copper deficiency results in neutropenia and hypochromic, microcytic anemia that does not lead to iron therapy. Many signs and symptoms of copper deficiency include osteoporosis, skin, and hair depigmentation, compromised immune system response, and possible neurological and cardiac anomalies.

INDICATIONS:

- Assist in the detection of Menkes Disease.
- Assist in the diagnosis of Wilson's Disease.
- Monitor patients receiving long-term parenteral nutrition therapy.

RESULT:

Increased in:
Anemias
Ankylosing spondylitis
Biliary cirrhosis
Collagen diseases
Complications of renal dialysis
Hodgkin's disease
Infections
Inflammation
Leukemia
Malignant neoplasms
Myocardial infarction
Pellagra
Poisoning from copper-contaminated solutions or insecticides
Pregnancy
Pulmonary tuberculosis
Rheumatic fever
Rheumatoid arthritis
Systemic lupus erythematosus
Thalassemias
Trauma
Thyroid disease (hypothyroid or hyperthyroid)
Typhoid fever
Use of the copper intrauterine device
Decreased in:
Burns
Infants (especially premature infants) taking milk deficient in copper
Chronic ischemic heart disease
Cystic fibrosis
Dysproteinemia
Iron-deficiency anemias (some)
Long-term total parenteral nutrition
Malnutrition
Menkes' disease
Malabsorption disorders (celiac disease, tropical sprue)
Nephrotic syndrome
Wilson's disease

IMPEDING FACTORS:

- Drugs that may increase the levels of copper include anticonvulsants and oral contraceptives.
- Drugs that may reduce copper levels include citrate, penicillamine, and valproic acid.
- Unnecessary therapeutic intake of zinc may interfere with copper intestinal absorption.

IRON (Fe)

SAMPLING: 1 mL of serum is collected in a red- or tiger-top tube.
TECHNIQUE: Spectrophotometry
NORMAL VALUE:

Age	Conventional Units	SI Units (Conversion Factor X0.179)
Newborn	100–250 µg/dL	17.9–44.8 µmol/L
Infant–9 y	20–105 µg/dL	3.6–18.8 µmol/L
10–14 y	20–145 µ g/dL	3.6–26.0 µmol/L
Adult		
Male	65–175 µg/dL	11.6–31.3 µmol/L
Female	50–170 µg/dL	9–30.4 µmol/L

EXPLAINATION:

Iron plays a key role in erythropoiesis. Iron is essential for the distribution and maturation of red blood cells and is needed for the synthesis of hemoglobin. The body normally has 4 g of iron, out of which nearly 65 percent of iron is hemoglobin and 3 percent is myoglobin. A small amount is also present in cellular enzymes that catalyze oxidation and reduce iron. Much of the iron is stored in the liver, bone marrow, and spleen as ferritin or haemosiderin. The iron found in the serum is in transit between the food tract, the bone marrow, and the sufficient sources of iron preservation. Iron moves through the bloodstream bound to transferrin, a protein produced by the liver. Usually, iron enters the body by oral ingestion; about 10% is consumed, but 20% can be ingested in patients with iron deficiency anemia. Freed iron is highly toxic, but there is usually an excess of transferrin available to prevent the build-up of unbound iron in circulation. Iron overload is as clinically considerable as iron deficiency, particularly in children's accidental poisoning caused by excessive intake of iron-containing multivitamins.

INDICATIONS:

- Assist in the diagnosis of blood loss caused by decreased serum iron.
- Help in the diagnosis of hemochromatosis or other diseases of iron metabolism and storage.
- Determine the presence of disorders involving decreased protein synthesis or iron absorption defect.

- Help to determine the differential diagnosis of anemia.
- Evaluate unintended iron deficiency.
- Evaluate iron toxicity in dialysis patients or patients with transfusion-dependent anemia.
- Evaluate thalassemia and sideroblastic anemia.
- Monitor hematological reactions during pregnancy when serum iron is normally lowered.
- Monitor exposure to anemia.

RESULT:

Increased in:
Pernicious anemias
Sideroblastic anemias
Thalassemia
Acute iron poisoning (children)
Acute leukemia
Acute liver disease
Aplastic anemia
Excessive iron therapy
Hemochromatosis
Hemolytic anemias
Lead toxicity
Nephritis
Transfusions (repeated)
Vitamin B6 deficiency
Decreased in:
Acute and chronic infection
Carcinoma
Hypothyroidism
Iron-deficiency anemia
Nephrosis
Postoperative state
Protein malnutrition (kwashiorkor)
Chronic blood loss (gastrointestinal, uterine)
Remission of pernicious anemia

CRITICAL VALUES:
Ingestion by the child of 30 mg/kg of elemental iron may be sufficient to induce toxicity. More than 400 g / dL is suggestive of possible toxicity. Intervention may include chelation therapy with deferoxamine mesylate (Desferal).

IMPEDING FACTORS:

- Medications that may raise iron levels include blood transfusions, chemotherapy, iron (intramuscular), iron dextran, iron-protein succinylate, methimazole, methotrexate, oral contraceptives, and rifampin.
- Products that may decrease iron levels include allopurinol, acetylsalicylic acid, cholestyramine, corticotropin, cortisone, deferoxamine, and metformin.
- Failure to withhold iron-containing medicine 24 hours before the check can falsely increase the value.

ZINC (Zn)

SAMPLING: 1 mL of serum is collected in a trace element–free, royal blue–top tube.

TECHNIQUE: Atomic absorption spectrophotometry

NORMAL VALUE:

Age	Conventional Units	SI Units (Conversion Factor 0.153)
Newborn–6 mo	26–141 g/dL	4.0–21.6 mol/L
6–11 mo	29–131 g/dL	4.5–20.1 mol/L
1–4 y	31–115 g/dL	4.8–17.6 mol/L
4–5 y	48–119 g/dL	7.4–18.2 mol/L
6–9 y	48–129 g/dL	7.3–19.7 mol/L
10–13 y	25–148 g/dL	3.9–22.7 mol/L
14–17 y	46–130 g/dL	7.1–19.9 mol/L
Adult	70–120 g/dL	10.7–18.4 mol/L

INDICATIONS:

- Aid in confirming acrodermatitis enteropathica.
- Evaluate nutritional deficiency.
- Evaluate possible toxicity.
- Monitor replacement therapy in individuals with identified deficiencies.
- Monitor therapy of individuals with Wilson's disease.

RESULT:

Increased in:

Coronary heart disease
Anemia
Arteriosclerosis
Decreased in:
Acrodermatitis enteropathica
Acute infections
Acute stress
Conditions that decrease albumin

Diabetes
Long-term total parenteral nutrition
Acquired immunodeficiency syndrome (AIDS)
Pulmonary tuberculosis
Pregnancy
Burns
Cirrhosis
Malabsorption
Myocardial infarction
Nephrotic syndrome
Nutritional deficiency

EXPLAINATION:

Zinc is found in all body tissues, but the highest concentration is present in the eye, bone, and male reproductive organs. Zinc is involved in RNA and DNA synthesis and is important for tissue repair. It is also needed for the growth of collagen and the production of active vitamin A (visual pigment rhodopsin). Zinc also serves as a chelating agent to protect the body from lead and cadmium toxicity. The small intestine absorbs zinc. Its absorption and excretion tend to be at the same sites as those for iron and copper. The body does not accumulate zinc, as it does copper and iron.

Untreated zinc deficiency in infants can result in a condition called enteropathic acrodermatitis. Symptoms cause growth retardation, diarrhea, impaired wound healing, and frequent infections.

Teenagers and adults with zinc deficiency have similar adverse effects on growth, sexual development, and immune function, as well as altered taste and smell, emotional instability, impaired tolerance to darkness, poor night vision, tremor, and a bullous, pustular rash over the extremities.

IMPEDING FACTORS:

- Medications that can improve zinc levels include auranofin, chlorthalidone, corticotropin, oral contraceptives, and penicillamine.
- Medications that may lower zinc levels include anticonvulsants, cisplatin, citrate, corticosteroids, estrogens, interferon, and oral contraceptives.

DRUGS AND TOXINS

LEAD - Pb

SAMPLING:
1 mL of whole blood is collected in a special lead-free royal blue– or tan-top tube. 1 mL plasma collected in a lavender-top (ethylenediaminetetraacetic acid [EDTA]) tube is also acceptable.

TECHNIQUE: Atomic absorption spectrophotometry

NORMAL VALUE:

	Conventional Units	SI (Conversion Factor X0.0483)
Children	0–9.9 µg/dL	0–0.48 µmol/L
Adults	0–25.0 µg/dL	0–1.20 µmol/L
OSHA action limit for occupational exposure	Up to 40 µg/dL	Up to 1.93 µmol/L

OSHA - Occupational Safety and Health Administration.

EXPLAINATION:
Lead is a heavy metal, a trace element. The respiratory and gastrointestinal systems absorb it. It can also be spread via the placenta from the mother to the fetus. Most parts of the body are affected when there is regular access to lead-containing items (e.g., paint, battery, fuel, pottery, firearms, printing materials) or professions (mining, automobile, publishing, and welding industries). Lead poisoning can cause severe behavioral and neurological effects. The blood test is considered to be the best predictor of lead poisoning and is confirmed by a lead mobilization test performed on a 24-hour urine specimen.

INDICATIONS: Aid in the diagnosis and treatment of lead poisoning.

RESULT:

Increased in:
• Anemia of lead intoxication
• Lead encephalopathy
• Metal poisoning
Decreased in: N/A

CRITICAL VALUES: N/A
IMPEDING FACTORS:
Exposure of the collection site and/or specimen with lead in dust can be avoided by taking special care to disinfect the surfaces around the collection site. Extra care can also be used to prevent contamination during practical venipuncture.

IMMUNOSUPPRESSANTS: CYCLOSPORINE, METHOTREXATE

Cyclosporine (Sandimmune), methotrexate (amethopterin, MTX, Folex, Rheumatrex), methotrexate sodium (Mexate)
SAMPLING:1 ml of whole blood is collected in a lavender-top tube for cyclosporine. 1 mL of serum is collected in a red-top tube for methotrexate.

Immunosuppressant	Route of Administration	Recommended Collection Time
Cyclosporine	Oral	12 hours after the dose
Methotrexate	Oral	Varies according to dosing protocol
	Intramuscular	Varies according to dosing protocol

NORMAL VALUES:

DRUG NAME	Therapeutic Dose		Half-Life		Volume of Distribution	Protein Binding	Excretion
	Conventional Units		SI Units (Conversion Factor 0.832)				
Cyclosporine	100–400 ng/mL Renal transplant		83–333 nmol/L		8–24 h	4–6 L/kg	90%	Renal
	100–300 ng/mL Cardiac transplant		83–250 nmol/L		8–24 h	4–6 L/kg	90%	Renal
	100–250 ng/mL Bone marrow transplant		83–208 nmol/L		8–24 h	4–6 L/kg	90%	Renal
Methotrexate	Dependent on therapeutic approach				8–15 h	0.4–1.0 L/kg	50–70%	Renal

EXPLAINATION:

Cyclosporine is an immunosuppressive drug used to regulate the rejection of organs, especially the rejection of the heart, liver, and kidneys. Its most serious side effects include kidney dysfunction or renal failure. Methotrexate is an extremely toxic drug that causes cell death by disrupting DNA synthesis. Several factors must be reflected in the successful dosing and control of therapeutic drugs, including patient age, weight, interacting medicines, protein levels, electrolyte balance, water balance, and illnesses that influence absorption and excretion, as well as foods, herbs, vitamins, and minerals that can either potentiate or impede the target dosage. Processing times should be carefully documented concerning the time of administration of the medication. This information must be communicated clearly and precisely to avoid a misapprehension of the dosage time concerning the collection time. Miscommunication between the person prescribing the drug and the individual extracting the test is the most frequent cause of sub-therapeutic levels, harmful amounts, and misleading information used in the measurement of potential doses.

INDICATIONS:

Cyclosporine:
- Assist in the management of therapies to prevent organ rejection.
- Toxicity control Methotrexate.
- Monitor the effectiveness of cancer treatment and some autoimmune disorders.
- Monitor for toxicity.

CRITICAL VALUES:

It is worth noting the adverse effects at sub-therapeutic levels. Care should be taken to examine the signs and symptoms of too little and too much medication.

Cyclosporine:

>400 ng/mL

Signs and symptoms of cyclosporine toxicity consist of increased severity of potential side effects, including nausea, stomatitis, vomiting, hypertension, anorexia, infection fluid retention, hypercalcemic metabolic acidosis, tremor, fits, headache, and flushing. Possible interventions require close monitoring of blood levels to make dosing changes, cause emesis (orally ingested), perform gastric lavage (orally ingested), delay treatment and initiate alternative therapy for a short period until the patient is stable.

Methotrexate:

Low-dose therapy------------>9.1 ng/mL
high-dose therapy------------- >454 ng/mL

Signs and symptoms of methotrexate toxicity consist of increased severity of potential side effects, including nausea, stomatitis, vomiting, anorexia, bleeding, infection, bone marrow dysfunction, and hepatotoxicity over a prolonged period of use. The influence of methotrexate on normal cells may still be reversed by the administration of 5-formyltetrahydrofolate (citrovorum or leucovorin). 5-Formyltetrahydrofolate requires higher doses of methotrexate to be given.

RESULTS:

Normal levels	Therapeutic effect
Toxic levels	Adjust dose as indicated
Cyclosporine	Renal impairment
Methotrexate	Renal impairment

IMPEDING FACTORS:
- Numerous drugs interact with and either raise cyclosporine levels or increase the risk of toxicity. These drugs include acyclovir, amiodarone, amphotericin B, anabolic steroids, cephalosporins, cimetidine, aminoglycosides, ketoconazole, melphalan, methylprednisolone, miconazole, nonsteroidal anti-inflammatory drugs (NSAIDs), danazol, erythromycin, furosemide, oral contraceptives, and trimethoprim-sulfamethoxazole.
- Products that may minimize cyclosporine levels include carbamazepine, ethotoin, mephenytoin, phenobarbital, phenytoin, primidone, and rifampin.
- Products that may raise the level of methotrexate or increase the risk of toxicity include NSAIDs, probenecid, salicylate, and sulfonamides.
- Antibiotics can reduce the absorption of methotrexate.

CARBOXYHEMOGLOBIN (Carbon monoxide, CO, COHb, COH)

SAMPLING: 1 mL of whole blood collected in a green-top (heparin) or lavender-top (ethylenediaminetetra-acetic acid [EDTA]) tube, depending on laboratory requirement. Specimens should be transported tightly capped (anaerobic) and in an ice slurry if blood gases are to be performed simultaneously. Carboxyhemoglobin is stable at room temperature.
TECHNIQUE: Spectrophotometry, co-oximetry

NORMAL VALUE:

	% Saturation of Hemoglobin	The fraction of Hemoglobin Saturation SI Units (Conversion Factor X0.01)
Newborns	10–12%	0.1–0.12
Nonsmokers	Up to 2%	Up to 0.02
Smokers	Up to 12%	Up to 0.12

EXPLAINATION:

Exogenous carbon monoxide (CO) is an odorless, colorless, tasteless by-product of incomplete combustion resulting from the burning of vehicles, coal and gas, and tobacco smoke. Endogenous CO is generated because of the catabolism of red blood cells. CO levels are increased in newborns due to the combined effects of high hemoglobin depletion and inefficiency of the infant's respiratory system. CO combines tightly to hemoglobin with an affinity 250 times higher than oxygen, competitively, and dramatically reducing the oxygen-carrying capacity of hemoglobin. The increase in the percentage of bound CO reflects the extent to which the natural flow of oxygen has been negatively affected.

Overexposure induces hypoxia, resulting in headache, nausea, vomiting, dizziness, collapse, or seizures.

Toxic exposure produces anoxia, increased levels of lactic acid, and permanent tissue damage, which may lead to coma or death. Acute exposure of cherry red to the lips, skin, and nail beds may be demonstrated; this finding may not be evident in cases of chronic exposure. There was a direct correlation between carboxyhemoglobin levels and signs of atherosclerotic disease, angina, and myocardial infarction.

INDICATIONS:

- Assist in the treatment of possible CO poisoning.
- Evaluate exposure to flames and smoke inhalation.
- Evaluate the effects of smoking on the patient.

RESULT:

Increased in:
• CO poisoning
• Hemolytic disease
• Tobacco smoking
Decreased in: N/A

CRITICAL VALUES:

Asymptomatic: 10 to 20 percent
Disturbance of judgment, dizziness, headache: 10 to 30 percent
Toxic concentration: >20 percent
Coma, respiratory arrest, and death: >50 percent

A possible intervention in mild CO poisoning is the use of additional oxygen under atmospheric pressure. Hyperbaric oxygen therapy might be used in extreme CO poisoning.

IMPEDING FACTORS: Sample should be collected before the administration of oxygen therapy.

Drug	Therapeutic Dose*	SI Units	Half-Life (h)	The volume of Distribution (L/kg)	Protein Binding (%)	Excretion
		(Conversion Factor 2.66)				
Haloperidol	5–20 ng/mL	13–53 nmo/L	15–40	18–30	90	Hepatic
		(Conversion Factor 1)				
Lithium	0.6–1.2 mEq/L	0.6–1.2 mmol/L	18–24	0.7–1.0	0	Renal

ANTIPSYCHOTIC DRUGS AND ANTIMANIC DRUGS: HALOPERIDOL, LITHIUM

SAMPLING: 1 mL of serum is collected in a red-top tube.

TECHNIQUE: Ion-selective electrode for lithium, Chromatography for haloperidol

EXPLAINATION:

Haloperidol is a drug that has antipsychotic properties. This tranquilizer is used for the following purposes: acute and chronic psychotic disorders, Tourette syndrome, and hyperactive adolescents with severe behavioral problems. Lithium is used for the management of manic depression. Other factors need to be considered for successful dosing and control of therapeutic drugs, including patient age, patient weight, interactive medicines, electrolyte balance, protein levels, water balance, conditions that affect absorption and excretion, and nutrients, herbals, vitamins, and minerals that can either potentiate or impede the target dosage. The optimum processing times should be carefully documented concerning the time of administration of the medication.

IMPORTANT NOTE:

Such details must be clearly and precisely conveyed to avoid a misapprehension of the dosage time concerning the collection time. Miscommunication between the person administering the drug and the individual extracting the test is the most frequent cause of sub-therapeutic levels, hazardous concentrations, and misleading information used in the measurement of potential doses.

INDICATIONS:
- Assist in the identification and prevention of toxicity.
- Monitor compliance with the therapeutic regimen.

RESULT

Level	Response
Normal levels	Therapeutic effects
Subtherapeutic levels	Adjust dose as indicated
Toxic levels	Adjust dose as indicated
Haloperidol	Hepatic impairment
Lithium	Renal impairment

CRITICAL VALUES:
It is essential to note the adverse effects at sub-therapeutic levels. Care should be taken to examine the signs and symptoms of inadequate treatment and too much medicine.

Haloperidol: >42 ng/mL

Signs and symptoms of haloperidol overdose include hypotension, respiratory depression, and extrapyramidal neuromuscular reactions. Necessary measures include emesis (contraindicated in the absence of gag reflex or central nervous system depression or excitation), ipecac cathartic administration, and gastric lavage accompanied by activated charcoal and saline cathartic administration.

Lithium: >1.5 mEq/L

Signs and symptoms of lithium toxicity involve ataxia, severe tremor, muscle weakness, vomiting, diarrhea, confusion, seizures, stupor, T-wave flattening, loss of consciousness, and potential coma. Possible interventions include the administering of activated carbon, gastric lavage, and the administration of intravenous fluids with diuresis.

IMPEDING FACTORS:
- Haloperidol can raise the level of tricyclic antidepressants and increase the risk of lithium toxicity.
- Products that may raise lithium levels include thiazide diuretics, angiotensin-converting enzyme inhibitors, and certain nonsteroidal anti-inflammatory drugs.
- Medications and compounds that may decrease lithium levels include acetazolamide, theophylline, osmotic diuretics, and caffeine.

ANTIDEPRESSANT DRUGS: AMITRYPTYLINE, DIAZEPAM, DOXEPIN, IMIPRAMINE, NORTRIPTYLINE, DESIPRAMINE

SAMPLING: 1 mL of serum is collected in a red-top tube.

TECHNIQUE: Chromatography for nortriptyline, diazepam, amitriptyline, and doxepin; immunoassay for imipramine and desipramine

NORMAL VALUE:

Drug	Therapeutic Dose (Conventional units.)	SI Units	Half-Life (h)	The volume of Distribution (L/kg)	Binding (%)	Excretion
			(Conversion Factor 3.61)			
Amitryptyline	120–250 ng/mL	433–903 nmol/L	17–40	10–36	85–95	Hepatic
			(Conversion Factor 3.8)			
Nortriptyline	50–150 ng/mL	190–570 nmol/L	20–90	15–23	90–95	Hepatic
			(Conversion Factor 0.0035)			
'Diazepam	100–1000 ng/mL	0.35–3.5 mol/L	20–50	1.0–1.5	96–99	Hepatic
			(Conversion Factor 3.58)			
Combined doxepin and desmethyl-	150–251 ng/mL	540–900 nmol/L	10–25	10–30	75–85	Hepatic

doxepin						
			(Conversion Factor 3.57)			
Imiprami ne	150–250 ng/mL	536–892 nmol/L	6–28	9–23	60–95	Hepati c
			(Conversion Factor 3.75)			
Desipram ine	75–300 ng/mL	281– 1125 nmol/L	6–28	9–23	60–95	Hepati c

DESCRIPTION

'Diazepam is a benzodiazepine derivative used for sedation. Other sedative medications are referred to as tricyclic antidepressants. MAO antagonists are classified as hydrazines and non-hydrazines. These are prescribed for the treatment of neurotic or atypical depressions. MAO inhibitors should be used with caution in patients with hyperthyroidism and in patients with diabetes who are taking insulin or antidiabetic medicines. Numerous drug interactions with cyclic antidepressants exist. Several factors need to be considered for successful dosing and control of therapeutic drugs, including patient age, patient weight, interactive drugs, protein levels, water balance, electrolyte balance, conditions that affect absorption and excretion, and herbals, vitamins, foods and minerals that can either potentiate or suppress the target dosage. The high and low processing periods should be carefully documented concerning the time of administration of the medication.

IMPORTANT NOTE:

This knowledge must be clearly and precisely conveyed to avoid a misapprehension of the dosage time concerning the collection time. Miscommunication between the person administering the drug and the individual extracting the test is the most frequent cause of sub-therapeutic levels, harmful tiers, and misleading information used in the measurement of potential doses.

INDICATIONS:

- Aid in the diagnosis and prevention of toxicity.
- Assess overdose, especially in combination with ethanol.
- Monitor compliance with the therapeutic regimen.

RESULT

Level	Response
Normal levels	Therapeutic effects
Subtherapeutic levels	Adjust dose as indicated
Toxic levels	Adjust dose as indicated
Amitriptyline	Hepatic impairment
Nortriptyline	Hepatic impairment
Diazepam	Renal or hepatic impairment
Doxepin	Hepatic impairment
Imipramine	Hepatic impairment
Desipramine	Hepatic impairment

CRITICAL VALUES:

It is important to note the harmful effects of sub-therapeutic levels of antidepressants. Care should be taken to examine the signs and symptoms of too little and too much medicine.

Benzodiazepine-Derivative Antidepressants:
- *Diazepam and N-desmethyldiazepam: >3000 ng/mL*
- *Diazepam and nordiazepam: >5000 ng/mL*

Signs and symptoms of diazepam or diazepam-derived toxicity include ataxia, convulsions, reduced reflexes, agitation, respiratory depression, slurred speech, somnolence, and potential coma. Possible interventions include the application of activated charcoal, saline or tap water gastric lavage, airway protection, central nervous system depression monitoring, and seizures prevention. Emetics are being contraindicated.

Tricyclic Antidepressants:
- *Amitriptyline: >500 ng/mL*
- *Nortriptyline: >500 ng/mL*
- *Combined doxepin and desmethyldoxepin: >500 ng/mL*
- *Imipramine: >500 ng/mL*
- *Desipramine: >400 ng/mL*

Signs and symptoms of tricyclic antidepressant toxicity cause anxiety, paranoia, confusion, seizures, arrhythmias, hyperthermia, flushing, pupil dilation, and probable coma. Likely interventions include administration of activated charcoal; emesis; saline gastric lavage; administration of physostigmine to prevent fits, hypertension, or respiratory depression; administration of bicarbonate, propranolol, lidocaine, or phenytoin to alleviate arrhythmias; and electrocardiographic monitoring.

IMPEDING FACTORS:
Cyclic antidepressants might potentiate the impacts of oral anticoagulants.

ANTICONVULSANT DRUGS: PHENOBARBITAL, PHENYTOIN, CARBAMAZEPINE, ETHOSUXIMIDE, PRIMIDONE, VALPROIC ACID

SAMPLING: 1 mL of sample is collected in a red-top tube.

Drug	Therapeutic Dose Conventional units.	SI Units	Half-Life (h)	The volume of Distribution (L/kg)	Protein Binding (%)	Excretion
(Conversion Factor 4.23)						
Carbamaz epine	4–12 µg/mL	17–51 µmol/L	15–40	0.8–1.8	60–80	Hepatic
(Conversion Factor 7.08)						
Ethosuxim ide	40–100 µg/mL	283–708 µmol/L	25–70	0.7	0–5	Renal
(Conversion Factor 4.31)						
Phenobar bital	Adult: 20–40 µg/mL Child: 15–30µ g/mL	Adult: 86–172 µmol/L Child: 65–129 µmol/L	50–140	0.5–1.0 L/kg	40–50	80% Hepatic 20% Renal
(Conversion Factor 3.96)						
Phenytoin	10–20 µ g/mL	40–79 µmol/L	Adult: 20–40 Child: 10	0.6–0.7	85–95	Hepatic
(Conversion Factor 4.58)						
Primidone	Adult: 5–12 µg/mL Child: 7–10 µg/mL	Adult: 23–55µ mol/L Child: 32–46 µmol/L	4–12	0.5–1.0	0–20	Hepatic
(Conversion Factor 6.93)						
Valproic Acid	50–100 µg/mL	347–693 µmol/L	8–15	0.1–0.5	85–95	Renal

EXPLAINATION:

Anticonvulsants are used to decrease the frequency and severity of seizures in patients with epilepsy. Carbamazepine is also used to regulate neurogenic pain in trigeminal neuralgia and diabetic neuropathy and to treat bipolar disorder and other neurological and psychiatric disorders. Other factors need to be considered for successful dosing and control of therapeutic drugs, including patient age, patient weight, interacting medicines, protein levels, water balance, electrolyte balance, conditions that influence absorption and excretion, and foods, vitamins, herbals, and minerals that can either potentiate or impede the target dosage.

INDICATIONS:

- Help in the diagnosis of and prevention of toxicity.
- Check compliance with the therapeutic regimen.

RESULT

CRITICAL VALUES:

It is important to remember the undesirable effects at sub-therapeutic levels. Care should be taken to examine the signs and symptoms of too little and too much medicine.

Carbamazepine: >12 µg/mL

Signs and symptoms of carbamazepine toxicity usually involve respiratory depression, seizure stupor, and potential coma. Possible interventions consist of gastric lavage (contraindicated if ileus is present); airway protection; administration of intravenous fluids and vasopressors to correct hypotension; control of seizure activity through diazepam, phenobarbital, or phenytoin; cardiac monitoring; monitoring of vital signs; and discontinuation of prescribed medicines. Emetics are also being contraindicated.

Ethosuximide: >150 µg/mL

Signs and symptoms of ethosuximide toxicity involve nausea, vomiting, and lethargy. Possible interventions consist of administration of activated charcoal, administration of saline cathartic and gastric lavage (contraindicated if ileus is suspected), protection of the airways, hourly evaluation of neurological function, and discontinuation of the medication.

Phenobarbital: >40 µg/mL

Signs and symptoms of phenobarbital poisoning include dry, pale skin; ataxia; central nervous system depression; hypothermia; Cheyne-Stokes respiration, hypotension, cyanosis, tachycardia; possible coma; and possible renal impairment. Possible interventions include gastric lavage, cathartic activated charcoal, airway protection, possible intubation, and mechanical ventilation (especially during gastric lavage when there is no gag reflex), monitoring for hypotension, and discontinuing of the medication.

Phenytoin: >40 µg/mL

Signs and symptoms of phenytoin toxicity include blurred vision, nystagmus, lethargy, central nervous system depression, and possible coma. Possible interventions include airway protection, electrocardiographic testing, administration of activated charcoal, gastric lavage with saline or tap water, administration of saline or cathartic sorbitol, and discontinuation of prescribed medication.

Primidone: >12 µg/mL

Signs and symptoms of primidone toxicity consist of ataxia, anemia, and agitation in the central nervous system. Possible interventions include airway safety, management of vitamin B12 and folate anemia, and discontinuation of the medicine.

Valproic Acid: >200 µg/mL

Signs and symptoms of valproic acid toxicity consist of numbness, tingling, fatigue, and mental illnesses. Possible interventions include the delivery of activated charcoal and naloxone and the discontinuation of treatment.

IMPEDING FACTORS

- Drugs that may raise carbamazepine levels or increase the risk of toxicity include cimetidine, erythromycin, isoniazid, propoxyphene, triacetyloleandomycin danazol, diltiazem, valproic acid, and verapamil.
- Drugs that may decrease carbamazepine levels consist of phenobarbital, phenytoin, and primidone.
- Drugs that may increase phenobarbital levels or raise the risk of toxicity include barbital drugs, salicylates, furosemide, primidone, and valproic acid.
- Phenobarbital may alter the metabolism of other drugs, increasing their effectiveness, such as chloramphenicol, corticosteroids, doxycycline, griseofulvin, beta-blockers, haloperidol, methylphenidate, phenothiazines, theophylline, phenylbutazone, propoxyphene, quinidine, tricyclic antidepressants, and valproic acid.
- Phenobarbital may alter the metabolism of other drugs, reducing their effectiveness, such as cyclosporine, ethosuximide, oral anticoagulants, oral chloramphenicol, contraceptives, theophylline, and phenytoin.
- Phenobarbital is the active metabolite of primidone, and levels of both drugs should be scrutinized while the patient is taking primidone to avoid either toxic or subtherapeutic levels of both medicines.
- Drugs that may raise phenytoin levels or increase the risk of phenytoin toxicity include chloramphenicol, disulfiram, ethanol, amiodarone, azapropazone, carbamazepine, cimetidine, imipramine, levodopa, miconazole, fluconazole, halothane, ibuprofen, metronidazole, nifedipine, phenylbutazone, trazodone, sulfonamides, tricyclic antidepressants, and trimethoprim. Small changes in the formulation (i.e., changes in the brand) also may increase phenytoin levels or increase the risk of phenytoin toxicity.
- Drugs that may lower phenytoin levels include folic acid, intravenous fluids containing glucose, nitrofurantoin, bleomycin, carbamazepine, cisplatin, disulfiram, oxacillin, rifampin, salicylates, and vinblastine.

- Primidone decreases the efficacy of oral anticoagulants.
- Drugs that may raise valproic acid levels or increase the risk of toxicity include dicumarol, phenylbutazone, and excessive doses of salicylate.
-Drugs that may lower valproic acid levels include carbamazepine, phenobarbital, phenytoin, and primidone.

ANTIBIOTIC DRUGS—AMINOGLYCOSIDES: AMIKACIN, TRICYCLIC
GLYCOPEPTIDE: GENTAMICIN, TOBRAMYCIN; VANCOMYCIN
SAMPLING:1 ml of serum is collected in a red-top tube.

Drug	Therapeutic dose Conventional units.	SI Units	Half-Life (h)	The volume of Distribution (L/kg)	Protein Binding (%)	Excretion
		(Conversion Factor 1.71)				
Amikacin						
Peak	20–30 µg/mL	34–51 µmol/L	4–8	0.4–1.3	50	90% renal
Trough	4–8 µg/mL	7–14 µmol/L				
		(Conversion Factor 2.09)				
Gentamicin						
Peak	6–10 µg/mL	12–21 µmol/L	4–8	0.4–1.3	50	90% renal
Trough	< 2 µg/mL	< 4 µmol/L				
		(Conversion Factor 2.14)				
Tobramycin						
Peak	6–10 µg/mL	13–21 µmol/L	4–8	0.4–1.3	50	90% renal

Trough	< 2 µg/mL	< 4 µmol/L				
		(Conversion Factor 0.69)				
Vancomycin						
Peak	20–40 µg/mL	14–28 µmol/L	4–8	0.4–1.3	50	90% renal
Trough	5–10 µg/mL	3–7 µmol/L				

Miscommunication between the person prescribing the drug and the individual extracting the test is the most frequent cause of sub-therapeutic levels, harmful amounts, and misleading information used in the measurement of potential doses.

Results:

Level	Result
Normal levels	Therapeutic effect
Subtherapeutic levels	Adjust dose as indicated
Toxic levels	Adjust dose as indicated
Amikacin	Renal, hearing impairment
Gentamicin	Renal, hearing impairment
Tobramycin	Renal, hearing impairment
Vancomycin	Renal, hearing impairment

EXPLAINATION:
Amikacin, gentamicin, and tobramycin antibiotics are used against certain gram-negatives (Acinetobacter, Citrobacter, Enterobacter, Providencia, Pseudomonas, Escherichia coli, Klebsiella, Proteus, Salmonella, Serratia, and Shigella) and certain gram-positive (Staphylococcus aureus) pathogenic microorganisms.
Aminoglycosides are weakly absorbed through the gastrointestinal tract and are most dispensed intravenously. Vancomycin is a tricyclic glycopeptide antibiotic utilized against many gram-positive microorganisms such as staphylococci, Streptococcus pneumoniae, A-β-hemolytic streptococci, enterococci, Corynebacterium, and Clostridium. Vancomycin was also used orally for the treatment of pseudomembranous colitis caused by Clostridium difficile infection. This method is less widely used because of the development of vancomycin-resistant enterococci.
Several factors must be considered for successful dosing and control of therapeutic drugs, including patient age, patient weight, interacting medicines, electrolyte balance, protein levels, water balance, conditions that affect absorption and excretion, and intake of substances (e.g., foods, herbals, vitamins, and minerals) that can either potentiate or impede the intended target dosage. Renal impairment and permanent ototoxicity (uncommon) are the most serious side effects of aminoglycosides and vancomycin. The peak and trough collection times should be carefully documented concerning the time of administration of the medication.

INDICATIONS:
- Assist in the diagnosis and inhibition of toxicity.
- Keep a check on renal dialysis patients or patients with rapidly changing renal function.
- Supervise therapeutic regimen

CRITICAL VALUES:
- The adverse effects at sub-therapeutic levels are critical.
- Care should be taken to examine the signs and symptoms of too little and too many medicines.
- Clinical presentations of toxic levels of these antibiotics are common, including hearing loss and decreased renal function.
- Precise therapeutic drug control is the most important intervention so that the treatment can be stopped before permanent damage is done.

Drug Name	Toxic Levels
Amikacin	Peak >35 µg/mL, trough >10 µg/mL
Gentamicin	Peak >10 µ g/mL, trough >2 µg/mL
Tobramycin	Peak >10 µg/mL, trough >2 µg/mL
Vancomycin	Peak >40 µ g/mL, trough >10 µg/mL

IMPEDING FACTORS

- Products that may decrease the potency of aminoglycoside include bleomycin, daunorubicin, doxorubicin, and penicillins (e.g., carbenicillin, piperacillin).
- Get society before and after the first dose of aminoglycosides.
- The concomitant use of aminoglycosides raises the risks of ototoxicity and nephrotoxicity.

ANTIARRHYTHMIC DRUGS: DIGOXIN, FLECAINIDE, LIDOCAINE, DISOPYRAMIDE, PROCAINAMIDE, QUINIDINE

SAMPLING:1 ml serum is collected in a red-top tube.

NORMAL values:

Drug (Indication)	Therapeutic Dose*	SI Units (Conversion Factor 1.28)	Half-Life (h)	Volume of Distribution (L/kg)	Protein Binding (%)	Excretion
Digoxin (arrhythmias)	1.5–2.0 ng/mL	1.9–2.6 nmol/L	20 – 60	7	20–30	60% renal 40% hepatic
Digoxin (CHF)	0.8–1.5 ng/mL	1.0–1.9 nmol/L				
		(Conversion Factor 2.95)				
Disopyramide (atrial arrhythmias)	2.8–3.2 g/mL	8.3–9.4 mol/L	4– 10	0.7–0.9	50–80	50% renal 50% hepatic
Disopyramide (ventricular arrhythmias)	3.3–7.5 g/mL	9.7–22.1 mol/L				

		(Conversion Factor 2.41)				
Flecainide	0.2–1.0 g/mL	0.5–2.4 mol/L	7–27	5–13	30–60	30% renal 70% hepatic
		(Conversion Factor 4.27)				
Lidocaine	1.5–6.0 g/mL	6.4–26 mol/L	1.5–2	1–1.5	60–70	90% hepatic
		(Conversion Factor 4.23)				
Procainamide	4–10 g/mL	17–42 mol/L	2–6	2–4	10–20	50% renal 50% hepatic
		(Conversion Factor 3.61)				
N-acetyl procainamide	5–30 g/mL	18–108 mol/L	8			
		(Conversion Factor 3.08)				
Quinidine	2–5 g/mL	6–15 mol/L	6–8	2–3	80–90	10–30% renal 60–80% hepatic

Results:

Level	Result
Normal levels	Therapeutic effect
Subtherapeutic levels	Adjust dose as indicated
Toxic levels	Adjust dose as indicated
Digoxin	Renal impairment, CHF, elderly patients
Disopyramide	Renal or hepatic impairment
Flecainide	Renal or hepatic impairment, CHF
Lidocaine	Hepatic impairment, CHF
Procainamide	Renal impairment
Quinidine	Hepatic impairment, CHF, elderly patients

EXPLAINATION:

Cardiac glycosides are used for prophylactic management and treatment of heart failure and ventricular and atrial arrhythmias.

Because these medications have narrow therapeutic windows, they need to be monitored closely. Signs and symptoms of toxicity are frequently difficult to distinguish from those of heart disease. Patients with toxic levels may have gastrointestinal, ocular, and central nervous system effects and potassium balance disorders.

Several factors need to be considered for successful dosing and control of therapeutic drugs, including patient age, patient weight, interacting medicines, electrolyte balance, protein levels, water balance, conditions that affect absorption and excretion, and intake of substances (e.g., foods, herbals, vitamins, and minerals) that can either potentiate or impede the intended target dosage. The peak and trough collection times should be carefully documented concerning the time of administration of the medication.

IMPORTANT NOTE:

This information must be communicated clearly and precisely to avoid a misapprehension of the dosage time concerning the collection time. Miscommunication between the person delivering the medicine and the individual extracting the test is the most frequent cause of sub-therapeutic levels, dangerous/toxic concentrations, and misleading information used in the estimation of possible doses.

INDICATIONS:

- Assist in the treatment and detection of toxicity.
- Check compliance with therapeutic regimen.
- Supervise patients who have a pacemaker, who have compromised renal or hepatic function, or who are taking digital medications.

CRITICAL VALUES:

The adverse effects of subtherapeutic levels are crucial. Care should be taken to probe the signs and symptoms of too little and too much medication.

Digoxin: >2.5 ng/mL

Signs and symptoms of digoxin toxicity show arrhythmias, anorexia, hyperkalemia, nausea, diarrhea, vomiting, psychiatric illnesses, and perceptual hallucinations (objects look yellow or have halos surrounding them). Possible treatments include drug discontinuation, continuous electrocardiogram (ECG) monitoring (prolonged P-R interval, widening QRS interval, Q-Tc prolongation, and atrioventricular block), transcutaneous pacing, activated charcoal administration (where the patient has a gag reflex and central nervous system function), electrolyte disruption treatment and care, and administration. The quantity of Digibind given depends on the degree of digoxin to be neutralized. Digoxin levels must be calculated before the administration of Digibind. Digoxin must not be used for several days following the administration of Digibind in patients with normal renal function (1 week or more in patients with reduced renal function). Digibind cross-reactions in the digoxin assay and which result in false elevations or decreases in values based on the specific assay used by the laboratory.

Disopyramide: >7 g/mL

Signs and symptoms of disopyramide toxicity consist of the prolonged QT interval, ventricular tachycardia, hypotension, and heart failure. Potential measures include medication discontinuation, airway support ECG, and blood pressure monitoring.

Flecainide: >1 g/mL

Signs and symptoms of flecainide toxicity include severe pharmacological effects resulting in arrhythmia. Possible interventions include discontinuation of treatment as well as continuous monitoring of ECG, respiratory, and blood pressure.

Lidocaine: >9 g/mL

Signs and symptoms of lidocaine poisoning include slurred speech, central nervous system depression, cardiovascular depression, vomiting, muscle twitches or cramps, and potential coma. Potential interventions include regular ECG screening, airway assistance, epilepsy protection, and daily temperature monitoring for hyperthermia.

Procainamide: >12 g/mL; Procainamide

N-acetyl Procainamide: >30 g/mL

N-acetyl procainamide (NAPA) is the active metabolite of procainamide. Signs and symptoms of procainamide toxicity consist of torsades de pointes (ventricular tachycardia), nausea, vomiting, agranulocytosis, and hepatic disorders. Possible interventions include airway safety, emesis, gastric lavage, and sodium lactate administration.

Quinidine: >8 g/mL

Signs and symptoms of quinidine toxicity consist of ataxia, nausea, vomiting, diarrhea, respiratory system collapse, hypotension, syncope, anuria, arrhythmias (heart block, QRS, and Q - T gap widening), asystole, paranoia, paresthesia, and irritability. Possible interventions include airway assistance, emesis, gastric lavage, activated carbon dioxide administration, sodium lactate administration, and emergency transcutaneous or transvenous pacemaker.

IMPEDING FACTORS:

- Medications that may raise digoxin levels or increase the risk of toxicity include amiodarone, amphotericin B, diltiazem, diclofenac, erythromycin, propantheline, quinidine, spironolactone, tetracycline, and verapamil.
- A pharmaceutical that can lower digoxin levels includes aluminum hydroxide (antacids), cholestyramine, colestipol kaolin-pectin, metoclopramide, neomycin, phenytoin, and sulfasalazine.
- Drugs that can increase disopyramide levels or increase the risk of toxicity include amiodarone and troleandomycin.
- Drugs that can reduce disopyramide levels include rifampin
- Drugs that can increase the levels of flecainide or raise the risk of toxicity include amiodarone and cimetidine.
- Drugs that can increase lidocaine levels or increase the risk of toxicity include anticonvulsants, beta-blockers, cimetidine, metoprolol, nadolol, and propranolol.
- Medications that may increase the level of procainamide or raise the risk of toxicity include amiodarone, other antiarrhythmic medications, cimetidine, ranitidine, and trimethoprim.
- Medications that can increase the amount of quinidine or raise the risk of toxicity include amiodarone, cimetidine, verapamil, and thiazide diuretics.
- Products that can decrease the levels of quinidine include disopyramide, nifedipine, phenobarbital, phenytoin, and rifampin.
- Digitoxin cross-reacts with digoxin; tests are wrongly improved when digoxin is tested while the patient is taking digitoxin.
- Digitalis-like immunoreactive agents are present in the sera of certain patients that do not take digoxin, resulting in false-positive tests. Patients whose sera include wireless immune-like compounds typically have a salt and fluid retention disorder, such as renal dysfunction, hepatic failure, low renin hypertension, and abortion.
- Unexpectedly, small levels of digoxin can be observed in patients with thyroid disease.
- Disopyramide can cause a drop in glucose levels. This can also improve the anticoagulating activity of warfarin.
- Long-term administration of procainamide can result in false-positive antinuclear antibody outcomes and the development of lupus-like syndrome in some patients.
- Quinidine can enhance the effectiveness of neuromuscular blocking drugs and warfarin anticoagulants.
- Simultaneous administration of quinidine and digoxin can rapidly raise digoxin to toxic levels. When all medications are to be prescribed simultaneously, the digoxin level will be assessed before the first dose of quinidine and again within 4 to 6 days.

ANALGESIC AND ANTIPYRETIC DRUGS: ACETAMINOPHEN, ACETYLSALICYLIC ACID

SYNONYMS/ACRONYM: Acetaminophen (Acephen, Apacet, Banesin, Dapa, Aspirin Free Anacin, Datril, Dorcol, Gebapap, Ty-Pap, Halenol, Liquiprin, Meda Cap, Panadol, Redutemp, Tempra, Tylenol, Uni-Ace); Acetylsalicylic acid (salicylate, aspirin, Anacin, Aspergum, Bufferin, Ecotrin, Empirin, Measuring, Synalgos, ZORprin, ASA).

TECHNIQUE: ImmunoassayG

SAMPLING: 1 ml serum is collected in a red-top tube.

NORMAL VALUE:

Drug	Therapeutic Dose*	SI Units	Half-Life	Volume of Distribution	Protein Binding	Excretion
Acetaminophen	10–30 g/mL	66–199 mol/L (Conversion Factor 6.62)	1–3 h	0.95 L/kg	20–50%	85–95% hepatic, metabo-lites, renal
Salicylate	15–20 mg/dL	1.1–1.4 mmol/L (Conversion Factor 0.073)	2–3 h	0.1–0.3 L/kg	90–95%	1 hepatic, metabo-lites, renal

EXPLAINATION:

Acetaminophen is commonly used for headache, fever, and pain relief, particularly for individuals who are unable to take salicylate as medications or who have bleeding disorders. It is an analgesic of choice for children under 13 years of age; salicylates are prevented in this age group due to the association of aspirin and Reye syndrome. Acetaminophen is promptly absorbed from the gastrointestinal tract and reaches a peak concentration within 30 to 60 minutes of the therapeutic dose. It may be a silent killer because the intoxication symptoms appear 24 to 48 hours after ingestion, and the antidote is ineffective. Acetylsalicylic acid (ASA) is also used to treat headaches, fever, and pain relief. Some patients with cardiovascular disease are taking small prophylactic doses. The main toxicity site for both drugs is the liver, particularly in the presence of liver disease or decreased drug metabolism and excretion. Many factors need to be considered when interpreting drug levels, including patient age, patient weight, drug interactions, electrolyte balance, protein levels, water balance, absorption and excretion conditions, and foods, herbals, vitamins, and minerals that can potentiate or inhibit the target concentration.

INDICATIONS:

- Suspected overdose
- Suspected toxicity
- Therapeutic monitoring

RESULT

Increased in:
• **Acetaminophen Toxicity**
• **Alcoholic cirrhosis**
• **Liver disease**
• **ASA Toxicity**
Decreased in:
• **Failure to comply with therapeutic regimen**

CRITICAL VALUES: Note: The harmful effects of subtherapeutic levels are also important. Care should be taken to explore the signs and symptoms of too little and too much medication.

Acetaminophen:

More than 150 mg / mL - Signs and symptoms of acetaminophen overdose arise in phases over some time. Stage I (0 to 24 hours after ingestion) effects may include gastrointestinal irritation, pallor, lethargy, diaphoresis, metabolic acidosis, and likely coma. In stage II (24 to 48 hrs after intake), signs and symptoms may include right upper abdominal quadrant pain, elevated liver enzymes, aspartate aminotransferase (AST) and alanine aminotransferase (ALT), and possibly decreased renal function. In stage III (72 to 96 hrs after intake), signs and symptoms may consist of nausea, vomiting, jaundice, depression, coagulation disorders, persistent elevation of AST and ALT, decreased renal function, and coma. Intervention may include gastrointestinal decontamination (stomach pumping) where the patient is present within 6 hours of ingestion or administration of acetylcysteine in acute intoxication in which the patient is present more than 6 hours after ingestion.

ASA:

Signs and symptoms of salicylate overdose include ketosis, convulsions, dizziness, nausea, vomiting, hyperactivity, hyperglycemia, hyperpnea, hyperthermia, respiratory arrest, and tinnitus. Possible interventions include administration of ipecac-like cathartic syrup to cause emesis if the patient is conscious of it, administration of activated carbonate following vomiting, alkalinization of the urine with bicarbonate, and a single dose of vitamin K (in rare cases of hypoprothrombinemia).

IMPEDING FACTORS:

- Medications that may increase the levels of acetaminophen include diflunisal, metoclopramide, and probenecid.
- Medications that may decrease acetaminophen levels include cholestyramine, magnesium, oral contraceptives, and propantheline.
- Medications that increase the ASA level include sulfinpyrazone.
- Medications that reduce ASA levels include dissolved carbon dioxide, antacids (aluminum hydroxide), and iron.

DRUGS OF ABUSE

Amphetamines, barbiturates, ethanol (alcohol, ethyl alcohol, EtOH), phencyclidine (PCP), opiates (heroin), tricyclic antidepressants (TCA), benzodiazepines (tranquilizers), cannabinoids (THC), cocaine

SAMPLING:

In the case of ethanol, serum (1 ml) obtained in a red-top tube or Plasma (1 mL) formed in the dark field (sodium fluoride/potassium oxalate). The tubing is appropriate as well.

In the case of a drug test, urine (15 ml) was obtained in a clean plastic jar. Gastric material (20 mL) can also be requested for review.

TECHNIQUE: immunoassay for drugs of abuse, Spectrophotometry for ethanol.

NORMAL VALUE:

Ethanol: None detected

Drug screen: None detected

EXPLAINATION:

Drug abuse continues to be one of the most serious social and economic challenges in the United States. NIDA or The National Institute for Drug Abuse has listed opioids, cocaine, cannabinoids, amphetamines, and phencyclidines (PCPs) as the most used illicit drugs.

Ethanol is the most widely used legal substance to induce abuse.

Chronic alcohol abuse can lead to high blood pressure, liver disease, heart disease, and birth defects.

INDICATIONS:

- Differentiate alcohol poisoning from a diabetic coma, brain trauma, or drug overdose.
- Investigate possible drug overdose.
- Investigate alleged drug overdose.
- Investigate suspected drug or alcohol misuse regimen.
- Monitor ethanol levels as applied to methanol intoxication.
- Routine workplace screening.

RESULT:

The urine panel only detects the presence of these compounds in urine: Does not signify the duration of exposure, quantity used, nature of the source used, and the degree of damage. Positive results should be deemed definitive. The drug-specific confirmatory process should be used to evaluate the doubtful results from a positive urine test.

Cutoff Values for Drugs of Abuse Recommended by NIDA

Amphetamines	1000 ng/mL
Barbiturates	300 ng/mL
Benzodiazepines	300 ng/mL
Cannabinoids	50 ng/mL
Cocaine	300 ng/mL
Opiates	300 ng/mL
Phencyclidine	25 ng/mL
Tricyclic antidepressants	1000 ng/mL

CRITICAL VALUES:

Due to constitutional variations, the toxicity of ethanol differs from State to State, but in most states, higher than 100 mg / dL is deemed stricken to prohibit driving. Rates of more than 300 mg / dL are correlated with amnesia, vomiting, blurred vision, hypothermia. Levels 400 to 700 mg / dL is consistent with a coma, and it could be fatal. Possible treatments for ethanol exposure include drinking/tap water or 3 % sodium bicarbonate lavage, respiratory support, and hemodialysis (usually only suggested if the amount reaches 300 (mg / dL)).

Barbiturate and benzodiazepine overdose are the causes of central nervous system (CNS) depression, which may advance to respiratory failure, hypotension, coma, and death. Do not induce vomiting because of the threat of aspiration. Possible interventions include airway safety, oxygen administration, water, or saline gastric lavage (up to 24 hours after ingestion), activated charcoal administration, and CNS depression monitoring.

PCP intoxication induces a variety of symptoms depending on the stage of intoxication. Level I involve psychiatric symptoms, muscle spasms, fever, tachycardia, flushing, swollen eyes, salivation, nausea, and vomiting. Stage II involves stupor, headaches, hallucinations, increased heart rate, and increased blood pressure. Stage III involves further rises in heart rate and blood pressure that may lead to cardiac and respiratory failure. Possible interventions may include the delivery of respiratory support, the administration of activated charcoal with a cathartic agent such as sorbitol, gastric lavage and suction, intravenous nutrition and electrolyte administration, and urinary acidification to help in excretion of the PCP.

Cocaine overdose induces short-term effects of CNS agitation, anxiety, tachypnea, mydriasis, and tachycardia. Possible interventions include emesis (if swallowed orally and if the patient has a gag reflex and proper CNS function), gastric lavage (if ingested orally), entire bowel irrigation (if ingested), airway protection, cardiovascular support, and application of diazepam or phenobarbital for convulsions. The use of beta-blockers is contraindicated.

Amphetamine intoxication causes paranoia, tremor, epilepsy, vomiting, tachycardia, dysrhythmia, impotence, stroke, and respiratory failure. Possible interventions include emesis (if ingested orally and if the patient has a gag reflex and normal CNS function), activated charcoal administration accompanied by magnesium citrate, excretion-promoting urinary acidification, and urinary-promoting fluid administration. Heroin is an opiate that causes bradycardia, flushing, itching, hypotension, hypothermia, and respiratory depression at toxic levels. Possible interventions consist of airway protection and the administration of naloxone (Narcan).

Tricyclic antidepressant overdose causes confusion, agitation, nausea, epilepsy, dysrhythmias, hyperthermia, pupil dilation, and coma. Possible interventions may consist of administration of activated charcoal, saline gastric lavage, intravenous administration of physostigmine (to combat coma, hypertension, respiratory depression, and seizures), bicarbonate (to control dysrhythmia), propranolol, lidocaine, or phenytoin for convulsion management, and cardiac function monitoring.

IMPEDING FACTORS:

- Codeine-containing cough medicines or antidiarrheal medicines, as well as intake of large amounts of poppy seeds, can result in false-positive opiate results.
- Adulterants such as bleach or other potent oxidizers can yield incorrect results on the urine drug screen results.
- Ethanol is a volatile substance, and experiments should be kept in a tightly closed container to avoid false values.

NOTES

MISCELLANEOUS

ALBUMIN AND ALBUMIN/ GLOBULIN RATIO (Alb, A/G ratio)

SAMPLING:1ml serum is collected in a red- or tiger-top tube. 1ml plasma collected in a green-top (heparin) tube is also standard.

TECHNIQUE: Spectrophotometry

NORMAL value: Usually, the albumin/globulin (A/G) ratio is >1.

Age	Conventional Units	SI Units (Conversion Factor 10)
Newborn–4 d	2.8–4.4 g/dL	28–44 g/L
5 d–14 y	3.8–5.4 g/dL	38–54 g/L
15–18 y	3.2–4.5 g/dL	32–45 g/L
19–60 y	3.4–4.8 g/dL	34–48 g/L
61–90 y	3.2–4.6 g/dL	32–46 g/L
>90 y	2.9–4.5 g/dL	29–45 g/L

EXPLAINATION:

For most, the body's total protein is a combination of albumin and globulin. Albumin, the protein present at the highest concentrations, is the main transport protein in the body. Albumin also retains oncotic plasma pressure.

Serum albumin values are affected by the synthesis, distribution, and degradation process. Low levels may be the consequence of either inadequate production or excessive losses. Albumin levels are more useful as a sign of chronic deficiency than short-term deficiency.

The amount of albumin is affected by posture. The findings of specimens collected in an upright position are higher than the samples collected in a supine posture.

The A/G ratio is helpful in the assessment of liver and kidney disease.

The ratio is analyzed using the following formula:

albumin/ (total protein-albumin), where globulin is the variation between the total protein value and the albumin value. For instance, with a total protein of 7 g / dL and albumin of 4 g / dL, the ratio of A/G is measured as 4/ (7–4) or 4/3= 1.33. The reverse of the ratio where globulin equals albumin (i.e., the ratio of < 1.0) is clinically significant.

INDICATIONS:

- Evaluate the nutritional status of hospitalized patients, especially geriatric patients
- Evaluate chronic illness
- Any condition that results in a decrease in plasma water (e.g., dehydration)
- Hyperinflation of albumin

Results:

Decreased in:
• Insufficient intake
• Malabsorption malnutrition
• Decreased synthesis by the liver
• Neoplasm
• Inflammation and chronic ailments
• Amyloidosis Bacterial Monoclonal gammopathies (e.g., multiple myeloma, Waldenström's macroglobulinemia)
• Parasitic infestations
• Peptic ulcer
• Sustained infections
• Immobilization
• Rheumatic diseases
• Severe skin disease
Acute and chronic liver ailments (e.g., alcoholism, cirrhosis, and hepatitis)
Increased loss over body surface:
• Rapid hydration or overhydration Burns
• Enteropathies due to vulnerability to swallowed substances (e.g., gluten allergy, Crohn's disease, ulcerative Colitis)
• Fistula (gastrointestinal or lymphatic)
• Decreased catabolism in Cushing's disease and Preeclampsia
• Hemorrhage
• Kidney diseaes
• Renal protein deficiency
• Recurrent thoracentesis or paracentesis
• Damage and crushing accidents
Increased in:
• Thyroid dysfunction
• Increased blood volume (hypervolemia)
• Congestive heart failure
• Pregnancy
• Monoclonal gammopathies (Waldenström's disease, myeloma)

IMPEDING FACTORS:

- Medications that may increase the level of albumin include enalapril.

- Drugs that may decrease albumin levels consist of acetaminophen (poisoning), dapsone, dextran, estrogens, prednisone (high doses), trazodone, ibuprofen, nitrofurantoin, oral contraceptives, phenytoin, and valproic acid.

- The effectiveness of drugs administered is affected by variations in albumin levels.

ALKALINE PHOSPHATASE AND ISOENZYMES

(ALP and fractionation, Alk Phos, heat-stabile ALP)

SAMPLING: 1 ml serum is collected in a red- or tiger-top tube. 1 ml plasma collected in a green-top (heparin) tube is also appropriate.

TECHNIQUE: Spectrophotometry for total alkaline phosphatase levels, inhibition/electrophoresis.

NORMAL VALUE:

Total ALP	Conventional Units	SI Units (Conversion Factor X0.017)	Bone Fraction	Liver Fraction
1-5 y				
Male	56–350 U/L	0.95–5.95 µKat/L	39–308 U/L	<8–101 U/L
Female	73–378 U/L	1.24–6.43 µKat/L	56–300 U/L	<8–53 U/L
6–7 y				
Male	70–364 U/L	1.19–6.19 µKat/L	50–319 U/L	<8–76 U/L
Female	73–378 U/L	1.24–6.43 µKat/L	56–300 U/L	< 8–53 U/L
8 y				
Male	70–364 U/L	1.19–6.19 µKat/L	50–258 U/L	<8–62 U/L
Female	98–448 U/L	1.67–7.62 µKat/L	78–353 U/L	<8–62 U/L
9–12 y				
Male	112–476 U/L	1.90–8.09 µKat/L	78–339 U/L	<8–81 U/L

Female	98–448 U/L	1.67–7.62 µKat/L	78–353 U/L	< 8–62 U/L
13 y				
Male	112–476 U/L	1.90–8.09 µKat/L	78–389 U/L	<8–48 U/L
Female	56–350 U/L	0.95–5.95 µKat/L	28–252 U/L	<8–50 U/L
14 y				
Male	112–476 U/L	1.90–8.09 µKat/L	78–389 U/L	<8–48 U/L
Female	56–266 U/L	0.95–4.52 µKat/L	31–190 U/L	<8–48 U/L
15 y				
Male	70–378 U/L	1.19–6.43 µKat/L	48–311 U/L	< 8–39 U/L
Female	42–168 U/L	0.71–2.86 µKat/L	20–115 U/L	< 8–53 U/L
16 yr				
Male	70–378 U/L	1.19–6.43 µKat/L	48–311 U/L	< 8–39 U/L
Female	28–126 U/L	0.48–2.14 µKat/L	14–87 U/L	<8–50 U/L
17 y				
Male	56–238 U/L	0.95–4.05 µKat/L	34–190 U/L	<8–39 U/L
Female	28–126 U/L	0.48–2.14 µKat/L	17–84 U/L	<8–53 U/L
18 y				
Male	56–182 U/L	0.95–3.09 µKat/L	34–146 U/L	<8–39 U/L
Female	28–126 U/L	0.48–2.14 µKat/L	17–84 U/L	<8–53 U/L
19 yr				

Male	42–154 U/L	0.71–2.62 µKat/L	25–123 U/L	<8–39 U/L
Female	28–126 U/L	0.48–2.14 µKat/L	17–84 U/L	<8–53 U/L
20 y				
Male	45–138 U/L	0.76–2.35 µKat/L	25–73 U/L	<8–48 U/L
Female	33–118 U/L	0.56–2.01 µKat/L	17–56 U/L	<8–50 U/L
Adult				
Male	35–142 U/L	0.60–2.41 µKat/L	11–73 U/L	0–93 U/L
Female	25–125 U/L	0.42–2.12 µKat/L		

EXPLAINATION:

ALP is an enzyme sited in the liver, in the Kupffer cells in the biliary tract, and the bones, intestines, and placenta. Additional sources of ALP include proximal renal tubules, pulmonary alveolar cells, germ cells, vascular beds, lactating mammary glands, and circulating blood granulocytes. ALP is described as alkaline because it functions optimally at a pH of 9.0. This method is most useful in determining the occurrence of liver or bone disease. Isoelectric concentrating techniques can be used to classify 12 ALP isoenzymes. Other tumors produce small amounts of isoenzymes of Regan and Nagao ALP.

Furthermore, four main ALP isoenzymes have clinical significance: ALP1 of liver origin, ALP2 of bone origin, ALP3 of intestinal origin (sometimes present in people with blood type O and B), and ALP4 of placental origin (third trimester). The level of ALP varies by age and gender. The values in infants are > in adults due to the level of bone growth and development. Immunoassay is available for measuring bone-specific ALP as a measure of high bone turnover and estrogen deficiency in postmenopausal women.

INDICATIONS:

- Assess signs and symptoms of various disorders associated with elevated rates of ALP, such as biliary obstruction, hepatobiliary illness, and bone disease, including malignancies.
- Distinguish obstructive hepatobiliary tract disorders from the hepatocellular disease.
- Determine the impacts of renal disease on bone metabolism.
- Determine bone growth or damage in children with abnormal growth patterns.

RESULT

Increased in:
Liver disease:
Biliary atresia
Biliary obstruction
Granulomatous or infiltrative liver diseases
Chronic active hepatitis
Cirrhosis
Diabetes mellitus (diabetic hepatic lipidosis)
Extrahepatic duct obstruction
Infectious mononucleosis
Viral hepatitis
Bone disease:
Healing fractures
Paget's disease (osteitis deformans)
Metabolic bone diseases (rickets, osteomalacia)
Metastatic tumors in bone
Osteogenic sarcoma
Osteoporosis
Other conditions:
Advanced pregnancy
Amyloidosis
Lung cancer
Pancreatic Carcinoma
Chronic renal failure
Congestive heart failure
Growing children
infarctions
Sarcoidosis
Ulcerative Colitis
Hodgkin's disease
Hyperparathyroidism (due to primary or secondary chronic renal disease)
Bowel perforation

Pulmonary and myocardial
Decreased in:
Anemia (severe)
Cretinism
Hypophosphatasia (congenital, rare)
Hypothyroidism
Kwashiorkor
Nutritional deficiency of zinc or magnesium
Scurvy

IMPEDING FACTORS:

- Medications that may increase ALP levels by causing cholestasis to consist of amitriptyline, anabolic steroids, androgens, benzodiazepines, chlorothiazide, chlorpropamide, nitrofurans, oral contraceptives, penicillin, phenothiazines, progesterone, propoxyphene, dapsone, erythromycin, estrogens, ethionamide, gold salts, imipramine, mercaptopurine, sulfonamides, tamoxifen, and tolbutamide.

- Medications that may increase ALP levels by causing hepatocellular damage include acetaminophen (toxic), anticonvulsants, asparaginase, acetylsalicylic acid, allopurinol, amiodarone, anabolic steroids, azithromycin, bromocriptine, captopril, cephalosporins, chloramphenicol, low-molecular-weight heparin, methyldopa, monoamine oxidase inhibitors, naproxen, nifedipine, clindamycin, clofibrate, danazol, enflurane, ethambutol, ethionamide, fenofibrate, fluconazole, interleukin-2, fluoroquinolones, foscarnet, gentamicin, indomethacin, interferon, levamisole, Levodopa, lincomycin, nitrofurans, oral contraceptives, probenecid, procainamide, quinine, ranitidine, retinol, ritodrine, sulfonylureas, tetracyclines, tobramycin, and verapamil.- Medications that may cause an overall decrease in ALP levels to include calcitriol, clodronate, clofibrate, cyclosporine, theophylline, etidronate, ipriflavone, norethisterone, oral contraceptives, pamidronate, tamoxifen, and ursodiol.

ALZHEIMER'S DISEASE MARKERS (CSF tau protein and β-amyloid 42, AD)

SAMPLING: 1 to 2 mL of Cerebrospinal fluid (CSF) is gathered in a simple plastic conical tube.

TECHNIQUE: Enzyme-linked immunosorbent assay

NORMAL VALUE: Tau protein and β-amyloid42 CSF tests are used in conjunction as biochemical markers for Alzheimer's disease (AD). Values are highly reliant on the reagents and criteria used in the study. The selection ranges between laboratories; the research laboratory should be consulted for the interpretation of the results.

EXPLAINATION:

AD or Alzheimer's Disease is the most common cause of dementia in the elderly. AD is a central nervous system disorder that results in a gradual and profound loss of memory, followed by a loss of cognitive abilities and death. It may undergo years of the progressive accumulation of amyloid plaques and brain tangles, or it may tend to be the early-onset form of the disease

. Neurofibrillary tangles and amyloid plaques observed in the brain are two recognized pathological characteristics of AD. Abnormal types of tau-associated microtubules are the main components of typical neurofibrillary tangles observed in patients with AD. The abundance of Tau protein is thought to reflect the number of neurofibrillary tangles and may signify the severity of the disease. β-Amyloid 42 is a free-floating protein commonly found in CSF. It is believed to collect in the central nervous system of patients with AD, causing amyloid plaques in brain tissue. As a result, these patients have lower CSF values compared to age-matched non-AD control subjects.

INDICATIONS:

- Assist in establishing a diagnosis of AD.

RESULT

Increased in:
• **Acquired immunodeficiency syndrome**
• **AD**
• **Cerebrovascular disease**
• **Creutzfeldt-Jakob disease**
• **Meningoencephalitis**
• **Pick's disease**

IMPEDING FACTORS:

- A few patients with AD may have normal levels of tau protein because of an inadequate number of neurofibrillary tangles.

AMINO ACID SCREEN, BLOOD

SAMPLING:1 ml of serum is collected in a red- or tiger-top tube. 1 ml of plasma collected in a green-top (heparin) tube is also acceptable.

TECHNIQUE: Chromatography

NORMAL VALUE:

There are several amino acids. The tables below include the most frequently screened amino acids for diagnostic purposes. The units are nanomoles per milliliter (nmol/mL).

Age	Alanine	β -Alanine	Anserine	α-Amino-adipic Acid	α-Amino-n-butyric Acid
Premature	212–504	0	—	0	14–52
Newborn–1mo	131–710	0–10	0	0	8–24
2 mo–2 y	143–439	0–7	0	0	3-26
2–18 y	152–547	0–7	0	0	4–31
Adult	177–583	0–12	0	0–6	5–41

AGE	γ - Amino butyric acid	β -Aminoiso-butyric Acid	Arginine	Asparagine	Aspartic Acid
Premature	0	0	34–96	90–295	24–50
Newborn–1 mo	0–2	0	6–140	29–132	20–129
2 mo–2 y	0	0	12–133	21–95	0–23
2–18 y	0	0	10–140	23–112	1–24
Adult	0	0	15–128	35–74	1–25
Age	Carnosine	Citrulline	Cystathionine	Cystine	Ethanolamine
Premature	—	20–87	5–10	15–70	—

Age				
Newborn–1 month	0–19	10–45	0–3	17–98	0–115
2 month–2 y	0	3–35	0–5	16–84	0–4
2–18 y	0	1–46	0–3	5–45	0–7
Adult	0	12–55	0–3	5–82	0–153

Age	Glutamic Acid	Glutamine	Glycine	Histidine	Homocysteine
Premature	107–276	248–850	298–602	72–134	3–20
Newborn–1 mo	62–620	376–709	232–740	30–138	0
2 mo–2 y	10–133	246–1182	81–436	41–101	0
2–18 y	5–150	254–823	127–341	41–125	0–5
Adult	10–131	205–756	151–490	72–124	0

Age	Hydroxylysine	Hydroxyproline	Isoleucine	Leucine	Lysine
Premature	0	0–80	23–85	151–220	128–255
Newborn–1 mo	0–7	0–91	26–91	48–160	92–325
2 mo–2 y	0–7	0–63	31–86	47–155	52–196
2–18 y	0–2	3–45	22–107	49–216	48–284
Adult	0	0–53	30–108	72–201	116–296

Age	Methionine	1-Methyl-histidine	3-Methyl-histidine	Ornithine	Phenylalanine
Premature	37–91	4–28	5–33	77–212	98–213

Newborn–1 mo	10–60	0–43	0–5	48–211	38–137
2 mo–2 y	9–42	0–44	0–5	22–103	31–75
2–18 y	7–47	0–42	0–5	10–163	26–91
Adult	10–42	0–39	0–8	48–195	35–85
Age	Phospho-ethanolamine	Phospho-serine	Proline	Sarcosine	Serine
Premature	5–35	10–45	92–310	0	127–248
Newborn–1 mo	3–27	7–47	110–417	0–625	99–395
2 mo–2 y	0–6	1–20	52–298	0	71–186
2–18 y	0–69	1–30	59–369	0–9	69–187
Adult	0–40	2–14	97–329	0	58–181

Age	Taurine	Threonine	Tryptophan	Tyrosine	Valine
Premature	151–411	150–330	28–136	147–420	99–220
Newborn–1 mo	46–492	90–329	0–60	55–147	86–190
2 mo–2 y	15–143	24–174	23–71	22–108	64–294
2–18 y	10–170	35–226	0–79	24–115	74–321
Adult	54–210	60–225	10–140	34–112	119–336

EXPLAINATION:

Screening for inborn amino acid metabolism abnormalities is generally performed on infants after the initial urine test is positive.

Other congenital enzyme defects interfere with healthy amino acid metabolism and cause excessive accumulation or loss of amino acid levels. Reduced growth rates, mental retardation, or other mysterious symptoms can occur unless an abnormality is identified and corrected early in life.

INDICATIONS:

- Assist in the detection of non-inherited disorders supported by elevated amino acid levels.

- Identify inborn errors of amino acid metabolism.

RESULT
Increased (total amino acids) in:
• Aminoacidopathies (usually hereditary; specific amino acids are involved)
• Fructose intolerance (hereditary)
• Malabsorption
• Renal failure (acute or chronic)
• Brain damage (severe)
• Burns
• Diabetes
• Eclampsia
• Reye's syndrome
• Acute liver damage
• Shock
Decreased (total amino acids) in:
• Adrenocortical hyperfunction
• Carcinoid syndrome
• Fever
• Glomerulonephritis
• Nephrotic syndrome
• Hartnup disease
• Huntington's chorea
• Malnutrition
• Pancreatitis (acute)
• Polycystic kidney disease
• Rheumatoid arthritis

IMPEDING FACTORS:
- Medications that may increase plasma amino acid levels include bismuth salts, glucocorticoids, levarterenol, 11-oxysteroids, and testosterone (older).
- Medications that may decrease plasma amino acid levels include cerulein, estrogens (males), epinephrine, leptin, oral contraceptives, progesterone (males), and secretin.

- Amino acids have a strong circadian rhythm; the values are highest in the afternoon and the lowest in the morning. The intake of protein does not control diurnal variation but significantly affects absolute concentrations. A quick 12-hour cycle before collection of specimens is needed.

AMINO ACID SCREEN, URINE

SAMPLING:10 ml of urine from a random or timed specimen collected in a clean and tidy plastic collection container and hydrochloric acid as a preservative.
TECHNIQUE: Chromatography
NORMAL VALUE: There are many amino acids. The tables below include the most frequently screened amino acids. The units are nanomoles per milligram (nmol/mg) creatinine.

Age	Alanine	β - Alanine	Anserine	α -Amino-adipic Acid	α - Amino-n-butyric Acid
Premature	1320–4040	1020–3500	—	70–460	50–710
Newborn–1mo	982–3055	25–288	0–3	0–180	8–65
2 mo–2 y	767–6090	0–297	0–5	45–268	30–136
2–18 y	231–915	0–65	0	2–88	0–77
Adult	240–670	0–130	0	40–110	0–90

Age	γ - Aminobutyric Acid	β - Aminoiso-butyric Acid	Arginine	Asparagine	Aspartic acid
Premature	20–260	50–470	190–820	1350–5250	580–1520
Newborn–1mo	0–15	421–3133	35–214	185–1550	336–810
2 mo–2 y	0–105	802–4160	38–165	252–1280	230–685
2–18 y	15–30	291–1482	31–109	72–332	0–120
Adult	15–30	10–510	10–90	99–470	60–240

Age	Carnosine	Citrulline	Cystathionine	Cystine	Ethanolamine
Premature	260–370	240–1320	260–1160	480–1690	—

Newborn–1month	97–665	27–181	16–147	212–668	840–3400
2mo-2 yr	203–635	22–180	33–470	68–710	0–2230
2yr–18 y	72–402	10–99	0–26	25–125	0–530
Adult	10–90	8–50	20–50	43–210	0–520

Age	Glutamic Acid	Glutamine	Glycine	Histidine	Homocysteine
Premature	380–3760	520–1700	7840–23,600	1240–7240	580–2230
Newborn–1mo	70–1058	393–1042	5749–16,423	908–2528	0–88
2 mo–2 y	54–590	670–1562	3023–11,148	815–7090	6–67
2–18 y	0–176	369–1014	897–4500	644–2430	0–32
Adult	39–330	190–510	730–4160	460–1430	0–32

Age	Hydroxy-lysine	Hydroxy-proline	Isoleucine	Leucine	Lysine
Premature	—	560–5640	250–640	190–790	1860–15,460
Newborn–1mo	10–125	40–440	125–390	78–195	270–1850
2 mo–2 y	0–97	0–4010	38–342	70–570	189–850
2–18 y	40–102	0–3300	10–126	30–500	153–634
Adult	40–90	0–26	16–180	30–150	145–634

Age	Methionine	1-Methyl-histidine	3-Methyl-histidine	Ornithine	Phenylalanine

Premature	500–1230	170–880	420–1340	260–3350	920–2280
Newborn–1mo	342–880	96–499	189–680	118–554	91–457
2 mo–2 y	174–1090	106–1275	147–391	55–364	175–1340
2–18 y	16–114	170–1688	182–365	31–91	61–314
Adult	38–210	170–1680	160–520	20–80	51–250

Age	ethanolamine	serine	Proline	Sarcosine	Serine
Premature	80–340	500–1690	1350–10,460	0	1680–6000
Newborn–1mo	0–155	150–339	370–2323	0–56	1444–3661
2 mo–2 y	108–533	112–304	254–2195	30–358	845–3190
2–18 y	18–150	70–138	0	0–26	362–1100
Adult	20–100	40–510	0	0–80	240–670

Age	Taurine	Threonine	Tryptophan	Tyrosine	Valine
Premature	5190–23,620	840–5700	0	1090–6780	180–890
Newborn–1mo	1650–6220	445–1122	0	220–1650	113–369
2 mo–2 y	545–3790	252–1528	0–93	333–1550	99–316
2–18 y	639–1866	121–389	0–108	122–517	58–143
Adult	380–1850	130–370	0–70	90–290	27–260

EXPLAINATION:

Screening for inborn amino acid metabolism defects is generally performed on infants after the initial urine test is positive. Such congenital enzyme defects interfere with normal amino acid metabolism and cause excessive accumulation or deficit of amino acid levels. Reduced growth rates, mental retardation, or other unexplained symptoms may result unless an abnormality is identified and corrected early in life.

INDICATIONS:

- Assist in recognition of non-inherited disorders demonstrated by elevated amino acid levels.
- Inspect for inborn errors of amino acid metabolism.

RESULT

Increased (total amino acids) in:
Primary causes (inherited):
• Aminoaciduria (specific)
• Cystinosis
• Fanconi's syndrome
• Fructose intolerance
• Galactosemia
• Hartnup disease
• Lactose intolerance
• Lowe's syndrome
• Maple syrup disease
• Tyrosinosis
• Wilson's disease
Secondary causes (non-inherited):
• Chronic renal failure
• Diabetic ketosis
• Hyperparathyroidism
• Hyperthyroidism
• Multiple myeloma
• Osteomalacia
• Liver necrosis and cirrhosis
• Muscular dystrophy (progressive)
• Thalassemia major
• Vitamin deficiency (B, C, and D)
• Viral hepatitis
Decreased in: Not any specific cause

IMPEDING FACTORS:
- Drugs that may upsurge urine amino acid levels include acetaminophen, amikacin, aminocaproic acid, amphetamine, ampicillin, cephalexin, colistin, corticotropin, dopamine, ephedrine, epinephrine, erythromycin, ethylenediamine, gentamicin, hydrocortisone, hydroxyaminobutyric acid, kanamycin, levarterenol, Levodopa, mafenide, metanephrine, methamphetamine, methyldopa, neomycin, normetanephrine, penicillamine, phenacetin, phenobarbital, phenylephrine, phenylpropanolamine, polymyxin, primidone, proSobee, pseudoephedrine, streptozocin, tetracycline, triamcinolone, and vigabatrin.
- Drugs that may reduce urine amino acid levels include insulin.
- Amino acids display a strong circadian rhythm; values are peak in the afternoon and lowest in the morning. Protein intake does not affect diurnal variation but significantly affects absolute concentrations, a 12- hour fast before specimen collection is required.
Dilute urine (specific gravity <1.010) should be refused for analysis.

AMNIOTIC FLUID ANALYSIS

SAMPLING:10 – 20 mL of Amniotic fluid is collected in clean amber glass or plastic containers.
TECHNIQUE: Macroscopic examination of fluid for color and appearance, electrophoresis for acetylcholinesterase, radioimmunoassay for fetoprotein, chromatography for lecithin/sphingomyelin [L/S] ratio, spectrophotometry for creatinine, bilirubin and also phosphatidylglycerol, dipstick for leukocyte esterase, tissue culture for chromosome analysis, and automated cell counter for white blood cell count and lamellar bodies.
NORMAL Value

Test	NORMAL Value
Color	Colorless to pale yellow
Appearance	Clear
-Fetoprotein	< 2.0 MoM
Acetylcholinesterase	Absent
Creatinine	1.8–4.0 mg/dL at term
Bilirubin	< 0.075 mg/dL in early pregnancy
	< 0.025 mg/dL at term pregnancy
L/S ratio	>2:1 at term
Phosphatidylglycerol	Present at term
Chromosome analysis	Normal karyotype
White blood cell count	None has seen

Leukocyte esterase	Negative
Lamellar bodies	30,000–50,000 platelet equivalents

EXPLAINATION:
Amniotic fluid is produced in a membrane sac that covers the fetus. The average volume of fluid over time is between 500 and 2500 ml. Throughout amniocentesis, the fluid is collected by ultrasound-guided aspiration from the amniotic sac. This procedure is usually done between 14 and 16 weeks of gestation, but it can also be performed between 26 and 35 weeks of gestation if fetal damage is suspected. Amniotic fluid is screened for developmental and neural tube defects, embryonic hemolytic disease, prenatal cancer, fetal renal failure, or fetal lung development.

INDICATIONS:
- Assist in detecting (in utero) metabolic disorders such as cystic fibrosis, or lipid, carbohydrate, or amino acid synthesis defects.
- Evaluate fetuses in families with a history of genetic disorders such as Down syndrome, Tay - Sachs disease, chromosome, or enzyme anomalies, or inherited hemoglobinopathies.
- Evaluate fetuses in mothers of advanced maternal age (some of those referred to above).
- Detection of secondary infection of ruptured membranes.
- Determination of fetal development where preterm birth is regarded. Fetal maturity is demonstrated by a ratio of L / S of 2:1 or greater.
- Determine fetal sex when a female is suspected of having a genetically related abnormal gene that could be transferred to a male offspring, such as hemophilia or Duchenne muscular dystrophy.
- Govern the presence of fetal distress in the late stage of pregnancy.

RESULT:
- Yellow-green, red, or brown fluid suggests the presence of bilirubin, blood (fetal or maternal), or meconium, suggesting fetal distress or death, hemolytic syndrome, or growth retardation.
- Elevated levels of bilirubin suggest fetal hemolytic disease or intestinal obstruction. Measurement of bilirubin is not usually done until 20 to 24 weeks of gestation because no action can be taken before that point. Optical density (OD) areas quantify the severity of hemolytic disease: 0.28 to 0.46 OD at 28 to 31 weeks of gestation indicates minimal hemolytic disease, which is unlikely to influence the fetus; 0.47 to 0.90 optical density (OD) specifies a moderate impact on the fetus, and 0.91 to 1.0 optical density (OD) shows a significant effect on the fetus. Increasing patterns with serial measurements can indicate the need for intrauterine transfusion or early delivery, depending on the fetal age. Between 32 to 33 weeks of gestation, early delivery is favored to intrauterine transfusion because early delivery is more effective in providing the neonate with the necessary care.

- Creatinine concentration > 2.0 mg / dL suggests fetal development (36 to 37 weeks) if maternal creatinine is also within the likely range. This value should be viewed following other parameters evaluated in the amniotic fluid. In particular, the L / S ratio as normal lung development can be influenced by normal renal development.
- L / S ratio < 2:1 and the lack of phosphatidylglycerol at term indicates fetal lung immaturity and likely respiratory distress syndrome. The expected L / S ratio of the fetus to the insulin-dependent diabetic mother is higher (3.5:1).
- Lamellar bodies are advanced alveolar cells in which the pulmonary surfactant is contained. These are about the thickness of the platelets. Their presence in sufficient quantities is a measure of fetal pulmonary maturity.
- Elevated α-fetoprotein levels and the presence of acetylcholinesterase indicate a defect in the neural tube.
- Abnormal karyotype indicates genetic abnormality (e.g., Tay - Sachs disease, mental retardation, DNA, or enzyme defects, and hereditary hemoglobinopathies).
- Elevated white blood cell count and elevated leukocyte esterase are markers of infection.

IMPEDING FACTORS:
- Bilirubin may be mistakenly elevated while maternal hemoglobin or meconium is present in the specimen; fetal acidosis may also lead to falsely raised bilirubin levels.
- Bilirubin may be decreased incorrectly if the sample is exposed to light or if the amount of amniotic fluid is high.
- Maternal serum creatinine should be measured at the same time as amniotic fluid creatinine for proper interpretation. Even in conditions where the maternal serum value is natural, the findings of amniotic fluid creatinine may be misleading. The high value of fluid creatinine in the fetus of a diabetic mother can reflect the increased muscle mass of a larger fetus. If the fetus is growing, creatinine may be strong, and the fetus may still have immature kidneys.
- Contamination of the specimen with blood or meconium or complications during pregnancy may result in incorrect L / S ratios.
- Fetoprotein and acetylcholinesterase may be falsely elevated if the sample is tainted with fetal blood.
- The karyotyping cannot be conducted under the following conditions:
  (1) failure to timely submit samples for chromosomal examination to the laboratory performing the test.
  (2) the insufficient incubation time of the sample causing cell death.
- Recent radioactive scans or contamination within one week of the test may conflict with the test results when radioimmunoassay is the test method.

- Amniocentesis is contraindicated in women who have a history of premature labor or an impaired cervix. It is also not indicated in the case of placenta previa or abruptio placentae.

C-REACTIVE PROTEIN (CRP)

SAMPLING: 1 mL of serum is collected in a red- or tiger-top tube.
TECHNIQUE: High-sensitivity immunoassay, nephelometry
NORMAL VALUE:

High-sensitivity immunoassay (cardiac applications)		0.08–3.10 g/mL
Nephelometry	Conventional Units	SI Units (Conversion FactorX10)
Cord	1–35 g/dL	10–350 g/L
Adult	6.8–820 g/dL	68–8200 g/L

EXPLAINATION:

C-reactive protein (CRP) is a glycoprotein produced by the liver in response to acute inflammation. The CRP assay is a non-specific test that determines the occurrence (not the cause) of inflammation; it is often conducted following the erythrocyte sedimentation rate (ESR). The CRP assay is a more sensitive and rapid predictor of inflammatory processes than the ESR. CRP disappears quickly from the bloodstream after the inflammation has subsided. The inflammatory process and its correlation with atherosclerosis allow the involvement of CRP, as measured by extremely sensitive CRP assay, a possible marker for coronary artery disease. It is suspected that the inflammatory process can contribute to the conversion of a stable plaque into a weakened plaque capable of breakup and occluding the artery. Several major studies are underway to validate the association and to create consistent NORMAL ranges for this reason.

INDICATIONS:
- Help in the differential diagnosis of appendicitis and acute pelvic inflammatory diseases>
- Aid in the differential diagnosis of Crohn's disease and ulcerative colitis.
- Help in the differential diagnosis of rheumatoid arthritis and simple systemic lupus erythematosus (SLE).
- Aid in the evaluation of coronary artery disease.
- Identifying the existence or exacerbation of inflammatory processes.
- Monitor responsiveness to autoimmune disorders therapy, such as rheumatoid arthritis.

RESULT:

Increased in:
Acute bacterial infections
Crohn's disease
Myocardial infarction
Pregnancy (second half)
Rheumatic fever
Rheumatoid arthritis
SLE
Inflammatory bowel disease
Decreased in: N/A

IMPEDING FACTORS:
- Medications that may reduce CRP include aurothiomalate, methotrexate, nonsteroidal anti-inflammatory drugs, oral contraceptives (progestogenic effect), penicillamine, pentopril, and sulfasalazine.
- Nonsteroidal anti-inflammatory drugs, salicylates, and steroids that induce false-negative effects due to the suppression of inflammation.
- Incorrectly elevated levels can occur when an intrauterine device is present.
- Lipemic samples which are turbid may be refused for review while nephelometry is the test method.

CHLORIDE, SWEAT

(Sweat test, pilocarpine iontophoresis sweat test, sweat chloride)
SAMPLING:0.1 mL minimum sweat is collected by pilocarpine iontophoresis.
TECHNIQUE: Ion-specific electrode or titration
NORMAL VALUE:

	Conventional Units	SI Units (Conversion Factor 1)
Normal	5–40 mEq/L	5–40 mmol/L
Intermediate	40–60 mEq/L	40–60 mmol/L

EXPLAINATION:

Cystic fibrosis (CF) is an inherited disease that affects the normal functioning of the exocrine glands, triggering large amounts of electrolytes to be excreted. Patients with CF have electrolyte sweat levels two to five times normal. Sweat test values, along with family history and signs and symptoms, are required to diagnose CF. CF is hereditary as an autosomal recessive trait characterized by abnormal exocrine secretions in the lungs, pancreas, small intestines, bile ducts, and skin. Clinical presentation may include chronic problems with the gastrointestinal and respiratory system. Testing stool samples for reduced trypsin content has been used as a CF check-in infants and children, but it is a much less trustworthy method than the sweat test.

The sweat test is a non-invasive analysis done to help detect CF while combined with other test results and physical assessments.

This test is usually performed in children, although adults may also be tested; it is not usually ordered in adults. The results can be highly variable and should be interpreted with caution. Sweat for the collection of specimens is induced by a small electrical current bearing the medicine pilocarpine.

The test assesses the concentration of chloride yielded by the skin's sweat glands. The presence of CF is indicated by a high concentration of chloride in the specimen. The sweat test is less commonly used to measure the concentration of sodium ions for the same purpose.

INDICATIONS:

- Assist with the detection of CF.
- Monitor for CF in people with a family history of illness.
- Check for suspected CF in children with chronic respiratory infections.
- Screen for suspected CF in babies with failure to thrive and infants who have passed meconium late.
- Screen for suspected CF in individuals with malabsorption syndrome.

RESULT:

	Increased in:
•	**Addison's disease**
•	**Alcoholic pancreatitis**
•	**Chronic pulmonary infections**
•	**Congenital adrenal hyperplasia**
•	**CF**
•	**Familial cholestasis**
•	**Familial hypoparathyroidism**
•	**Fucosidosis**
•	**Glucose-6-phosphate dehydrogenase deficiency**
•	**Hypothyroidism**

• **Mucopolysaccharidosis**	
• **Nephrogenic diabetes insipidus**	
Decreased in:	
• **Edema**	
• **Hypoaldosteronism**	
• **Hypoproteinemia**	
• **Sodium depletion**	

CRITICAL VALUES:

20 years or younger: >60 mmol/L considered diagnostic of CF
Older than 20 years: >70 mmol/L considered diagnostic of CF

The validity of the test result is greatly affected by the proper collection and handling of specimens. it is important to perform repeat checks on patients whose results are within the diagnostic or intermediate range. A negative test should be done again if the results of the test do not reflect the clinical picture.

IMPEDING FACTORS:

- Insufficient sweating will yield incorrect results. Sweat screening of children < 1 month of age is not advised because they are often unable to provide an adequate sample of sweat.

- This procedure should not be performed in patients with skin disorders (e.g., rash, eczema, erythema).

- Improper clean-up of the skin or improper application of the gauze pad or filter paper for processing impacts the tests' results.

- High environmental temperatures can reduce the concentration of sodium chloride in sweat; cool environmental temperatures can reduce the amount of sweat produced.

- If the sample container that stores the gauze or filter paper is handled without gloves, the test results could indicate a false improvement in the final weight of the collection container.

- Testing for CF can be performed using a silver nitrate test paper, and a positive test can be performed with pilocarpine iontophoresis.

CHROMOSOME ANALYSIS, BLOOD

SAMPLING: 2 mL of whole blood is collected in a green-top (sodium heparin) tube.

TECHNIQUE: Tissue culture and microscopic analysis

NORMAL VALUE: No chromosomal abnormalities were identified.

Syndrome	Chromosome Defect	Features
Beckwith-Wiedemann	Duplication 11p15	Macroglossia, omphalocele, ear lobe creases
Cat's eye	Trisomy 2q11	Anal atresia, coloboma
Cri du chat	Deletion 5p	Catlike cry, microcephaly, hypertelorism, mental retardation, retrognathia
Down's	Trisomy 21	Epicanthal folds, simian crease of the palm, congenital heart disease mental retardation, flat nasal bridge,
Edwards'	Trisomy 18	Micrognathia, congenital heart disease, clenched third/fourth fingers with the fifth finger overlapping, rocker-bottom feet, mental retardation,
Pallister-Killian	Trisomy 12p	Psychomotor delay, micrognathia, sparse anterior scalp hair, hypotonia

Patau's	Trisomy 13	Microcephaly, polydactyly, mental retardation, cleft palate or lip, congenital heart disease
Warkam	Mosaic trisomy 8	Malformed ears, bulbous nose, deep palm creases, absent or hypoplastic patellae

Wolf-Hirschhorn	Deletion 4p	Microcephaly, growth retardation, mental retardation, carp mouth
Syndrome	**Sex-Chromosome Defect**	**Features**
XYY	47, XYY	Tall, increased risk of behavioral problems
Klinefelter's	47, XXY	Hypogonadism, infertility, underdeveloped secondary sex characteristics, learning disabilities
Triple X	47, XXX	Increased risk of infertility and learning disabilities
Ullrich-Turner	45, X	Short, gonadal dysgenesis, webbed neck, low posterior hairline, renal and cardiovascular abnormalities

EXPLAINATION:

Screening for birth defects, as well as mental and physical retardation, can be carried out using several technologies. Chromosome examination by the phytohemagglutinin test is used to identify Down Syndrome and improper sexual development. Fluorescence in situ hybridization (FISH) testing helps detect microdeletion syndromes (e.g., Beckwith-Wiedemann, Prader-Willi, Angelman, Smith-Magenis, DiGeorge, Williams, Miller-Dieker) and other acquired chromosome changes associated with hematological disorders. Amniotic blood, chorionic villus screening, and fetal tissue cells or conception may also be tested for chromosome abnormalities.

INDICATIONS:

- Evaluate disorders linked to cryptorchidism, hypogonadism, chronic amenorrhea, and infertility.
- Evaluate congenital defects, delayed development (physical or mental retardation, and undefined sexual organs.
- Investigate the status of carriers of patients or relatives with known genetic abnormalities.
- Investigate the cause of multiple miscarriages.
- Provide prenatal care or genetic counseling.

CRYOGLOBULIN (Cryo)

SAMPLING: 1 mL of serum is collected in a red-top tube.

TECHNIQUE: Visual observation for changes in appearance

NORMAL VALUE:

Negative.

EXPLAINATION:

Cryoglobulins are abnormal proteins in serum that cannot be identified by electrophoresis.

Cryoglobulins cause vascular complications, as they can precipitate in the blood vessels of the fingers when exposed to air, causing Raynaud's phenomenon. They are usually associated with immunological diseases. The laboratory procedure for the detection of cryoglobulins is a two-step process. The serum sample is observed in cold precipitation after 72 hours of storage at 4°C. Real cryoglobulins vanish when heated to room temperature so that the sample is reheated in the second step of the procedure to check the reversibility of the reaction.

INDICATIONS:

- Aid in the diagnosis of neoplastic diseases, acute and chronic illnesses, and collagen diseases.
- Predict cryoglobulinemia in patients with symptoms that suggest or resemble Raynaud's disease.
- Monitor the progression of collagen and rheumatic disorders.

RESULT:

Increased in case of:
• **Type I cryoglobulin (monoclonal)**
• **Multiple myeloma**
• **Lymphoma**
• **Chronic lymphocytic leukemia**
• **Type II cryoglobulin (combinations of monoclonal immunoglobulin M [IgM] & polyclonal IgG)**
• **Waldenström's macroglobulinemia**
• **Rheumatoid arthritis**
• **Sjögren's syndrome**
• **Autoimmune hepatitis**
• **Type III cryoglobulin (combinations of polyclonal IgM and IgG)**
• **APGN or Acute post-streptococcal glomerulonephritis**
• **Chronic infection (especially hepatitis C)**
• **Cirrhosis**
• **Endocarditis**

• **Infectious mononucleosis**
• **Polymyalgia rheumatica**
• **Rheumatoid arthritis**
• **Sarcoidosis**
• **Systemic lupus erythematosus**
Decreased in: N/A

IMPEDING FACTORS:
- Testing the specimen prematurely (before total precipitation) can result in incorrect findings.
- Failure to maintain the sample at normal body temperature before centrifugation may have an impact on the results.
- A recent fatty meal can increase blood turbidity and decrease visibility.

CULTURE AND SMEAR, MYCOBACTERIA

(tuberculosis (TB) culture and smear, Acid-fast bacilli (AFB) culture and smear, *Mycobacterium* culture and smear)

SAMPLING: 5 to 10 mL of sputum, bronchopulmonary lavage, material from fine-needle aspiration, tissue, bone marrow, gastric aspiration, cerebrospinal fluid (CSF), urine, and stool.

TECHNIQUE: Culture on specified media microscopic examination of sputum using acid-fast or auramine-rhodamine fluorochrome stain). Rapid methods include chemiluminescent-labeled DNA probes targeting mycobacterium ribosomal RNA, radiometric identification of 14C-labelled media, polymerase chain reaction/amplification techniques.

NORMAL VALUE:
Culture: No growth
Smear: Negative for AFB

EXPLAINATION:
A culture and smear test are seen capable of detecting Mycobacterium tuberculosis, which is a tubercular bacillus. The cell wall of this mycobacterium includes complex lipids and waxes that do not contain ordinary stains. Cells that are resistant to acid alcohol decolorization are called Acid fast. There are only a few acid-fast bacilli (AFB) groups; this feature is useful for rapid identification so that treatment can be started promptly. Smears may be -ve in 50% of the time, even if the culture develops growth 3 to 8 weeks later. AFB cultures are used to validate positive and negative AFBs. M. Tuberculosis is slowly growing in culture. Automated liquid cultivation devices, such as Bactec and MGIT, have a processing time of approximately 10 days for results of tests using polymerase chain reaction. By using these methods, results are available within 36 to 48 hours.

M. Tuberculosis is spread to the lungs via the airborne route. It induces areas of granulomatous inflammation, cough, fever, and hemoptysis. It may remain dormant in the lungs for long periods. The incidence of tuberculosis has risen since the late 1980s in deprived inner-city areas, prison populations, and human immunodeficiency virus (HIV)-positive patients. The growth in antibiotic-resistant strains of M. tuberculosis is of great concern. HIV-positive patients often become ill due to concomitant infections caused by M. Tuberculosis and Mycobacterium avium intracellular.

M. Avium intracellular is acquired through the gastrointestinal tract through the ingestion of contaminated food or water. The waxy cell wall of the organism protects it from acids in the human digestive tract. The presence of mycobacteria in the stool does not mean that the patient has tuberculosis in the intestines because mycobacteria in the stool are most often found in the sputum that has been swallowed.

INDICATIONS:

- Aid in the diagnosis of mycobacteriosis.
- Help in the diagnosis of presumed pulmonary tuberculosis secondary to acquired immunodeficiency syndrome (AIDS).
- Assist in the distinction of tuberculosis from carcinoma or bronchiectasis.
- Evaluate suspected pulmonary tuberculosis.
- Monitor responsiveness to pulmonary tuberculosis treatment.

Results:

Identified Organism	Specimen Source	Condition
Mycobacterium avium intracellulare	Sputum, urine, CSF, semen, lymph nodes	Opportunistic pulmonary infection
M. fortuitum	Surgical wound, sputum, joint, bone, tissue	Opportunistic infection (usually pulmonary)
M. leprae	Skin scrapings, CSF, lymph nodes	Hansen's disease (leprosy)
M. kansasii	Skin, joint, sputum, lymph nodes	Pulmonary tuberculosis
M. marinum	Joint	Granulomatous skin lesions
M. tuberculosis	Sputum, urine, CSF, gastric washing	Pulmonary tuberculosis
M. xenopi	Sputum	Pulmonary tuberculosis

CSF=cerebrospinal fluid.
CRITICAL VALUES:
Smear: Positive for AFB
Culture: Growth of pathogenic bacteria
IMPEDING FACTORS:
- The collection of specimens after initiation of treatment with antituberculosis drug therapy can result in slowed or no growth of organisms.
- The contamination of sterile containers with organisms from an exogenous source can yield misleading results.
- Specimens obtained on a dry swab should be refused: a dry swab indicates that the sample is unlikely to have been correctly extracted or is unlikely to produce enough relevant species for proper assessment.
- Incomplete or inaccurate (e.g., saliva) tests should be rejected.

CULTURE, FUNGAL
SAMPLING: Hair, nail, pus, skin, sterile fluids, bronchial washings, sputum, blood, bone marrow, stool, or tissue samples collected in a sterile plastic, tight lid container.
TECHNIQUE: macroscopic and microscopic examination; Culture on specific media.
NORMAL VALUE: No fungi detected.
EXPLAINATION:
 Fungi, organisms that usually live in soil, can be transmitted to humans by unintended inhalation of spores or by trauma leading to the inoculation of spores into tissues. Individuals more vulnerable to fungal infection are typically affected by chronic disease, have extended antibiotic therapy, or have compromised immune systems. Fungal diseases may be categorized according to the type of tissue involved: dermatophytosis includes superficial and cutaneous tissue; subcutaneous and systemic mycoses are also present.
INDICATIONS:
- Help to determine the antimicrobial sensitivity of the organism.
- Isolate and identify organisms responsible for nail diseases or anomalies.
- Isolate and identify organisms responsible for skin rash, drainage, or other signs of infection.

RESULT

	Positive findings in:
•	Blood
•	*Candida albicans*
•	*Histoplasma capsulatum*
•	Cerebrospinal fluid
•	*Coccidioides immitis*
•	*Cryptococcus neoformans*
•	Members of the order Mucorales
•	*Paracoccidioides brasiliensis*
•	*Sporothrix schenckii*
•	Hair
•	*Epidermophyton*
•	*Microsporum*
•	*Trichophyton*
•	Nails
•	*Candida albicans*
•	*Cephalosporium*
•	*Epidermophyton*
•	*Trichophyton*
•	Skin
•	*Actinomyces israelii*
•	*Candida albicans*
•	*Coccidioides immitis*
•	*Epidermophyton*
•	*Microsporum*
•	*Trichophyton*
•	Tissue
•	*israelii*
•	*Aspergillus*
•	*Candida albicans*
•	*Nocardia*
•	*P. brasiliensis*

IMPEDING FACTORS:
Prompt and proper collection, storage, and analysis of specimens are important for achieving accurate results.

CULTURE, VIRAL

SAMPLING: Urine, blood, semen, body fluid, stool, tissue, or swabs from the affected site.
TECHNIQUE: Culture in special media, direct fluorescent antibody techniques, enzyme-linked immunoassays, latex agglutination, immunoperoxidase techniques
NORMAL VALUE: No virus isolated.
EXPLAINATION:
Viruses, the most common source of human infection, are submicroscopic organisms that invade living cells. These may be listed as either RNA-or DNA-type viruses. Viral titers are strongest in the early stages of the disease before the host begins to produce sufficient antibodies to the invader. Specimens must be obtained as soon as possible during the disease process.
INDICATIONS: Aid in the identification of viral infection.
RESULT:

Positive findings in:
• **Acquired immunodeficiency syndrome**
• **Human immunodeficiency virus (HIV)**
• **Acute respiratory failure**
• **Hantavirus**
• **Anorectal infections**
• **Herpes simplex virus (HSV)**
• **Human papillomavirus**
• **Bronchitis**
• **Parainfluenza virus**
• **Respiratory syncytial virus (RSV)**
• **Condylomata**
• **Human papilloma DNA virus**
• **Conjunctivitis/keratitis**
• **Adenovirus**
• **Epstein-Barr virus**
• **HSV**
• **Measles virus**
• **Parvovirus**

- Rubella virus
- Varicella zoster virus
- Croup
- Parainfluenza virus
- RSV
- Cutaneous infection with rash
- Enteroviruses
- HSV
- Varicella zoster virus
- Encephalitis
- Enteroviruses
- Flaviviruses
- HSV
- HIV
- Measles virus
- Rabies virus
- Togaviruses
- Febrile illness with rash
- Coxsackieviruses
- Echovirus
- Gastroenteritis
- Norwalk virus
- Rotavirus
- Genital herpes
- HSV-1
- HSV-2
- Hemorrhagic cystitis
- Adenovirus
- Hemorrhagic fever
- Ebola virus
- Hantavirus
- Lassa virus
- Marburg virus
- Herpangina

- Coxsackievirus (group A)
- Infectious mononucleosis
- Cytomegalovirus
- Epstein-Barr virus
- Meningitis
- Coxsackieviruses
- Echovirus
- HSV-2
- Lymphocytic choriomeningitis virus
- Myocarditis/pericarditis
- Coxsackievirus
- Echovirus
- Parotitis
- Mumps virus
- Parainfluenza virus
- Pharyngitis
- Adenovirus
- Coxsackievirus (group A)
- Epstein-Barr virus
- HSV
- Influenza virus
- Parainfluenza virus
- Rhinovirus
- Pleurodynia
- Coxsackievirus (group B)
- Pneumonia
- Adenovirus
- Influenza virus
- Parainfluenza virus
- RSV
- Upper respiratory tract infection
- Adenovirus
- Coronavirus
- Influenza virus

• Parainfluenza virus
• RSV
• Rhinovirus

CRITICAL VALUES: Positive RSV culture should be immediately reported to the patient health care practitioner.

IMPEDING FACTORS: Viral samples are not stable. Prompt and proper collection, storage, and analysis of specimens are important for the achievement of accurate results.

CYTOLOGY, SPUTUM

SAMPLING:10 to 15 mL of sputum is collected on 3 to 5 consecutives, the first morning, deep-cough expectorations.

TECHNIQUE: Macroscopic and microscopic examination.

NORMAL VALUE:

Negative for abnormal cells, ova, fungi, and parasites.

EXPLAINATION:

Cytology is a study of cell origin, structure, function, and pathology. Cytological tests are generally performed in clinical practice to diagnose changes in cells arising from neoplastic or inflammatory conditions. Sputum specimens for cytological analyses may be obtained by expectoration alone, by suction, by lung biopsy, by bronchoscopy, or by expectoration after bronchoscopy.

INDICATIONS:
- Aid in establishing the diagnosis of lung cancer.
- Support in the diagnosis of Pneumocystis carinii in individuals with acquired immunodeficiency syndrome (AIDS).
- Detection of known or suspected fungal or parasitic infections affecting the lung.
- Detection of known or suspected pulmonary viral disease.
- Screen tobacco smoking for neoplastic (nonmalignant) cell changes.
- Screen patients with a history of acute or chronic inflammatory or contagious lung disorders that may contribute to mild atypical or metaplastic changes.

RESULT:

The method of reporting the results of the cytology studies varies depending on the laboratory doing the examination.

Words used to report results may include negative (no abnormal cells seen), infectious, benign atypical, suspicious of neoplasm, and positive for neoplasm.

Positive findings in:
- Infections induced by fungi, ova, or parasites.
- Lipoid or aspiration pneumonia when lipid droplets in macrophages are seen.

- Viral infections and lung disease.
- Neoplasms.

CRITICAL VALUES:
If the patient is hypoxic or cyanotic, immediately remove the catheter and give it oxygen. If the patient has asthma or chronic bronchitis, look for aggravated bronchospasms with normal saline or acetylcysteine in the aerosol.

IMPEDING FACTORS:
- Inadequate fixation of specimens may be the source of rejection of samples.
- The inadequate technique used to achieve bronchial washing can lead to the rejection of the specimen

---

CYTOLOGY, URINE

SAMPLING: Urine up to 180 mL for an adult or minimum of 10 mL for a child is collected in a clean wide-mouth plastic container.

TECHNIQUE: Microscopic examination

NORMAL VALUE: No abnormal cells or inclusions are seen.

EXPLAINATION:
Urinary tract epithelial lining cells can be found in the urine. Testing of these cells for anomalies is valuable for suspected infection, inflammatory conditions, or malignancy.

INDICATIONS: Help diagnose urinary tract diseases, such as cancer, cytomegalovirus, and other inflammatory conditions.

RESULT:

Positive findings in:
• **Cancer of the urinary tract**
• **Cytomegalic inclusion disease**
• **Inflammatory disease of the urinary tract**
Negative findings in N/A

BACTERIAL CULTURE, URINE

SAMPLING: 5 mL of urine collected in a sterile plastic collection container.

TECHNIQUE: Culture on selective and enriched media

NORMAL VALUE:

Negative: no growth.

EXPLAINATION:
Urine culture involves collecting a sample of urine so that the disease-causing agent can be detected and identified. Urine may be obtained by urinary catheterization, clean catch, or suprapubic aspiration. The gravity of the infection or contamination of the specimen may be determined by knowing the type and number of pathogens (colonies) present in the specimen.

The laboratory shall initiate sensitivity testing if the test results are suggested.

Sensitivity testing detects drugs that are vulnerable to organisms to ensure an effective treatment plan.

Commonly detected species are those typically found in the genitourinary tract, including enterococci, Escherichia coli, Klebsiella, Proteus, and Pseudomonas. A culture that shows multiple species suggests a contaminated sample.

Colony counts of $\geq$100,000 / mL are suggestive of urinary tract infection (UTI). Colony counts of 1000 / mL or less indicate contamination resulting from poor collection techniques.

Colony counts in the middle of 1000 and 10,000 / mL may be important depending on a variety of factors, e.g., the age of the patient, gender, number of types of organism's present, form of specimen collection, and usage of antibiotics.

INDICATIONS:
- Help in the diagnosis of suspected UTI.
- Establish the sensitivity of significant organisms to antibiotics.
- Monitor the response to UTI treatment.

RESULT

Positive findings in:
UTIs
Negative findings in:
Not any disease

IMPEDING FACTORS:
- Antibiotic treatment started before the Collection of specimens can yield false-negative outcomes.
- Improper collection methods end in contamination of the test.
- Storage of samples more than 30 minutes at room temperature or 24 hours at refrigerated temperatures will end in bacterial overgrowth and false positive outcomes.
- Urine culture findings are also viewed in combination with routine urinalysis performance.
- Differences between culture and urinalysis can be a reason to recollect the specimen.

BACTERIAL CULTURE, THROAT OR NASAL PHARYNGEAL

Routine throat culture.
SAMPLING: Throat or nasal pharyngeal swab.
TECHNIQUE: Aerobic culture
NORMAL VALUE: No growth.

EXPLAINATION:

A routine throat culture is a commonly ordered screening test for the presence of Group A-hemolytic streptococci. S. Pyogenesis, the body that most commonly causes acute pharyngitis. Further severe sequelae of scarlet fever, rheumatic heart disease, and glomerulonephritis are less commonly observed due to early care of pharyngitis infection. A variety of other bacterial agents are responsible for pharyngitis. Different cultures may be formed to identify certain pathogens, such as Bordetella, Corynebacteria, Haemophilus, or Neisseria if they are detected or by special request from the health care provider. Corynebacterium diphtheriae is a causative agent for diphtheria. Neisseria gonorrhea is a sexually transmitted pathogen. Among infants, Neisseria's positive throat culture usually indicates sexual abuse. Whether test results are indicated, the laboratory must begin antibiotic sensitivity tests. Susceptibility testing identifies drugs that are susceptible to pathogens to ensure an effective treatment plan.

INDICATIONS:

- Aid in the diagnosis of bacterial infections such as tonsillitis, diphtheria, gonorrhea, or pertussis.
- Help in the diagnosis of upper respiratory infections resulting in bronchitis, pharyngitis, croup, and influenza.
- Isolate and recognize Group A-β-hemolytic Streptococci as the source of strep throat, acute glomerulonephritis, scarlet fever, or rheumatic fever.

RESULT:

Culture results that are positive for Group A-β-hemolytic Streptococci are generally available within 24 to 48 hours. Cultures that document normal respiratory flora are given after 48 hours. Culture findings of no growth for Corynebacterium allow 72 hours to record; 48 hours to report negative Neisseria cultures.

IMPEDING FACTORS:

- Contamination with oral flora can discredit the result.
- The acquisition of specimens after antibiotic therapy has been started may result in inhibition or non-growth of pathogens.

BACTERIAL CULTURE, STOOL

SAMPLING: Fresh random stool stored in a clean plastic container.

TECHNIQUE: Culture on selective media for detection of pathogens usually to include Salmonella, Shigella, Escherichia coli O157: H7, latex agglutination or enzyme immunoassay for Clostridium A and B toxins, Yersinia enterocolitis, and Campylobacter.

NORMAL VALUE:

Negative: No growth of pathogens.

Natural fecal flora is 96 to 99 percent anaerobic and 1 to 4 percent aerobic. Normal flora present may include Bacteroides, Enterococcus, E. Coli, Candida albicans, Clostridium, Proteus, Pseudomonas, and Staphylococcus aureus.

EXPLAINATION:

Stool culture involves collecting a stool sample so that the pathogens present can be separated and identified. Some bacteria are usually present in the feces. Nevertheless, when these species become overgrown or pathogenic, diarrhea, or other signs and symptoms of systemic infection arise. These effects are the result of damage to the intestinal tissue of pathogenic organisms. Routine stool culture usually screens a limited number of common pathogens, such as Campylobacter, Salmonella, and Shigella. Identification of other bacteria shall be initiated by special request or consulting with a microbiologist, where special circumstances are identified. If the test results are indicated, the laboratory will begin antibiotic sensitivity testing. Sensitivity testing recognizes drugs that are vulnerable to organisms to ensure an effective treatment plan.

INDICATIONS:

- Aid in establishing a diagnosis for diarrhea of unknown cause.
- Identify pathogenic organisms producing gastrointestinal disease and carrier states.

RESULT:

Positive findings in:

- Bacterial infections: Aeromonas spp., Bacillus cereus, Campylobacter, Clostridium, E. Coli including O157:H7 serotype, Plesiomonas shigelloides, Salmonella, Shigella, Yersinia, and Vibrio. Staphylococcus aureus isolation can indicate an infection or a carrier condition.
- Botulism: Clostridium botulinum (the organism must also be extracted from the diet or the existence of reported toxins in the stool specimen).

IMPEDING FACTORS:

- A rectal swab does not provide enough specimen for evaluating the carrier state and should be avoided in pNORMAL of a regular stool specimen.
- For Clostridium toxin tests, a rectal swab should never be requested. Samples for Clostridium toxins should be refrigerated if they are not instantly shipped to the laboratory because toxins decay rapidly.
- A rectal swab for Campylobacter culture should never be sent. Unnecessary exposure of the sample to air or room temperature can kill this type of bacteria to not grow in culture.
- Antibiotic therapy before the collection of specimens can decrease the type and number of bacteria.
- Failure to convey the culture within 1 hour of the sample collection or contamination of the urine may have an impact on the results.
- Barium and laxatives, if used < 1 week before the test, can reduce the growth of bacteria.

BACTERIAL CULTURE, SPUTUM

Routine culture of sputum.

SAMPLING: Sputum (10 to 15 mL).

EXPLAINATION:

This test involves the collection of a sputum specimen so that the pathogen can be isolated and detected. The test results will indicate the type and number of organisms present in the specimen, as well as the antibiotics to which the pathogenic organisms identified are susceptible. Sputum collected by anticipation or suction with catheters and bronchoscopy cannot be cultivated for anaerobic organisms; instead, trans-tracheal aspiration or lung biopsy must be used. If the test results are indicated, the laboratory will initiate antibiotic sensitivity testing. Sensitivity testing identifies antibiotics that are susceptible to organisms to ensure an effective treatment plan.

INDICATIONS:

Culture:

Help in the establishment of the diagnosis of respiratory infections, as indicated by the presence or absence of organisms in culture.

Gram Stain:

- Assist in the separation of gram-positive and gram-negative bacteria in respiratory infection.
- Assist in the distinction of sputum from upper respiratory tract secretions, which are demonstrated by abundant squamous cells or loss of polymorphonuclear leukocytes.

RESULT:

- The main challenge in evaluating the results is the difference between pathogens infecting the lower respiratory tract and species that have colonized but not invaded the lower respiratory tract. The Gram stain analysis assists in this process. The occurrence of more than 25 squamous epithelial cells per low-power field (lpf) suggests oral infection, and the specimen should be discarded. The appearance of many polymorphonuclear neutrophils and few squamous epithelial cells suggests that the specimen has been collected from the area of infection and is suitable for further study.
- Streptococcus pneumoniae may cause Bacterial pneumonia, Haemophilus influenzae, staphylococci, and some gram-negative bacteria. Certain pathogens established by culture include Corynebacterium diphtheriae, Klebsiella pneumoniae, and Pseudomonas aeruginosa. Several infectious agents, including C. Diphtheriae, are more accelerated in their growth requirements and cannot be cultured and identified without special treatment. Suspicion of contamination by less commonly identified and/or fastidious pathogens must be conveyed to the laboratory to ensure that the appropriate method for diagnosis is selected.

IMPEDING FACTORS:
- Contamination of oral flora can invalidate the result.
- The collection of specimens after the start of antibiotic therapy can result in slowed or no growth of organisms.

BACTERIAL CULTURE, BLOOD

SAMPLING: 10 to 20 mL for adult patients or 1 to 5 mL for pediatric patients. Whole blood is collected in bottles comprising standard aerobic and anaerobic culture media.

TECHNIQUE: Growth of bacteria in standard culture media detected by radiometric or infrared automation, or by the manual reading of subculture.

NORMAL VALUE:

Negative: no growth of pathogens.

EXPLAINATION:

Blood cultures are obtained if bacteremia or septicemia is reported. While mild bacteremia is present in many infectious diseases, chronic, constant, or recurring bacteria indicate a more serious infection that may need immediate treatment. Early discovery of pathogens in the blood may help with clinical and etiological diagnosis. Blood culture involves the introduction of a blood specimen into an artificial aerobic and anaerobic culture medium. The colony is incubated for a specific duration, at a specific temperature and under certain conditions suitable for the growth of pathogenic microorganisms. Pathogens enter the bloodstream from soft tissue infection sites, infected intravenous tubes, or surgical procedures (e.g., surgery, tooth extraction, cystoscopy). An antimicrobial removal system (ARD) can also be used to cultivate blood. It involves transferring some of the blood samples to a special vial containing absorbent resins that extract drugs from the sample before the culture is done. When test results are indicated, the laboratory must start antibiotic sensitivity testing. Susceptibility testing identifies antibiotics that are susceptible to pathogens to ensure an effective treatment plan.

INDICATIONS:

- Determine neonatal sepsis due to prolonged labor, early membrane rupture, maternal infection, or neonatal aspiration.
- Evaluate chills and fever in patients with bacterially infected burns, urinary tract infections, postoperative wound, sepsis, rapidly developing tissue infection, and indwelling venous or arterial catheter.
- Evaluate irregular or constant temperature spike of unknown origin (pyrexia of unknown origin).
- Evaluate persistent or new heart murmur that appears along with fever.
- Evaluate rapid heartbeat and temperature changes with or without chills and diaphoresis.
- Evaluate suspicion of bacteremia after invasive procedures.
    - Identify the reason for a shock in the postoperative period.

RESULT

Positive findings in suspected Bacteremia or septicemia:

- Aerobacter, Brucella, Escherichia coli, Bacteroides, and other coliform bacilli, Clostridium perfringens, enterococci, Listeria monocytogenes, Pseudomonas aeruginosa, Haemophilus influenzae, Klebsiella, Salmonella, Staphylococcus aureus, Staphylococcus epidermidis, and β-hemolytic Streptococcus.
- Plague
- Typhoid fever
- Malaria (on special request, a stained capillary smear would be examined)
- A yeast, Candida albicans, that can cause infection and can be isolated by blood culture.

CRITICAL VALUES:

Positive findings must be immediately conveyed to the primary health care practitioner.

IMPEDING FACTORS:

- Pre-test antimicrobial therapy may slow or inhibit the growth of pathogens.
- The contamination of the specimen by the resident flora of the skin can invalidate the interpretation of the test results.
- The insufficient amount of blood or the number of blood samples taken for analysis can invalidate the interpretation of the results.
- Specimens tested more than 1 hour after sampling can result in decreased growth or non-growth of species.
- The negative findings do not guarantee that there is no infection.

BACTERIAL CULTURE, ANAL/ GENITAL, SKIN, EAR, EYE, AND WOUND

SAMPLING: Sterile fluid or swab from the affected area placed in the transport media tube provided by the laboratory.

TECHNIQUE: DNA probe assays are available for the identification of Neisseria gonorrhoeae, culture aerobic and/or anaerobic organisms on selected media.

NORMAL VALUE:

Negative: no growth of pathogens.

EXPLAINATION:

Anal cultures may be used to identify the organism responsible for sexually transmitted diseases, as suggested by the patient's history.

Ear and eye cultures are used to distinguish the organism responsible for the chronic or acute ear and eye infections.

Skin and soft tissue extracts from infected sites must be carefully collected to prevent contamination of natural skin flora in the surrounding area. Both aerobic and anaerobic species can cause skin and tissue infections.

A portion of the sample should, therefore, be put in aerobic and anaerobic transport media. Care must be taken to use the transport media accredited by the laboratory conducting the tests

A wound culture requires collecting a specimen of exudate, discharge, or tissue so that the causative organism can be separated, and pathogens can be identified. Specimens can be collected from deep and shallow wounds.

Samples should be collected optimally before antibiotic application. The system used to cultivate and expand the agent depends on the suspicious infectious organism. Transport media, specifically for bacterial agents, are available. The laboratory must select appropriate media for suspected pathogens. If the test results are indicated, the laboratory will begin antibiotic sensitivity testing. Susceptibility testing identifies antibiotics that are susceptible to organisms to achieve an accurate treatment plan.

INDICATIONS:

Anal/genital:
- Aid in the treatment of sexually transmitted diseases.
- Determine the cause of genital discomfort or purulent discharge.
- Determine effective antimicrobial therapy relevant to the pathogen detected.

Ear:
- Isolate and identify the organisms responsible for ear pain, discharge, or hearing changes.
- Isolate and identify the organisms responsible for the outer, middle, or inner ear infection.
- Assess successful antimicrobial therapy specific to the pathogen detected.

Eye:
- Isolate and identify pathogenic microorganisms responsible for eye infection.
- Determine appropriate antimicrobial therapy according to identified pathogens.

Skin:
- Isolate and identify pathogens responsible for skin rashes, drainage, or other signs of infection.
- Determine successful antimicrobial therapy specific to the pathogen detected.

Sterile fluids:
- Isolate and identify organisms before surrounding tissues are affected.
- Determine successful antimicrobial therapy specific to the pathogen detected.

Wound:

- Predict abscess or deep-wound infectious infection.
- Determine whether an infectious agent induces wound redness, swelling or edema with leakage at the location.
- Determine the presence of infectious agents at stage 3 and stage 4 of the decubitus ulcer.
- Isolate and identify the organisms responsible for the presence of pus or other exudates in the open wound.
- Determine successful antimicrobial therapy relevant to isolated pathogen.
- Predict abscess or deep-wound infectious infection.
- Determine whether an infectious agent induces wound redness, swelling or edema with leakage at the location.
- Determine the presence of infectious agents at stage 3 and stage 4 of the decubitus ulcer.
- Isolate and identify the organisms responsible for the presence of pus or other exudates in the open wound.
- Determine successful antimicrobial therapy relevant to cultured pathogen.

RESULT:
Positive findings in:
Anal/Endocervical/Genital
Infections or carrier conditions caused by the following organisms: Gardnerella vaginalis, N. Gonorrhea, toxin-producing strains of Staphylococcus aureus, and Treponema pallidum.
Ear
Commonly identified bacteria include Escherichia coli, Proteus spp., Pseudomonas aeruginosa, Staphylococcus aureus, and β- hemolytic Streptococcus.
Eye
Commonly identified organisms are Haemophilus influenzae, H. Aegypt, N. Gonorrhea, Pseudomonas aeruginosa, Staphylococcus aureus, and Streptococcus pneumoniae.
Skin
Generally identified organisms comprised of Bacteroides, Clostridium, Pseudomonas, Staphylococci, Corynebacterium, and group A Streptococci.
Sterile fluids
Commonly recognized pathogens include Bacteroides, Pseudomonas aeruginosa, Enterococcus spp., E. coli, and Peptostreptococcus spp.
Wound
In wound culture samples, both aerobic and anaerobic microorganisms can be established. Commonly identified bacteria include Clostridium perfringens, Klebsiella, Proteus, Pseudomonas, Staphylococcus aureus, and Streptococcus group A.
IMPEDING FACTORS:

- Failure to collect adequate specimens, improper collection or storage techniques, and failure to transport specimens promptly is grounds for refusal of specimens.
- Pre-test antimicrobial therapy may slow or inhibit the growth of pathogens.
- Processing specimens more than 1 hour after collection can result in decreased growth or non-growth of species.

KETONES, BLOOD, AND URINE
Ketone bodies, acetoacetate, acetone
SAMPLING: 1 mL of serum is collected from a red- or tiger-top tube. 5 mL of urine random or timed specimen is collected in a clean plastic collection container.
TECHNIQUE: Colorimetric nitroprusside reaction
NORMAL VALUE: Negative.
EXPLAINATION:
Ketone bodies refer to three intermediate oxidation products: acetone, acetoacetic acid, and β-hydroxybutyrate. Although-hydroxybutyrate is not a ketone; it is usually referred to as ketone. In healthy individuals, ketones are developed and fully metabolized by the liver so that quantifiable levels are not normally present in the serum. Ketones present in the urine before a large serum level is measured. If the patient has excess fat metabolism, ketones are found in the blood and urine.
Excessive fat metabolism can occur if the patient has impaired ability to metabolize carbohydrates, inadequate intake of carbohydrates, inadequate insulin levels, excessive carbohydrate loss, or increased demand for carbohydrates. A moderately positive result of acetone without extreme acidosis, followed by normal glucose, electrolyte, and bicarbonate levels, is indicative of isopropyl alcohol poisoning. A low-carbohydrate or low-fat diet may result in a positive acetone test. Ketosis in diabetics is generally accompanied by increased glucose and reduced bicarbonate and pH. Incredibly high levels of ketone will result in a coma.
INDICATIONS:
- Assist in the detection of malnutrition, fatigue, depression, reported isopropyl alcohol consumption, glycogen storage problems, and other metabolic disorders.
- Monitor and monitor the treatment of diabetic ketoacidosis.
- Diabetes management tracking.
- Ketonuria screening to aid in the evaluation of inborn metabolism defects.
- Ketonuria test to help diagnose possible isopropyl alcohol poisoning.
- Ketonuria screening due to acute disease or stress in non-diabetic patients.
RESULT:

Increased in:
• **Glycogen storage diseases**
• **Hyperglycemia**

• **High-fat or high-protein diet**
• **Acidosis**
• **Branched chain ketonuria**
• **Fasting or starvation**
• **Gestational diabetes**
• **Ketoacidosis of alcoholism and diabetes**
• **Illnesses with marked vomiting and diarrhea**
• **Isopropyl alcohol ingestion**
• **Methylmalonic aciduria**
• **Postanesthesia period**
• **Propionyl coenzyme A carboxylase deficiency**
• **Carbohydrate deficiency**
• **Eclampsia**
Decreased in: N/A

CRITICAL VALUES:
The elevated level of ketone bodies is evidenced by a fruity-smelling odor, acidosis, ketonuria, and a decreased level of consciousness. Insulin administration and repeated blood glucose monitoring may be suggested.

IMPEDING FACTORS:
- Medicines that may cause an increase in serum ketone levels include acetylsalicylic acid (if the medication results in acidosis, especially in children), fenfluramine, albuterol, levodopa, nifedipine, and paraldehyde.
- Medications that may decrease serum ketone levels include acetylsalicylic acid and valproic acid. Increases were shown in hyperthyroid patients receiving propranolol and propylthiouracil.
- Drugs that may increase urinary ketone levels include acetylsalicylic acid (if treatment results in acidosis, especially in children), ether, ifosfamide, insulin, captopril, dimercaprol, levodopa, mesna, metformin, methyldopa, N-acetylcysteine, niacin, phenazopyridine, phenolphthalein, paraldehyde, penicillamine, phenolsulfonphthalein, pyrazinamide, streptozocin, sulfobromophthalein, and valproic acid.
- Medications that may decrease urinary ketone levels include acetylsalicylic acid and phenazopyridine.
- Urine should be tested within 60 minutes of collection time.
- Bacterial contamination of urine may result in false-negative results.
- Failure to keep the reagent strip tightly closed will lead to false-negative results.
- Light and moisture have an impact on the ability of the chemicals in the strip to perform as expected.
- False-negative or weakly false-positive test results may be obtained when β-hydroxybutyrate is the predominant ketone body in cases of lactic acidosis.

LACTIC ACID (Lactate)

SAMPLING: 1 mL of plasma is collected in a gray-top (sodium fluoride) or a green-top (lithium heparin) tube. Samples should be transported tightly capped and in an ice slurry.

TECHNIQUE: Spectrophotometry/enzymatic analysis

NORMAL VALUE:

Conventional Units	SI Units (Conversion Factor X0.111)
3–23 mg/dL	0.3–2.6 mmol/L

EXPLAINATION:

Lactic acid (present in the blood as lactate) is a by-product of carbohydrate metabolism. Typically, the concentration of lactate in the liver is based on the rate of output and metabolism. Levels rise during strenuous exercise, which results in an insufficient supply of oxygen to the tissues. Pyruvate, the usual end product of glucose metabolism, is converted to lactate in emergencies where energy is needed. Still, there is not sufficient oxygen in the body to support the aerobic and classical energy cycles. When hypoxia or circulatory collapse increases the production of lactate, or when the hepatic system does not metabolize lactate adequately, the amount of lactate increases. The lactic acid test may be performed in conjunction with the pyruvic acid test to monitor the oxygenation of the tissues. Lactic acidosis can be distinguished from ketoacidosis by a lack of ketosis and highly elevated glucose levels.

INDICATIONS:

- Evaluate tissue oxygenation.
- Evaluate acidosis.

RESULT:

Increased in:
• Cardiac failure
• Diabetes
• Hemorrhage
• Hepatic coma
• Lactic acidosis
• Pulmonary embolism
• Pulmonary failure
• Reye's syndrome
• Shock
• Strenuous exercise
• Intake of large doses of ethanol or acetaminophen
Decreased in: N/A

CRITICAL VALUES:
More than or equal to 45 mg / dL, scrutinize the patient for signs and symptoms of raised levels, such as Kussmaul's breathing and increased pulse rate. Generally, there is an inverse relationship between highly elevated lactate levels and recovery.

IMPEDING FACTORS:
- Products that may increase lactate levels include albuterol, anticonvulsants (long-term use), epinephrine, intravenous glucose, lactose, oral contraceptives, sodium bicarbonate, and sorbitol.
- Falsely low lactate levels are observed in samples with elevated levels of the enzyme lactate dehydrogenase (LDH) because the enzyme interacts with the accessible lactate substrate.
- Using a tourniquet or directing the patient to clench his or her fist during venipuncture can cause high levels.
- Participating in strenuous physical activity (i.e., any activity in which blood flow and delivery of oxygen cannot keep pace with increased energy needs) before the processing of specimens can lead to increased outcomes.
- Delay in the transfer of the specimen to the laboratory shall be avoided. For analysis, specimens not separated by centrifugation in a tightly closed collection container within 15 minutes of sampling should be rejected. It is better to transport specimens to the laboratory in an ice slurry to delay further cell metabolism, which may change the lactate levels in the sample before analysis.

β2-MICROGLOBULIN (β2-M)

SAMPLING:1 mL of serum is collected in a red-top tube or 5 mL of urine from a scheduled collection in a clean, plastic container as well as for 1N NaOH as a preservative.

TECHNIQUE: Immunoassay for serum sample, radioimmunoassay for the urine sample

NORMAL VALUE:

	Conventional SI Units	Sample Units (Conversion Factor X10)
Serum		
Newborn	< 0.3 mg/dL	< 3 mg/L
Adult	< 0.2 mg/dL	< 2 mg/L
Urine	0.03–0.37 mg/24 h	

EXPLAINATION:

β2-Microglobulin is an amino acid peptide part of human leukocyte antigen (HLA) complexes. β2-Microglobulin rises in inflammatory conditions and when lymphocyte turnover increases, such as in lymphocytic leukemia or when T-lymphocyte helper (OKT4) cells are invaded by human immunodeficiency virus (HIV). Serum β2-microglobulin increases with malfunctioning glomeruli but decreases with malfunctioning tubules because it is metabolized through renal tubules. Conversely, urinary β2-microglobulin reduces with malfunctioning glomeruli but increases with malfunctioning tubules.

INDICATIONS:

- Diagnosis of aminoglycoside toxicity (becomes elevated before creatinine).
- Detection of chronic lymphocytic leukemia, multiple myeloma, lung cancer, hepatoma, or breast cancer.
- Detection of HIV infection.
- Evaluation of renal disease to differentiate glomerular from tubular dysfunction.
- Monitoring of antiretroviral therapy.

RESULT:

Increased in:
• **Aminoglycoside toxicity**
• **Amyloidosis**
• **Acquired immune deficiency syndrome (AIDS)**
• **Autoimmune disorders**
• **Breast cancer**
• **Crohn's disease**
• **Felty's syndrome**
• **Hepatitis**
• **Hepatoma**
• **Hyperthyroidism**
• **Lung cancer**
• **Lymphoma**
• **Multiple myeloma**
• **Poisoning with heavy metals, like mercury or cadmium**
• **Inflammation of all types**
• **Leukemia (chronic lymphocytic)**
• **Renal dialysis**
• **Renal disease (glomerular): serum only**
• **Renal disease (tubular): urine only**
• **Viral infections (e.g., cytomegalovirus)**
• **Sarcoidosis**
• **Systemic lupus erythematosus**
• **Vasculitis**
Decreased in:

•	Response to zidovudine (AZT)
•	Renal disease (glomerular): urine only
•	Renal disease (tubular): serum only

IMPEDING FACTORS:

- Medications and proteins that may raise serum levels of β2-microglobulin include cefuroxime, cyclosporine A, gentamicin, interferon-β, pentoxifylline, and tumor necrosis factor.

-Medications that may reduce serum β2-microglobulin levels include zidovudine.

- Medications that may raise β2-microglobulin levels in urine include azathioprine, cisplatin, cyclosporine A, furosemide, gentamicin, mannitol, nifedipine, sisomicin, and tobramycin.

- Medications that may reduce β2-microglobulin levels in the urine include cilostazole.

- Urinary β2-microglobulin is unstable at < 5.5pH.

- Recent radioactive scans or radiation exposure within one week of the test may conflict with the test results, while radioimmunoassay is the test method.

TOTAL PROTEIN AND FRACTIONS

(TP, SPEP (fractions consist of albumin, α1-globulin, α2-globulin, β-globulin, and δ-globulin)

SAMPLING:1 mL of serum is collected in a red- or tiger-top tube.

TECHNIQUE: Electrophoresis for protein fractions, Spectrophotometry for total protein,

NORMAL VALUE:

TOTAL PROTEIN:

Age	Conventional Units	SI Units (Conversion Factor X10)
Newborn–5 d	3.8–6.2 g/dL	38–62 g/L
1–3 y	5.9–7.0 g/dL	59–70 g/L
4–6 y	5.9–7.8 g/dL	59–78 g/L
7–9 y	6.2–8.1 g/dL	62–81 g/L
10–19 y	6.3–8.6 g/dL	63–86 g/L
Adult	6.0–8.0 g/dL	60–80 g/L

PROTEIN FRACTION:

	Conventional Units	SI Units (Conversion Factor X10)
Albumin	3.4–4.8 g/dL	34–48 g/L
α1-Globulin	0.2–0.4 g/dL	2–4 g/L
α2-Globulin	0.4–0.8 g/dL	4–8 g/L

β-Globulin	0.5–1.0 g/dL	5–10 g/L
δ-Globulin	0.6–1.2 g/dL	6–12 g/L

EXPLAINATION:

Protein is essential to all physiological functions. The proteins are formed of amino acids, building blocks in blood and body tissue. Protein is also necessary for the regulation of metabolic processes, immunity, and the proper balance of water. Full protein is made up of albumin and globulins. α1-Globulin contains α1-antitrypsin, α1-fetoprotein, α1-acid glycoprotein, α1-antichymotrypsin, inter-α1-trypsin inhibitor, high-density lipoproteins, and a group-specific portion (vitamin D-binding protein). α2-Globulin contains haptoglobin, ceruloplasmin, and α2-macroglobulin. β-Globulin contains transferrin, hemopexin, very low-density lipoproteins, low-density lipoproteins, β2-microglobulin, fibrinogen, complement, and C-reactive Protein. δ-Globulin contains immunoglobulin G (IgG), IgA, IgM, IgD, and IgE. Many of the liver-derived proteins rise following acute infection or damage, while albumin decreases; these conditions may not indicate irregular total protein determination.

INDICATIONS:

- Assessment of edema as seen in patients with low total protein and low albumin levels.

- Estimation of nutritional status.

RESULT:

Increased:
• α1-Globulin proteins in acute & chronic inflammatory diseases
• α2-Globulin proteins occasionally in diabetes, pancreatitis, and hemolysis
• β-Globulin proteins in hyperlipoproteinemias and monoclonal gammopathies
• δ-Globulin proteins in chronic liver diseases, chronic infections, autoimmune disorders, hepatitis, cirrhosis, and lymphoproliferative disorders
• Total protein:
• Dehydration
• Monoclonal and polyclonal
• Gammopathies
• Myeloma
• Sarcoidosis
• Some types of chronic liver disease
• Tropical diseases (e.g., leprosy)
• Waldenström's macroglobulinemia
Decreased:
• α1-Globulin proteins in hereditary deficiency

- α2-Globulin proteins in nephrotic syndrome, malignancies, various subacute and chronic inflammatory diseases, healing stage of severe burns
- β-Globulin proteins in hypo-lipoproteinemia and IgA deficiency
- δ-Globulin proteins in immune deficiency or suppression
- **Total protein**
- **Administration of intravenous fluids**
- **Burns**
- **Chronic alcoholism**
- **Chronic ulcerative colitis**
- **Cirrhosis**
- **Crohn's disease**
- **Glomerulonephritis**
- **Heart failure**
- **Hyperthyroidism**
- **Malabsorption**
- **Malnutrition**
- **Neoplasms**
- **Nephrotic syndrome**
- **Pregnancy**
- **Prolonged immobilization**
- **Protein-losing enteropathies**
- **Severe skin disease**
- **Starvation**

IMPEDING FACTORS:

- Drugs that may raise protein levels include amino acids (if administered intravenously), anabolic steroids, angiotensin, anticonvulsants, carbenicillin, corticosteroids, corticotropin, digitalis, furosemide, insulin, isotretinoin, levonorgestrel, oral contraceptives, progesterone, radiographic agents, and thyroid agents.

- Medications and substances that may reduce protein levels include arginine, acetylsalicylic acid, benzene, carvedilol, citrate, floxuridine, laxatives, oral contraceptives, pentastarch, mercury compounds, phosgene, pyrazinamide, rifampin, trimethadione, and valproic acid.

- Levels of recumbent cases are significantly lower (5 to 10%).

- Hemolysis can mistakenly increase the results.

- Venous stasis can wrongly increase the results; the tourniquet should not be left on the arm for more than 60 seconds.

PRE-ALBUMIN

SYNONYM/ACRONYM: Transthyretin.

SAMPLING: 1 mL of serum is collected in a red- or tiger-top tube.

TECHNIQUE: Nephelometry

NORMAL VALUE:

Age	Conventional Units	SI Units (Conversion Factor X 10)
Newborn–1 mo	7.0–39.0 mg/dL	70–390 mg/L
1–6 mo	8.3–34.0 mg/dL	83–340 mg/L
6 mo–4 y	2.0–36.0 mg/dL	20–360 mg/L
5–6 y	12.0–30.0 mg/dL	120–300 mg/L
6 y–adult	12.0–42.0 mg/dL	120–420 mg/L

EXPLAINATION:

Prealbumin is a protein produced mainly by the liver. It is the main transport protein for triiodothyronine and thyroxine. It is also critical for the metabolism of retinol-binding protein required for the transport of vitamin A (retinol).

Prealbumin has a brief biological half-life of 2 days. It makes it a good measure of protein status and a good marker for malnutrition. Prealbumin is often measured at the same time as transferrin and albumin.

INDICATIONS: Evaluate nutritional status

RESULT:

Increased in:
• Alcoholism
• Chronic renal failure
• Patients receiving steroids
Decreased in:
• Diseases of the liver
• Hepatic damage
• Malnutrition
• Tissue necrosis
• Acute-phase inflammatory response

IMPEDING FACTORS:

- Medications that may raise prealbumin rates include anabolic steroids, anticonvulsants, danazole, oral contraceptives, prednisolone, prednisone, and propranolol.

- Medications that may lower prealbumin rates include amiodarone and diethylstilbestrol.

- Fasting 4 hours before the collection of specimens is highly recommended. NORMAL ranges are often focused on fasting samples to provide some degree of standardization for comparison. The concentration of lipids in the blood may also interfere with the test method; fasting removes this possible source of error, especially if the patient has elevated lipids.

PROTEIN, URINE: TOTAL QUANTITATIVE AND FRACTIONS

SAMPLING: 5 mL of urine from an unpreserved random or timed specimen is collected in a clean, plastic collection container.

TECHNIQUE: Electrophoresis for protein fractions, Spectrophotometry for total protein

NORMAL VALUE:

	Conventional Units	SI Units (Conversion Factor X 0.001)
Total protein	10–140 mg/24 h	0.01–0.14 g/24 h

Electrophoresis for fractionation is qualitative: no monoclonal gammopathy has been observed. (Urine protein electrophoresis and serum protein electrophoresis should be ordered.)

EXPLAINATION:

All proteins, except immunoglobulins, are produced and metabolized in the liver, wherever they are split down into amino acids. Amino acids have been decomposed into ammonia and ketoacids. Ammonia has been transformed into urea by the urea cycle. Urea is excreted through the urine.

INDICATIONS:

- Assist in the treatment of myeloma, Waldenström macroglobulinemia, lymphoma and amyloidosis.
- Assist in the identification of Bence Jones proteins (light chains).
- Evaluate kidney function.

RESULT:

Increased in:
• **Diabetic nephropathy**
• **Fanconi's syndrome**
• **Heavy metal poisoning**
• **Malignancies of the urinary tract**
• **Postexercise period**
• **Monoclonal gammopathies**
• **Multiple myeloma**
• **Nephrotic syndrome**
• **Sarcoidosis**
• **Sickle cell disease**

• Urinary tract infections	
• Other myeloproliferative and lymphoproliferative disorders	
Decreased in: N/A	

IMPEDING FACTORS:
- Medications and substances that may raise protein levels in urine include acetaminophen, aminosalicylic acid, amphotericin B, ampicillin, antimony compounds, antipyrin, arsenic, ascorbic acid, bacitracin, bismuth subsalicylate, bromate, capreomycin, cephaloridine, chlorpromazine, carbenoxolone, carbutamide, cephaloglycin, doxycycline, enalapril, gentamicin, radiographic agents, rifampin, sodium bicarbonate, streptokinase, sulfisoxazole, suramin, tetracyclines, thallium, phenols, phenolphthalein, phensuximide, mercury compounds, methicillin, methylbromide, meziocillin, mitomycin, nafcillin, naphthalene, gold, hydrogen sulfide, iodoalphionic acid, iodopyracet, iopanoic acid, corticosteroids, cyclosporine, demeclocycline, 1,2-diaminopropane, diatrizoic chlorpropamide, chlorthalidone, mefenamic acid, melarsonyl, melarsoprol, oxacillin, paraldehyde, penicillamine, penicillin, chrysarobin, colistimethate, colistin, captopril, carbamazepine, carbarsone, dihydrotachysterol, iophenoxic acid, ipodate, kanamycin, corn oil (Lipomul), lithium, neomycin, nonsteroidal anti-inflammatory drugs, phosphorus, picric acid, piperacillin, plicamycin, polymyxin, probenecid, promazine, pyrazolones, quaternary ammonium compounds thiosemicarbazones, tolbutamide, tolmetin, triethylenemelamine, and vitamin D.
- Medications that may reduce urinary protein levels include captopril, cyclosporine, diltiazem, enalapril, fosinopril, interferon, lisinopril, prednisolone, and quinapril.
- All urine that has been voided for the specified collection period must be included in the sample.

METANEPHRINES

SAMPLING: 25 mL of urine from a timed specimen is collected in a clean amber, plastic collection vessel with 6N hydrochloride as a preservative.

NORMAL VALUE:

Age	Conventional Units	SI Units
Normetanephrine		
		(Conversion Factor X5.46)
0–3 mo	47–156 µg/24 h	257–852 nmol/24 h
4–6 mo	31–111 µg/24 h	171–607 nmol/24 h
7–9 mo	42–109 µg/24 h	230–595 nmol/24 h
10–12 mo	23–103 µg/24 h	127–562 nmol/24 h

1–2 y	32–118 µg/24 h	175–647 nmol/24 h
2–6 y	50–111 µg/24 h	274–604 nmol/24 h
6–10 y	47–176 µg/24 h	255–964 nmol/24 h
10–16 y	53–290 µg/24 h	289–1586 nmol/24 h
Adult	82–500 µg/24 h	448–2730 nmol/24 h
Metanephrines		
		(Conversion Factor X.07)
0–3 mo	5.9–37 µg/24 h	30–188 nmol/24 h
4–6 mo	6.1–42 µg/24 h	31–213 nmol/24 h
7–9 mo	12–41 µg/24 h	61–210 nmol/24 h,
10–12 mo	8.5–101 µg/24 h	43–510 nmol/24 h
1–2 y	6.7–52 µg/24 h	34–264 nmol/24 h
2–6 y	11–99 µg/24 h	56–501 nmol/24 h
6–10 y	54–138 µg/24 h	275–701 nmol/24 h
10–16 y	39–243 µg/24 h	200–1231 nmol/24 h
Adult	45–290 µg/24 h	228–1470 nmol/24 h

EXPLAINATION:

Metanephrine is an inactive metabolite of epinephrine and norepinephrine. Metanephrine is either excreted or further metabolized into vanillylmandelic acid. The release of metanephrines in the urine is indicative of disorders associated with excessive development of catecholamines, especially pheochromocytoma. Vanillylmandelic acid and catecholamines are usually measured with urinary metanephrines. Creatinine is usually measured simultaneously to ensure sufficient accumulation and to determine the metabolite-creatinine excretion ratio.

INDICATIONS:

- Assist in the detection of presumed pheochromocytoma.
- Assist in the discovery of the cause of hypertension.
- Check suspicious tumors associated with excessive catecholamine secretion.

RESULT

Increased in:
Pheochromocytoma
Ganglioneuroma
Neuroblastoma
Severe stress
Decreased in: N/A

IMPEDING FACTORS:

- Medications that may increase the levels of metanephrine include labetalol, monoamine oxidase inhibitors, oxprenolol, oxytetracycline, and prochlorperazine.

-Methylglucamine in x-ray contrast media can produce false-negative results.

BLOOD GROUPS AND ANTIBODIES
(blood group antibodies, type and crossmatch, ABO group and Rh typing, type, and screen)
SAMPLING:2 mL of serum is collected in a red-top tube. 2 mL of whole blood collected in a tube with lavender-top (ethylenediamine tetra-acetic acid [EDTA]).
TECHNIQUE: FDA-licensed reagents along with glass slides, glass tubes, or automated systems) Compatibility (no clumping or hemolysis)
NORMAL VALUE:

Blood Type	Rh Type (with any ABO)	Other Antibodies That React at 37°C or with Antiglobulin	Other Antibodies That Respond at Room Temperature or Below
A	Positive	Kell	Lewis
B	Negative	Duffy	P
AB		Kidd	MN
O		S	Cold agglutinins
		s	
		U	

EXPLAINATION:
Blood typing is a sequence of tests, including the ABO and Rh blood group schemes, conducted to identify surface antigens in red blood cells through agglutination and compatibility tests to detect antibodies to these antigens. A and B are the main antigens in the ABO system, while AB and O are also important phenotypes. The A-antigen patient has blood type A; the B-antigen patient has blood type B. Patients with both A and B antigens have AB blood type (universal recipient); patients with neither A nor B antigens have an O blood type (universal donor). The origin of blood is genetically determined. After six months of age, persons develop serum antibodies that respond with an A or B antigen missing from their red blood cells. They are called anti-A and anti-B antibodies. In ABO blood sorting, the patient's red blood cells are combined with anti-A and anti-B sera, a process known as a forward grouping. The cycle is then reversed, and the patient's serum is combined with type A and B cells in the opposite classification.

Generally, only blood with the identical ABO and Rh group as the recipient transfused as anti-A and anti-B antibodies are potent agglutinins that cause rapid, complementary death of incompatible cells. ABO and Rh examinations are also conducted as a prenatal screening of pregnant women to identify the risk of fetal hemolytic disease. Although most anti-A and anti-B activity is in the immunoglobulin M (IgM) class of immunoglobulins, some activity remains with IgG. Anti-A and anti-B antibodies of the IgG family bind red blood cells without having an immediate effect on their viability. These can easily cross the placenta, resulting in newborn hemolytic disease. People with type O blood often have more IgG anti-A and anti-B; thus, hemolytic ABO disease of the newborn may affect babies of type O mothers nearly entirely (unless the newborn is also of type O).

The main antigens in the Rh system are D (or Rho), C, E, c, and e. Individuals whose red blood cells have a D antigen are considered Rh-positive; those who lack a D antigen are called Rh-negative, irrespective of what other Rh antigens are present. Individuals who are Rh-negative develop anti-D antibodies when exposed to Rh-positive cells by either transfusion or pregnancy. Such anti-D antibodies cross the placenta to the fetus and may cause newborn hemolytic disease or transfusion reactions if Rh-positive blood is given.

INDICATIONS:

- Help to determine ABO and Rh compatibility of donor and recipient before transfusion.
- Assess anti-D antibody titer of Rh-negative mothers following pregnancy sensitization of Rh-positive fetus.
- Evaluate the need for immunosuppressive therapy (e.g., with RhoGAM) when a Rh-negative woman delivers or aborts Rh-positive fetus.
- Identify ABO and Rh blood type donors for stored blood.
- Detect maternal and infant ABO and Rh blood types to predict the risk of newborn hemolytic disease.
- Identify ABO and Rh blood type patients, particularly before a blood loss or blood replacement intervention may be required.

RESULT:

• ABO system: A, B, AB, and/or O specific antigens to the person
• Rh system: positive or negative specific to the person
• Cross-matching: determining compatibility between donor and recipient
• Incompatibility specified by clumping (agglutination) of red blood cells

Group and Type	Incidence (%)	Substitute Transfusion Group and Type of PACKED CELL UNITS in Order of PNORMAL If Patient's Own Group and Type Not Accessible
O Positive	37.4	O Negative
O Negative	6.6	None
A Positive	35.7	A Negative, O Positive, O Negative
A Negative	6.3	O Negative, O Positive, A Positive
B Positive	8.5	B Negative, O Positive, O Negative
B Negative	1.5	O Negative, O Positive, B Positive
AB Positive	3.4	AB Negative, A Positive, B Positive, A Negative, B Negative, O Positive, O Negative
AB Negative	0.6	A Negative, B Negative, O Negative, AB Positive, A Positive, B Positive, O Positive
Rh Type		
Rh Positive	85–90	
Rh-Negative	10–15	

CRITICAL VALUES:
Signs and symptoms of blood transfusion reactions vary from slightly febrile to anaphylactic. They may include chills, dyspnea, fever, headache, nausea, vomiting, palpitations and tachycardia, chest or back pain, anxiety, flushing, hives, angioedema, diarrhea, hypotension, oliguria, hemoglobinuria, renal failure, sepsis, shock, and jaundice. Complications of disseminated intravascular coagulation (DIC) may also occur. Possible interventions in mildly febrile outcomes would include reducing the rate of administration, then testing and comparing the identification of patients, the requisitioning of transfusions, and the marking of blood bags. The patient should be closely monitored for further development of signs and symptoms.

Epinephrine administration may be ordered.

Probable interventions in a more severe transfusion reaction may comprise an immediate cessation of infusion, notification to the health care provider, keeping the intravenous (IV) line open with saline or lactated Ringer solution, collection of red and lavender tubes for post-transfusion work-up, urine collection, monitoring of vital signs every 5 minutes, ordering additional tests if DIC is suspected, maintain airway and blood pressure, and administer mannitol if required.

IMPEDING FACTORS:
- Drugs like levodopa, methyldopa, and methyldopa hydrochloride induce false-positive Rh typing.
- Recent administration of blood, blood components, dextran, or IV contrast media causes cell accumulation that resembles agglutination in ABO typing.
- Abnormal proteins, cold agglutinins, and bacteremia can interfere with the analysis.
-Screening does not detect any antibody and may skip the presence of a weak antibody.

Made in the USA
Las Vegas, NV
18 October 2024

96936401R00261